"This book is the authoritative source on on underappreciated thinkers in mental health in world-class expert who trained in Sullivan's m: principles for his entire illustrious career. As in the first edition, Evans provides a thorough treatment of Sullivan's thinking about development, psycho-pathology, assessment, psychotherapy, and broader social problems. In this new edition, he elaborates significantly on how Sullivan's approach to clinical and social issues can be understood through a contemporary lens and inform current practice. A must read for anyone who wants to understand this central player in the story of medicine and social science and situate their clinical work in the historically rich and eminently humane context offered by interpersonal theory."

**Christopher Hopwood, Ph.D.**, *Professor of Psychology,*
*University of Zurich*

"Evans' book on Harry Stack Sullivan is the best summary of Sullivan's work on the market today. It clearly describes all his basic concepts and their clinical implications. And this second edition contains clinical material illustrating an interpersonal approach to trauma work. Patients re-enact their traumas in therapy in order to tell the history of their interpersonal suffering. And if the therapist can listen with a relational ear, he can provide a climate of safety where the unsayable in the past can be said in the present. If for no other reason, the interpersonal understanding of anxiety and the strategies of self-other protection alone will reward the reader with new vistas of understanding."

**Jon Frederickson, MSW**, *Faculty, Washington School of Psychiatry; Author,*
*Co-Creating Change and Co-Creating Safety*

"In this engaging new edition of his 1996 book, Barton Evans shows himself to be the pre-eminent authority on all things Sullivanian. Readers will be intrigued as Evans connects Sullivan's life story to his interpersonal theory and then traces the influence of Sullivan's concepts on modern psychotherapy, psychological assessment, social psychology, and psychiatry. Sullivan remains an underappreciated genius, and Evans helps us recognize his immense and far-reaching impact. Readers interested in Collaborative/Therapeutic Assessment (C/TA) will especially appreciate Evans' discussion of current interpersonal models of psychological assessment."

**Stephen E. Finn, Ph.D.**, *President, Therapeutic Assessment Institute; Clinical*
*Associate Professor of Psychology, University of Texas at Austin*

"Dr. Evans succeeds in this masterful effort to 're-collect' the silent, forgotten, and sometimes maligned contributions of the genius Harry Stack Sullivan. Evans' scholarly research and skillful explanation of Sullivan's largely unacknowledged imprint on contemporary developments in psychoanalysis, theories of anxiety and psychopathology, and the vicissitudes of child development reminds us of how his ideas never really disappeared. In this gem of a book, Evans makes clear that at the heart of Sullivan's theories was the enduring strength of interpersonal connections, which can 'heal the developmental warps' that unfortunately occur in some. In Evans' beautiful words, it is the 'love between humans which ultimately liberates us.' These words have never been more important than they are now."

**James H. Kleiger, Psy.D., ABPP, ABAP**, *Independent Practice Bethesda, MD; Past President, Baltimore-Washington Psychoanalytic Institute*

# Harry Stack Sullivan

This book covers the works and life of Harry Stack Sullivan (1892–1949), who has been described as "the most original figure in American psychiatry."

Challenging Freud's psychosexual theory, Sullivan founded the interpersonal theory of psychiatry, which emphasizes the role of interpersonal relations, society, and culture as the primary determinants of personality development and psychopathology. This concise and coherent account of Sullivan's work and life invites the modern audience to rediscover the provocative, ground-breaking ideas embodied in Sullivan's interpersonal theory and psychotherapy that continue to advance. This revised second edition is updated to reflect new research and ideas - such as an expanded section on Sullivan's groundbreaking ideas about homosexuality and new sections on his concept of anxiety in infancy and on psychological trauma and how interpersonal theory impacts attachment theory, human sexuality, psychopathology, personality assessment, psychotherapy, and social issues.

This book, which has been a primary resource on Sullivan's works for over 25 years, will continue to be of interest to a range of psychotherapy professionals and practitioners including beginning and experienced psychotherapists, psychological assessment practitioners, interpersonal researchers, and teachers of personality theory.

**F. Barton Evans III** is a retired clinical and forensic psychologist, former Professor of Psychiatry at East Tennessee State University, and a Clinical Professor of Psychiatry at George Washington University. He is a Life Fellow of the American Psychological Association and the Society for Personality Assessment.

# Makers of Modern Psychotherapy

Series Editors: Laurence Spurling and Clea Mcenery-West

*This series of introductory, critical texts looks at the work and thought of key contributors to the development of psychodynamic psychotherapy. Each book shows how the theories examined affect clinical practice, and includes biographical material as well as a comprehensive bibliography of the contributor's work.*

The field of psychodynamic psychotherapy is today more fertile but also more diverse than ever before. Competing schools have been set up, rival theories and clinical ideas circulate. These different and sometimes competing strains are held together by a canon of fundamental concepts, guiding assumptions and principles of practice.

This canon has a history, and the way we now understand and use the ideas that frame our thinking and practice is palpably marked by how they came down to us, by the temperament and experiences of their authors, the particular puzzles they wanted to solve and the contexts in which they worked. These are the makers of modern psychotherapy. Yet despite their influence, the work and life of some of these eminent figures is not well known. Others are more familiar, but their particular contribution is open to reassessment. In studying these figures and their work, this series will articulate those ideas and ways of thinking that practitioners and thinkers within the psychodynamic tradition continue to find persuasive.

**Titles in the Series:**

**R. D. Laing and the Paths of Anti-Psychiatry**
*Zbigniew Kotowicz*

**Anna Freud: A View of Development, Disturbance and Therapeutic Techniques**
*Rose Edgcumbe*

**Jacques Lacan and the Freudian Practice of Psychoanalysis**
*Dany Nobus*

**Harry Stack Sullivan: Interpersonal Theory and Psychotherapy, 2nd edition**
*F. Barton Evans III*

# Harry Stack Sullivan

## Interpersonal Theory and Psychotherapy
Second Edition

## F. Barton Evans III

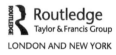
Routledge
Taylor & Francis Group

LONDON AND NEW YORK

Designed cover image: With permission from the Washington School of
Psychiatry

Second edition published 2024
by Routledge
4 Park Square, Milton Park, Abingdon, Oxon, OX14 4RN

and by Routledge
605 Third Avenue, New York, NY 10158

*Routledge is an imprint of the Taylor & Francis Group, an informa business*

First edition published by Routledge 1996

*British Library Cataloguing-in-Publication Data*
A catalogue record for this book is available from the British Library

ISBN: 978-1-032-30564-6 (hbk)
ISBN: 978-1-032-30561-5 (pbk)
ISBN: 978-1-003-30571-2 (ebk)

DOI: 10.4324/9781003305712

Typeset in Times New Roman
by MPS Limited, Dehradun

To
Judy
(Always Judy)

# Contents

# Preface to Revised Edition

It has been over 25 years since the publication of *Harry Stack Sullivan: Interpersonal Theory and Psychotherapy*. These 25 years have been gratifying to me in many ways. This was my first book and a labor of love to accomplish what several of my teachers, most notably Robert Kvarnes, had not been able to do. An audience for Sullivan's groundbreaking work suffered from books about him that did not fully understand the meaning and scope of his work and I set out to correct that as best I could. In addition to trying to summarize his work in a readable form, I also wanted to tie his ideas about psychological theory to research and to the many clinical practice areas his ideas spurred. The result was quite successful.

While the 1996 edition of this book stands on its own as a concise introduction the work of Harry Stack Sullivan, much has happened since its publication. Harry Stack Sullivan's contributions remain at the vanguard of modern thinking in a wide variety of areas. Much has happened that shows a continuing influence of his contributions since the original publication. For example, Sullivan's cutting-edge ideas about child development continue to be validated by research and application of his work in clinical practice has developed as well. His early work of human sexuality continues to be surprisingly contemporary and has spurred interesting perspectives about homosexuality.

Together with Routledge editors Sara Gore and Grace McDonnell, we arrived at an approach to the Revised Edition of this book. First, all chapters were reviewed and edited for clarity and expression and any additions that arise in the process. As a picky writer, I welcomed the opportunity to take "another bite of the apple" and clarify less than clear passages that grated on me over the years. Of course, a revised edition needed to include new material and update previous information. Specifically, the number of chapters was expanded by two to capture the newer material available.

Chapters 1 and 2 remain essentially the same with the advantage of another editing for clarity and readability and some minor corrections.

Chapter 3 elaborates Sullivan's basic concepts and includes an expanded section on Sullivan's wholly original concept of the theorem of anxiety as the particular human need for interpersonal relatedness. Sullivan's foundational thinking here is not well understood, in no small part because of his own lack of clarity. This chapter includes a significantly updated discussion on the literature on John Bowlby's and Mary Ainsworth's attachment theory, which better defines and elaborates our built-in need and capacity for human connectedness. The child development conceptual thinking and research literature on attachment has literally exploded since this book was published in 1996, which needed to be added to this book. I used Robert Marvin's and colleagues' Circle of Security model (Marvin, Cooper, Hoffman & Powell, 2002), a powerful approach to dealing with children's attachment difficulties, to illustrate attachment theory. The relationship between Sullivan's theorem of anxiety and Bowlby and Ainsworth's attachment theory was further discussed and considered in light of these new findings.

Chapter 4 explores Sullivan's writings about infancy as the seminal developmental period within his epochs of development stand on their own as a superb set of observations and theorizing about the young infant's emergence into the interpersonal world. His clear thinking on the development of self and other personifications provides a clear path to understanding the infants' interpersonal world and their budding cognitive structures of interrelationship that, to my mind, transcends British object relations theory and adds to the much sturdier concept of internal working model in attachment theory.

Chapter 5 in the original book took a broad sweep through Sullivan's remaining epochs of development. Rather than to leave Chapter 5 in its longer entirety, I chose to divide the chapter into Sullivan's thinking about Childhood and the Juvenile Era and create a new Chapter 6 focused exclusively on his ideas about the stages of Adolescence. Chapter 5 includes an updated review of relevant child development literature on Sullivan's ideas about peer relationships and the interpersonal aspects of child development up to adolescence.

In retrospect, I think a separate chapter, now Chapter 6, should have been devoted to the Adolescent Eras in 1996, if for no other reason than to emphasize Sullivan's unique contributions about adolescence. Before Sullivan, there was preciously little serious consideration of adolescence in psychoanalytic theory. His emphasis on interpersonal processes provided a new and lively perspective on adolescence. The new Chapter 6 is an updated review of relevant child development literature on the interpersonal aspects of adolescence, including Sullivan's ideas about peer relationships and formation of interpersonal intimacy. Further, I include an expanded section on Sullivan's truly cutting-edge thoughts about homosexuality that are surprisingly contemporary to our current understanding. Sullivan bucked the psychiatric, medical, and societal thinking about homosexuality as a perversion beginning back in the mid-1920s (Sullivan, 1926). Sullivan's remarkable writings about human sexuality presaged by nearly 70 years the American Psychiatric Association's completely dropping mentions of homosexuality, transvestism, etc. from the *Diagnostic and Statistical Manual of Mental Disorders* (4th ed.) (DSM IV: American Psychiatric Association, 1994). Additionally, I will critique the more recent literature on "the gay Sullivan" (Allen, 1995; Wake, 2008) on the cultural importance of his sexual orientation.

Chapter 7, Interpersonal Theory of Mental Disorder expands Sullivan's critique of Kraepelin in light of the modern neo-Kraepelinian direction in modern psychiatry focus on the medical model as seen in the DSM IV and DSM 5. I discuss what is lost in dropping an interpersonal focus in looking at individuals' "problems of living," especially with the growing research on the interpersonal underpinnings in schizophrenia and bipolar disorder. Also, I added a new discussion of psychological trauma to the "dynamisms of difficulty" section with a focus on how modern trauma theory and treatment is fundamentally interpersonal in ways that Sullivan's theory foretold. As part of this, I will discuss dissociative disorders and Sullivan's concept of the "not me" that is so much a part of the work of Putnam and now Brand.

Chapters 8 and 9 are divided in this revision from what was the previous Chapter 7 New Chapter 8 starts with Sullivan's concept of the psychiatric interview, but now includes an updated section on Sullivan's impact on modern personality assessment. The chapter adds Stephen Finn's work on therapeutic assessment, Christopher Hopwood and Aaron Pincus's work on the interpersonal circumplex, and my work on the interpersonal approach to the Rorschach to illustrate Sullivan's modern influence in personality assessment. On the advice of Laurence Spurling and Clea McEnery-West, co-editor of the Makers of Modern Psychotherapy series, I added an illustrative case example of my approach to the psychiatric interview.

The new Chapter 9 focuses exclusively on Sullivan's interpersonal approach to psychotherapy. In addition to the original ideas expressed in the previous book, this chapter reviews the influence of Sullivan's work on modern interpersonal and relational psychoanalysis as well as Jon Frederickson's interpersonally focused approach to intensive short-term dynamic psychotherapy (Frederickson, 2013, 2020).

Chapter 10 expands the previous Chapter 8's meagre four pages on Sullivan's work on interpersonal theory and social science, picking up and expanding his work on repressive sexual attitudes, prejudice, racism, and international conflict and world peace. I also include the influence of Sullivan's interpersonal theory on forensic psychology, especially understanding the impact of torture individually and socially.

# Acknowledgments for the Revised Edition

So much has happened in the past 25 years in terms of the many exceptional teachers and colleagues who guided me earlier in my career and specifically through the writing of the original edition of this book. Many of my most important influences have passed away, leaving me as the "old man" who passes along the traditions they shared with me. My appreciation for them remains alive in my work and in my heart.

In terms of the current edition of this book, I would like to express my special appreciation to the following:

Jon Frederickson – dear friend, "grokker" extraordinaire, and inspiration for what interpersonal psychodynamic assessment and treatment can truly be. I remember well our secret two-person club called the Wild Analysts in Washington, DC, where we shared forbidden ideas about psychotherapy. It is a joy to see so many of these ideas move the mainstream. His encouragement is priceless and his edits for this book have been enormously helpful.

Chris Hopwood is an inspiration for interpersonal theorists and therapists, young and old, keeping Sullivan alive now and into the future. and provided excellent feedback for this book.

Steve Finn and I met as a result of the publication of the first edition of this book, which in turn led to our rich collaboration over the years, including learning his Therapeutic Assessment model. His edits on this section of the book were quite helpful.

Thanks to Lawrence Raymond for sharing his work on Sullivan and Boisen in its formative phase and inviting me into it. Raymond is an inspiration for those working late into life and I appreciated his encouragement for this old warhorse to take another lap around the paddock.

To my many colleagues and friends from the International Society for the Rorschach and the Society for Personality Assessment for their support, collaboration, and encouragement- the late Bruce L. Smith, Odile Hussain, Irving Weiner, James Kleiger, Ali Khadivi, Giselle Hass, David Nichols, Ety Berant, Howard Lerner, Nancy Kaser-Boyd, and Judy Armstrong. Over the years, Bethany Brand and Judge Lori Rosenberg have been good friends and thoughtful collaborators. I treasure Bill Ryan as a valued friend, intellectual provocateur, and important part of my life. What a delight Rick Ferris has been in my recent years, constantly questioning and challenging, all the while providing steadfast friendship.

Naturally, my friends, colleagues, and teachers should be held accountable only for whatever improvements they made; any intellectual lapses, defects, or errors expressed in this book are solely my own.

I was most fortunate to make acquaintance with British Routledge editors Sara Gore and Grace McDonnell who helped me develop a reasonable proposal. Grace (how aptly named) especially collaborated with me throughout and offered good advice as well as strong support and encouragement. Laurence Spurling and Clea McEnery-West, co-editors of the *Makers of Modern Psychotherapy* series also provided advice that improved this book.

My greatest love and thanks go to my dearest dear, Judy Maris. It is a true blessing to have a loving, supportive wife and best friend, who is also an excellent editor with a strong mind.

# Preface to the Original Edition

Harry Stack Sullivan is the most original figure in American psychiatry.

(Havens, 1973: 183)

The idea for this book was originally conceived in 1980 by Dr. Robert Kvarnes, who was at that time Director of the Washington School of Psychiatry and a supervisee of Sullivan. As part of the Washington School's Advanced Psychotherapy Training Program, Dr. Kvarnes gave an exceptional semester-long seminar on interpersonal theory, which brought Sullivan's ideas to life. It was increasingly clear to Dr. Kvarnes and Dr. Alec Whyte, his teaching partner in the seminar, that an introductory book of manageable size, summarizing and translating Sullivan's often turgid ideas, could be of great value to students interested in Sullivan's work. I wholeheartedly agreed with Dr. Kvarnes and offered to work with him. Unfortunately, after considerable effort, Dr. Kvarnes was unable to obtain funding to support the writing of the book. When Dr. Kvarnes passed away several years later, so apparently did the book. My life was far too full of professional and family responsibilities to take on such a task by myself. Little did I know that the book was simply undergoing a long period of hibernation.

In the Spring of 1993, Dr. David Scharff, then Director of the Washington School of Psychiatry, with whom I had worked closely in the previous year in my role as Conference Chair of the Sullivan Centennial Conference, approached me with a letter that he had received from Dr. Laurence Spurling. Dr. Spurling inquired of Dr. Scharff about someone to write a book on Harry Stack Sullivan for Routledge's "Masters of Modern Psychotherapy" series. I contacted Dr. Spurling and the rest is history. I am delighted to have the opportunity to complete this task laid before me over a decade earlier.

The purpose of this book is to "re-collect" Sullivan, that is to reintroduce his work to a modern audience. While important comparative studies of psychoanalytic theory (see Greenberg and Mitchell, 1983; Mitchell, 1988) stressed Sullivan's importance in the history and development of psychoanalytic theory, books surveying the breadth of his work are few and far between. To my knowledge, except for Chatelaine's (1992) brief, edited course notes, there has been no published book summarizing Sullivan's many contributions in 20 years. Such a summary has been badly needed as much of Sullivan's writings appear remote and inaccessible to many readers, even though Sullivan's ideas are surprisingly contemporary. This gap in the literature on psychodynamic theory has badly needed filling, all the more in light of the modern emphasis on object relations theories. I hope to demonstrate in this book that Sullivan was ahead of his time in the richness, complexity, and accuracy of his thinking about the human condition and truly merits Greenberg and Mitchell's belief that Sullivan was, and still is, one of the great masters of psychodynamic theory and psychotherapy.

The other not-so-secret goal of this book is to encourage modern readers to take on the really not-so-onerous task of reading Sullivan in the original. Sullivan's ideas have been passed along by a largely oral tradition (with some notable exceptions), a tradition in which I have had the good fortune of participating as a student, supervisee, client, and now teacher and supervisor. My hope is that this book will serve as a "road map" to navigate through some of Sullivan's denser ideas, with the hope of bringing good things to light. Throughout the book, I tried (mainly) to stay close to Sullivan's original ideas, hopefully providing an advertisement for reading his works in the original. If I am successful in my task, I wish to remind the reader that the very best of Sullivan's writings (*The Interpersonal Theory of Psychiatry, The Psychiatric Interview,* and *Clinical Studies in Psychiatry*) were not his writings at all. Sullivan was a notoriously malignant self-critic when it came to writing. Fortunately, we are indebted to the William Alanson White Psychiatric Foundation Committee on Publication of Sullivan's Writings and its editorial consultant Helen Swick Perry who toiled many years to construct these three books from recorded lectures and written lecture notes. Following the advice of the late Robertson Davies (1992) to reject modern teaching against "subvocalizing" when reading, I encourage the reader to "listen" to Sullivan's books as if you were attending one of his lectures, which separates better the rich Sullivan wheat from the abrasive chaff. In doing so, one can experience Sullivan alive- a charming, witty, pompous, and intellectually challenging old cuss who has much to share about the human condition.

The book is organized as follows.

The first section, Historical Context, has two parts. Chapter 1 is a critical essay that I wrote for the 1992 Washington School of Psychiatry Sullivan Conference, which attempts to establish Sullivan's place in modern psychoanalytic theory and psychology as well as contribute some thoughts about why his many extraordinary contributions have been forgotten. Chapter 2 presents a brief biography of Sullivan with an emphasis on the social context in which his career, his ideas, and (as befits the interpersonal model) his personality developed.

Section II, Sullivan's Interpersonal Theory is in many ways the heart of this book, as it was the heart of Sullivan's work. The interpersonal theory of psychiatry was Sullivan's personality theory, though conceived in a most unique way. All things flowed from Sullivan's then novel conception of humans as social beings and the often-perilous course of their development. Chapter 3 reviews Sullivan's basic concepts found throughout the rest of his writings and this book. I have paid particular attention to his theory of anxiety, which was not well elucidated, and how it fits with Bowlby's attachment theory. As Sullivan's conceptualization of infancy commands such a large part of *The Interpersonal Theory of Psychiatry* as well as his later thinking on schizophrenia and severe mental disorder, Chapter 4 is devoted to summarizing his ideas on this epoch of development in some detail. Chapter 5 covers Sullivan's developmental theory from childhood through late adolescence. Sullivan went well beyond psychoanalytic concepts of the Oedipus complex into fresh perspectives on the importance of the role of peer relations in personality development, a unique and valuable contribution which has spurred considerable empirical research.

Section III turns to the application of Sullivan's interpersonal theory to psychopathology, psychotherapy, and social psychiatry. Chapter 6 presents his ideas about "problems in living," Sullivan's iconoclastic answer to the question of what constitutes psychopathology. His focus on interpersonal process over clinical entities raises provocative questions which remain unanswered by descriptive psychiatry still. Chapter 7 attempts to describe Sullivan's ideas about psychotherapy in terms of a basic stance toward assessment and treatment. His remarkable ideas about the psychiatric interview will be reviewed as well as his influence on the modern field of psychotherapy. With Chapter 8, we come full circle with a very brief review of some of Sullivan's ideas about the relation between psychiatry and society. Sullivan conceived psychiatry as a social science, which at its core should critique and offer solutions to society's many dilemmas, such as peace and international conflict, racism, sexism, and homosexuality. Sullivan's belief that psychiatry should ultimately focus on the prevention of the conditions which lead to disturbed lives is a testament to how seriously he took the implications of his ideas.

Throughout this book, within the scope of a general introduction to Sullivan's work, I shall draw parallels to past and present psychoanalytic thinkers. Because, as Greenberg and Mitchell (1983) so aptly pointed out, Sullivan's interpersonal theory and Freud's drive theory are the two most significant conceptual models of object relations in psychoanalytic theory, emphasis in this book will be placed on comparisons of interpersonal theory to drive theory. Additionally, as space permits, I shall endeavor to back up my claim that much of Sullivan's thinking is alive and well (if unacknowledged) in modern psychoanalysis, psychology, and psychotherapy. I believe that Sullivan's interpersonal theory (along with Bowlby's attachment theory) provides the outline for a more powerful model of personality than other psychoanalytic theories and integrates well what we know about the best of modern psychotherapy. I regret that I cannot fully give this topic the full treatment it deserves as such an analysis lies outside the goals and purposes of this book.

# Acknowledgments to Original Edition

Appreciation is expressed to W. W. Norton & Company for their permission to allow me to quote liberally from all seven of the books of Sullivan's work which they published and to the Washington School of Psychiatry and The William Alanson White Psychiatric Foundation for permission to use to the cover photograph.

I have been privileged to have the opportunity to work with many fine colleagues, teachers, and students in the Advanced Psychotherapy Training Program at the Washington School of Psychiatry (of which I am proudly a graduate and now teach Sullivan). The intellectual beginnings of this intelligently multi-theoretical and multi-disciplinary psychodynamic psychotherapy training program hearken back to the days and spirit of Sullivan. It is one of the places, to quote Martin Buber, that still keeps the questions open. In particular faculty who gave me an excellent background in psychodynamic and psychoanalytic thought include Margaret Rioch, Morris Parloff, Robert Kvarnes, Gerald Perman, Gordon Kirshner, Jack Fearing, Arnold Meyersburg, Henry Segal, Joseph Lichtenberg, David Scharff, Alec Whyte, John Zinner, Susannah Gourevitch, Rochelle Kainer, Christopher Bever, Stanley Greenspan, David Feinsilver, Bernardo Hirschman, and Stanley Palumbo. While many of these faculty disagree with Sullivan's point of view, I have always found it possible to work side by side with them.

I wish also to express deep gratitude to Morris Parloff, Jack Fearing, Lois Showalter, and Roger Harder for their special contributions to my personal and professional development.

I wish to thank Robert Jenkins, the Director of the Clinical Psychology Internship Program at the George Washington University School of Medicine for backing my idea for a course on Sullivan and for relieving me from significant faculty duties in support of writing this book.

Special thanks go to David Scharff, former Director of the Washington School of Psychiatry for providing me the opportunity to chair the Sullivan Centennial Conference in 1992 and for nominating me to write this book for Routledge House.

I am grateful for the help and support of my good friends and colleagues who took the time to help me in my first endeavor as a book author: Benjamin Schutz, Jon Frederickson, Roger Fallot, Maxine Harris, and Linda Blick.

Two of my teachers, now friends and colleagues, must be given special thanks. I have had the privilege to know Morris Parloff in a variety of professional roles over the years. Morris Parloff's penetrating and uncompromising intellect as a scholar is superseded only by his generous and kind spirit as a person. He critiqued several chapters of this book and made important suggestions about the book that improved it greatly. Thanks also go to Gloria Parloff for her editorial suggestions in Chapter 1.

One can consider oneself blessed to sit in the presence of greatness, if only for a moment. Over the past 24 years, I have had the opportunity to bask in it. Through her extraordinary teaching and supervision, Margaret Rioch introduced me to Sullivan's ideas, among many other important inspirations, and taught me how to live by them. She was instrumental in helping me in countless ways in the early stages of this book. Margaret Rioch's confidence, encouragement, and Zen teaching are at the center of this book, my work as a psychotherapist, and my life.

Naturally, my friends, colleagues, and teachers should be held accountable only for whatever improvements they made; any intellectual lapses, defects, or errors expressed in this book are solely my own.

Many thanks must go to Dr. Laurence Spurling, Series Editor, for his recognition of the importance of Sullivan's place in the history of psychodynamic psychotherapy and his editorial assistance and humane encouragement from across ocean; and to Edwina Welham, Commissioning Editor at Routledge House, for being the voice of reality (never an easy job), an act of kindness that was instrumental to finishing this book.

I also wish to acknowledge the warmth, understanding, and loving support of my brother Robert Evans and sisters Halee Cordray and Susan Whilden through the emotional period of the past year and a half. Writing this book was more or less bracketed by the deaths of our parents, Joanna Garner Evans and Frank Barton Evans, Jr. I regret that they are not with us to share the joy of its publication.

My final and greatest love and thanks go to Joanne Evans and our children Rebecca and Samuel for their devotion, patience, and love throughout my writing of this book. They unselfishly put aside many of their own needs to allow me to complete this work and still remained supportive and understanding throughout.

# Section I

# Historical Perspectives

# Historical Perspective

# Chapter 1

# Introduction

Sullivan's professional fate has been similar to that of many another innovator. The conservative community responded to his ideas at first by ignoring them, then by attacking them, and finally by so assimilating them that their innovative nature is forgotten.

(Yalom, 1975: 22)

Harry Stack Sullivan, an American psychiatrist working in the 1930s and 40s, was the founder and chief proponent of a branch of psychodynamic/psychoanalytic thinking called variously interpersonal psychiatry or interpersonal psychoanalysis. Along with Erich Fromm and Karen Horney, Sullivan is perhaps best known for his social and psychologically based critique of Sigmund Freud's psychoanalytic drive theory. Challenging the central role of infantile sexual drives in Freud's theory, Sullivan and other social psychoanalytic theorists emphasized the role of culture and society as a primary determinant of personality development and psychopathology. During the 1940s, these interpersonal theories, sometimes called the "Neo-Freudian theories," greatly influenced psychoanalytic theory and practice, as evidenced by their inclusion in most survey books on psychoanalysis and personality theory. Yet, their acknowledged impact on current mainstream thinking in psychoanalysis has been minimal until recently.

Harry Stack Sullivan occupies a unique and puzzling place in both the historical and current thinking of psychodynamic theory and psychotherapy. On one hand, his interpersonal theory has been regarded by many (perhaps most) mainstream psychoanalytic writers as superficial or incorrect, as they believe Sullivan totally disregarded the importance of intrapsychic experience. The critiques of Edith Jacobson (1955) and Otto Kernberg (1976) are most representative of this point of view.

On the other hand, recent works by important scholars of comparative psychodynamic theory have claimed that Sullivan's radical and iconoclastic departure from classical psychoanalytic drive theory and technique is one of the two most important streams of thought in psychoanalytic theory, along

DOI: 10.4324/9781003305712-2

with Freud. Leston Havens (1973) has long noted the importance of Sullivan's contributions, calling him "the most original figure in American psychiatry," and stating that his thinking "secretly dominates" modern psychodynamic psychiatry in the United States (Havens & Frank, 1971). In their groundbreaking book on object relations theory, Greenberg and Mitchell (1983) consider Sullivan's interpersonal theory and Freud's drive theory to be the two most significant conceptual models of object relation theory. Greenberg and Mitchell (1983: 81) stated that Sullivan presented ideas that "have resurfaced, at times in strikingly unaltered form, within the most important and popular Freudian authors of the past decade. Yet he (Sullivan) is rarely credited with originating these approaches and ideas."

A measure of the robustness of a theory is its capacity to survive over time and be confirmed by other theorists and researchers. It can be readily argued that much of Sullivan's thought has met this standard. As will be argued in the next section, Sullivan's main ideas have survived, though unacknowledged, within psychoanalysis in British objects relations theory, self psychology, and Erikson's psychosocial theory.

To broaden the question further about the validity of Sullivan's work, it might be valuable to briefly review some important modern currents in psychiatry, academic psychology, and social science to determine if Sullivan's ideas have survived in either acknowledged or unacknowledged forms. Sullivan's ideas undeniably presaged other developments in psychiatry, psychology, and social science in ways perhaps even more significant than his influence on psychoanalysis. In psychiatry and psychotherapy, as Leon Salzman (1966) noted, Sullivan's work on obsessional states contributed greatly to popular modern ideas about personality disorders. Klerman et al. (1984) interpersonal psychotherapy of depression, one of the most empirically effective treatments for depression, and Strupp and Binder (1984) openly acknowledged the importance of Sullivan's thinking in the development of brief psychotherapy. In a personal conversation, Jay Haley (1979), the famous American family therapist, stated that Sullivan, through his influence on another family psychotherapy pioneer (and supervisee of Sullivan) Don D. Jackson (1968), was one of Haley's two major models for the development of systems-oriented family therapy. Yalom (1975) credits Sullivan's theory as one of the most important contributions leading to the field of group psychotherapy. It is little known that Jerome Frank, Morris Parloff, and Florence Powdermaker's (Powdermaker & Frank, 1953) original and groundbreaking study of group psychotherapy was conducted under the auspices of the Washington School of Psychiatry in 1947 (see Rioch, 1948).

Interestingly, perhaps the most scientifically robust support for Sullivan's work comes from the research on experimental analysis of behavior and social learning theory (see Rychlak, 1979 for a discussion of the similarity of interpersonal theory and behaviorism). Ferster and Skinner's (1957) *Schedules of Reinforcement* empirically validates suppositions about the impact of learning by reward and punishment which Sullivan (1953) stated in *Interpersonal Theory of Psychiatry*. The social learning experiments of Bandura (1977) confirm Sullivan's notions about the importance of modeling and vicarious learning in child development. In addition to the validation from behavioral psychology, Sullivan's ideas on developmental theory have impacted other child development researchers. For example, child development research (Buhrmester & Furman, 1987; Furman & Buhrmester, 1985; Hartup, 1993, 1992, 1989, 1979; Youniss, 1980; Youniss & Smollar, 1985) on childhood and adolescent social networks explicitly addresses many aspects of Sullivan's developmental theory. In his integration of psychoanalysis and developmental psychology research, Stern (1985) acknowledges and supports Sullivan's ideas about the essentially interpersonal nature of humans, subjective relatedness (i.e., personifications), development of self, and anxiety.

In the areas of social psychology and social science, Sullivan's influence was considerable and many of his concepts have been strongly supported. It has been largely forgotten that Sullivan historically played a pioneering role in establishing an active research collaboration between psychiatrists and social scientists. As early as 1927, W. I. Thomas, President of the American Sociological Society, described the importance of Sullivan's work for sociology (see Volkart, 1951). Sullivan's work with scholars from the University of Chicago's historically seminal Department of Sociology and Anthropology led to his mutual collaboration with, and significant influence on, anthropologist Edward Sapir (e.g., Sapir, 1936/1937) and political scientist Harold Lasswell (1930), the founder of the field of political psychology (see Perry, 1964). In 1938, Sullivan (1964) personally participated in field research, and collaborated, with noted black sociologist Charles S. Johnson, which led to Johnson's (1941) important book on personality development and difficulties with Southern rural black youth. His collaboration with Charles Johnson was indeed pioneering in that psychoanalysts of that time were nearly or exclusively all white and mainly male and there is no other collaboration from that period in which a prominent psychoanalyst worked across racial lines. As social psychologist Gordon Allport stated (see Perry, 1964), "Sullivan, perhaps more than any other person, labored to bring about the fusion of psychiatry and social science."

Sullivan's theoretical ideas appear well-represented and well-supported in modern social science as well. For example, much theory building and empirical work in social psychology on interpersonal competition, social attribution, and face-saving (see Jones et al., 1971) have confirmed Sullivan's notions of security operations, interpersonal cooperation and conflict, and social construction of reality (see Berger & Luckman, 1966). The works of Stanton and Schwartz (1954), Goffman (1961), and Levinson and Gallagher (1964) on the importance of the socialization of the patient role in mental hospitals are but a few of the important empirical and observational studies that confirm Sullivan's observations on social psychiatry in the 1920s and 30s with regard to his schizophrenic ward at Sheppard Pratt Hospital (see Sullivan, 1962). These direct influences of, and concurrent findings supporting, Sullivan's work further attest to its importance and validity, indicating that his intellectual influence has been far greater than is usually acknowledged. As such, I believe that we must consider other factors if we are to answer the question of why the perhaps greatest American contributor to psychiatry is largely forgotten.

## Comparison of Sullivan to Modern Psychoanalytic Theories

Let us first turn to the question of the importance and significance of Sullivan's work as perceived within psychodynamic/psychoanalytic mainstream. As mentioned above, perhaps most influential to modern psychoanalysts have been the critiques of Sullivan by Edith Jacobson (1955) and Otto Kernberg (1976). Jacobson, and later Kernberg, faulted Sullivan for what they perceived as his lack of concern for intrapsychic phenomena and exclusive concentration on external factors, especially interpersonal relations, as well as his abandonment of Freud's drive theory and structural model (id, ego, and superego) of the mind. Clearly, Sullivan's work seriously challenged the validity of Freud's structural model, calling into question whether reified, static explanatory concepts like id, ego, and superego contribute to the understanding of human experience and processes that are essentially dynamic (Sullivan, 1953). Also, Sullivan (1953) relegates biological drive or instinct (which he calls the tension of needs) to a much more limited role than Freud does, while emphasizing the importance of interpersonal connectedness and learning in personality development. While both of his criticisms are true divergences from classical psychoanalytic theory, they are hardly unique to Sullivan, both inside and outside psychoanalytic circles. Most curious is Jacobson's and Kernberg's insistence that Sullivan's emphasis on interpersonal relations is necessarily superficial, lacking depth, and interested in only the surface areas of personality. As I have stated elsewhere (Evans, 1992), Jacobson's and Kernberg's criticisms arise from a puzzling misreading of Sullivan's work.

Jacobson and Kernberg have serious bones to pick with Sullivan because of his abandonment of drive theory and structural models of the mind, again both of which are hardly unique to Sullivan. Jacobson and Kernberg most criticize Sullivan for his lack of concern for intrapsychic phenomena. The belief that Sullivan's theory ignores intrapsychic phenomena is what one usually hears from psychoanalytic colleagues, indicating that it is deeply in the lore of the psychoanalytic community. Yet, as Greenberg and Mitchell (1983) state, the criticism that Sullivan favored interpersonal over intrapsychic phenomena is largely due to a misreading or lack of understanding of Sullivan. Regarding the so-called debate between interpersonal versus intrapsychic models, Sullivan pointed out that human experience is a dynamically unfolding interaction between interpersonal, environmental influences and the internal (i.e., intrapsychic) meaning system of personifications of self and other, which have a powerful influence on how one perceives, interprets and responds to these external experiences.

While nobody disputes that Sullivan introduced, and was fundamentally interested in, the importance of interpersonal relationships in personality theory, his centrally important concepts of meaning and personification, Sullivan's "intrapsychic" equivalents, do not seem to be understood by Jacobson, Kernberg, and others. Though a detailed discussion of these concepts will come later in this book, a quick summary of Sullivan's thinking on the matter is in order. According to Sullivan, understanding an individual's "real" interpersonal relationships is only part of the picture. Sullivan was equally interested in the way a person interprets his or her experience, i.e., what the experience *means* to the person. This in turn is influenced by the ways the person comes to know the world, through the formulation of a set of internal assumptions, ideas, and fantasies about people and the self, based on developmental experience, which he calls personifications. To quote Sullivan ...

> But I would like to make it forever clear that the relation of personifications to that which is personified is always complex and sometimes multiple; and that personifications are not adequate descriptions of that which is personified.
>
> (Sullivan, 1953: 167)

Personification is quite akin to the psychoanalytic concept of inner objects, which is the basis for understanding intrapsychic experience. Where Sullivan parted company with psychoanalysis was not that inner life is unimportant. Quite to the contrary, he believed that it is so important that we must be especially careful, attentive, and detailed in our exploration of the patient's inner experience. Again to quote Sullivan ...

> There are no purely objective data in psychiatry, and there are no valid subjective data, because the material becomes scientifically usable only in the shape of a complex resultant inference.
>
> (1953: 15)

Thus, part of the skill of interviewing comes from a sort of quiet observation all along: "Does this sentence, this statement have unquestionable meaning? Is there any certainty to what this person means?" (1954: 8). He also believed that inner life and real interpersonal experience exist in constant dynamic relation, with each influencing the other. He was especially adamant that the psychotherapist cannot assume to know the patient's inner experience except by a careful, detailed analysis of what the patient tells him.

Sullivan had little patience with psychotherapists who stretch their patients on the Procrustean bed of the therapists' abstract, unexplored inferences and, in case conferences, he often exacted Theseus' cure for Procrustean hospitality (see Kvarnes & Parloff, 1976). There is little doubt that Jacobson's and Kernberg's criticisms were based on poor understanding of Sullivan's writings, yet their criticism has been broadly held within psychoanalytic circles.

To broaden the question of Sullivan's role in modern psychoanalytic theory, Havens, and Greenberg and Mitchell have pointed to the unacknowledged similarity to, and influence on, psychoanalytic thought of Sullivan's ideas. One needs only turn to the relational writings of the British Object Relations Theorists (Fairbairn, 1952; Guntrip, 1969, 1971; Winnicott, 1958, 1965); the self psychology (Kohut, 1971, 1977); and Erikson's psychosocial developmental theory (Erikson, 1950) to illustrate these similarities.

Suffice it to say that the British Object Relations Theorists place great importance on object relations in the formation of personality and psychopathology. These theorists shifted the theoretical focus in psychoanalytic theory from Freud's vicissitudes of instinctual life to the influence of early mother-child relations on the development of internal representations of self and others and how these representations determine relatedness to others in later life. For the British Object Relations Theorists, the person becomes an object (or person) seeking human rather than the pleasure-seeking creature of classical psychoanalysis. Although I think Sullivan would greatly disapprove of the word 'object' used for a person, there is much correspondence between the basic thrust of the British Object Relations Theorists and Sullivan's essential interest in human development, interpersonal relations, and the linking concept of personification which was elaborated earlier. Indeed, Harry Guntrip (1971) stated ...

> I remember discussing Sullivan with Fairbairn around the early 1950s, and he stated how close he felt that he and Sullivan were in this basic matter, of moving beyond the impersonal to the personal levels of abstraction, from mechanistic to motivational concepts ... Fairbairn owed more to Freud than Sullivan did, but they both moved beyond classical psychoanalysis at the same point.
>
> (Guntrip, 1971:43)

Complementing the British Object Relations Theorists, Heinz Kohut's (1971, 1977) major contribution to psychoanalysis was to posit a line of development separate from drives, the development of *normal narcissism*, as he called it in his early work. Later, as he abandoned the language of drive theory, Kohut interestingly substituted the term *development of the self* for normal narcissism. Kohut believed that the development and preservation of a viable sense of self was critical for human psychological development and that much of what is termed psychopathology comes from maintaining this positive sense of self in the face of serious past and present challenges. From my perspective, Kohut's concept of the self does not differ fundamentally from one of Sullivan's core contributions, the concept of the *self-system* and its role in *problems of living* (as Sullivan preferred to call psychopathology). When Kohut's complex structural psychoanalytic language is stripped away, many of Kohut's concepts (e.g., transmuting internalization and narcissistic injury) are directly parallel to Sullivan's more elegantly expressed ideas about the development of the self through reflected appraisals of others as the way of learning from experiences of tenderness, empathy, and anxiety. Kohut did not acknowledge Sullivan's writings, which is puzzling. It is a well-known phenomenon in science for similar ideas to be developed concurrently by different thinkers without awareness of each other's work, perhaps in the way Fairbairn's ideas developed contiguously with, but separately from, Sullivan's ideas. Yet it is difficult to see how this phenomenon could have operated in Kohut's writings since he wrote considerably after Sullivan's publications. Additionally, Kohut's ideas were developed in large measure while working in Chicago, where Sullivan had deep intellectual roots and modern ties.

Erik Erikson's psychosocial theory of ego development (Erikson, 1950) matches Sullivan's epochs of development (Sullivan, 1947, 1953) quite closely. Erikson was the first mainstream psychoanalytic writer to specifically complement Freud's psychosexual stages with a theory of childhood psychosocial development, as well as to extend psychoanalytic developmental theory beyond childhood into adolescence and adulthood. Erikson and Sullivan were both active in American psychoanalytic circles at approximately the same time, as Sullivan was the supervising psychoanalyst, taught in the Baltimore-Washington Psychoanalytic Institute, and was active in the American Psychoanalytic Association (see Perry, 1982). Both were active at Yale University contemporaneously, where Sullivan was invited to lecture on Interpersonal Theory through his relationship to Edward Sapir and Erikson who was active in the Yale Psychiatry Department through his connection with the Western New England Psychoanalytic Association. When Erikson (1950, 1959) first explication of his theory of psychosocial development, he referenced Sullivan's Interpersonal Theory of Psychiatry and his ideas about the self, though did not mention Sullivan's epochs of interpersonal development. It is highly puzzling that Erikson did not notice, and therefore reference and acknowledge, the very close similarity of his psychosocial theory to Sullivan's interpersonal developmental theory.

Clearly, Harry Stack Sullivan's main thinking is alive and well in psychoanalysis, even if it is unacknowledged or presented in a different language. In the parlance of modern object relations theory, there also seems to be some splitting going on, i.e., half Sullivan's theory appears to reside in British Object Relations Theory and the other half in self psychology (with perhaps a "third half" in Erikson's psychosocial theory). Naturally, a psychodynamic theory of personality that could incorporate and integrate much of the best thought from various important modern psychoanalytic theories would be considered an intellectual tour de force. It is my thesis that the work of Harry Stack Sullivan does just that. While the purpose of this book will be to literally "re-collect" Sullivan, that is to reintroduce his work to a modern audience, I shall first explore the question of why Sullivan's work has been forgotten.

## Why Has Sullivan Been Forgotten?

Why has Sullivan not received more explicit notice by modern psychoanalytic writers or not been credited for greatly similar ideas that are clearly within the Sullivan corpus? While there has been the beginning of a Sullivan renaissance with the work of Leston Havens and Greenberg and Mitchell, many psychoanalysts and psychotherapists are surprised to hear about how close Sullivan's interpersonal theory is to modern interest in "object relations" and self psychology. Additionally, although Harry Stack Sullivan founded the prestigious Washington School of Psychiatry in Washington, DC, it has been of considerable interest to me for years that many psychotherapists, students, and faculty have little acquaintance with his work, even on the faculty of the Washington School of Psychiatry. My curiosity has deepened by the fact that Sullivan has been credited by scholars, such as Greenberg and Mitchell, Guntrip, and Havens, with being a most important contributor to the advancement of the interpersonal/object relations branch of psychodynamic/psychoanalytic theory. In my personal experience, the unique character of the Washington School of Psychiatry's interpersonal orientation and long history of an attitude welcoming serious students of human behavior and psychodynamic psychotherapy regardless of their profession, gender, or theoretical orientation is deeply grounded in Sullivan's original vision. Why then has Sullivan largely been forgotten?

There are four factors that may account for Sullivan's seemingly limited influence, despite his very important contributions to psychoanalysis, psychiatry, psychology, and social science. First, Parloff (1994) has posited that, paradoxically, Sullivan's central contributions are too widely incorporated into all psychological theories. The second factor is that Sullivan wrote relatively little compared to other great thinkers and, on the whole, did not write very well, making it hard for his work to be adequately disseminated. The third limitation to the recognition of Sullivan's work is that he attacked cherished psychoanalytic canon, spoke disdainfully about psychoanalysts and psychiatrists, and gave up working within the psychoanalytic establishment. Perhaps Sullivan's followers have not directly challenged the clear failure of important psychoanalytic writers to acknowledge Sullivan's contribution or similarity to their work because of ambivalence inspired by his problematic relations with these followers. Last, it is abundantly clear that Sullivan was personally a very difficult man, one who inspired rumors of myriad devian-cies. I strongly believe that these last two factors have made it difficult for many of those who knew Sullivan to wholeheartedly carry on his work in his name.

First, Parloff (1994) has raised the novel and paradoxical perspective that Sullivan's theory has been the victim of its own success. Parloff believes that one reason for Sullivan's seeming lack of recognition is that "his contributions about the interpersonal nature of human development, personality, and psychopathology have become integral and almost 'self-evident' aspects of all current psychological theory." As much as Shakespeare's plays are dismissed by new students as trite and full of cliches, Sullivan's original formulations about self concept and self esteem, as well as how interpersonal experience shapes our view of ourselves and others, may similarly fall under the category of "that's nothing new." Of course, these ideas were new to psychiatry and psychoanalysis when Sullivan introduced them, but they have made so much good sense that they have been widely appropriated. Certainly, while Parloff's perspective is strongly supported by the previously cited broad influence of Sullivan's previously cited in this chapter, this perspective cannot fully account for Sullivan's relative anonymity.

Secondly, as Greenberg and Mitchell have stated, a major reason for Sullivan's relative lack of acknowledgment in modern theory is that his original writings are difficult to understand. Sullivan was an overly self-critical, obtuse, and relatively unproductive writer, who by default left the survival of his most advanced ideas to the talented and dedicated William Alanson White Psychiatric Foundation Committee on Publication of Sullivan's Writings (Mabel Blake Cohen, David Rioch, Janet Rioch, Clara Thompson, Dexter Bullard, and later Otto Will and Donald Burnham) under the able editorship of Helen Swick Perry. From recorded lectures, journal articles, and Sullivan's written notes, this group worked many years to assemble five of the seven books that comprise Sullivan's published works. These included his two most important works *The Interpersonal Theory of Psychiatry* (1953) and *The Psychiatric Interview* (1954). Of the two books actually written by Sullivan himself, only one was published in his lifetime, *Conceptions of Modern Psychiatry* (1940/1953), a hastily prepared transcription of five lectures prepared for the February 1940 issue of Psychiatry, and later privately reprinted in a hard-bound copy for informal distribution, selling a remarkable 20,000 copies. This book was so popular at the time that it was used as a textbook in several social science departments and was reviewed in the *New York Times Book Review* in 1947, where its reviewer Lloyd Frankenberg pointed out that it was a difficult book to read.

Despite the success of Sullivan's initial exposure to the world beyond the Washington School of Psychiatry, Sullivan did not keep up the momentum with further books. Basically, Sullivan's publications during his lifetime consisted of a number of journal articles, mostly in his own journal, *Psychiatry*, and the book, *Conceptions of Modern Psychiatry*, of which he said, "The here reprinted lectures fail of close correspondence with my current views in the following more significant respects." (Sullivan, 1940/1953: ix). He went on to say that the concepts of anxiety, self-dynamism, and selective inattention are not adequately presented in this book. Anyone remotely familiar with his work will quickly realize that these are three of his most important concepts. His trouble with writing was a quite striking contradiction for a prolific lecturer, dynamic speaker, and founder of a school of psychiatry and a journal. Sullivan's own description of his difficulties with writing was quite telling. With reference to his discussion on internal self-criticism, which he called *supervisor patterns*, he referred in the following way to the supervisory pattern that he called his *reader* ...

> Thus when I attempt to use the written language to communicate serious thought, I am unhappily under constant harassment to so hedge the words around that the most bitterly critical person (his reader) will be unable to grossly misunderstand them, and, at the same time, to make them so clear that this wrongheaded idiot will grasp what I'm driving at. The result is, as I say, that I write almost nothing. I usually give up in the process of revising it.
> (1953: 240)

In addition, as Parloff (1994) pointed out, for a man who emphasized the essential importance of language and communication in his theory, Sullivan had a persistent tendency to invent terms for recognized psychoanalytic constructs, some of which approximated neologisms. Taking a moment to compare Sullivan with Freud, it is easy to see how Freud's influence would be vastly greater, independent even of the validity of his ideas, because of both the quantity and quality of his writing. Because of Sullivan's difficulties with writing style (which alternates between being obtuse and eloquent) and infrequent publication, Sullivan's ideas were basically transmitted through an oral tradition. Without a knowledgeable translator, one imbued with the oral tradition of interpersonal theory, the meaning of many of Sullivan's important points remains obscure. Fortunately, over time, more translators of Sullivan have appeared, for example, Havens (1973, 1976) and Greenberg and Mitchell (1983), but more elucidation of his concepts is definitely needed if his work is to be properly summarized.

Certainly, this problem of communication of Sullivan's main ideas may be responsible in large part for why his contributions are not better acknowledged. Yet, given the tendency toward pyrotechnic abstraction of many critical psychoanalytic thinkers such as Hartmann (1939), Kernberg, and early Kohut, the problem of Sullivan's writing style hardly seems like a fully adequate explanation for the lack of transmission of his ideas. One need only look to Freud and the development of his psychoanalytic school in modern times to realize that the dissemination of important and controversial ideas requires loyal disciples who carry these ideas into the future. I will now explore two hypotheses about why many of Sullivan's followers may have been ambivalent disciples – 1. his often disdainful challenge to cherished psychoanalytic canon and his irascibility towards psychoanalysts and psychiatrists and 2. rumors of Sullivan's personal deviance. i.e., his homosexuality or bisexuality.

Perhaps Sullivan's greatest political, and possibly intellectual, mistake in furthering his ideas was his remarkable and seemingly disciplined exclusion of significant references to Freud's work. For example, in the Indices of his two most important books, *The Interpersonal Theory of Psychiatry* and *The Psychiatric Interview*, there is only one reference to Freud. While Sullivan does indirectly refer to Freud's notions of regression, defense, sexuality, and structural (id, ego, and superego) concepts, such references tend to be dismissive. Sullivan does not acknowledge his similarities and differences with Freud's work, but rather largely ignores the prevailing psychoanalytic theory and canon of the day, while working, at least initially, within the framework of psychoanalysis. This need to separate himself from Freud was perhaps so great that he persistently invented new, sometimes obtuse, terms for concepts already well expressed by Freud. While Sullivan's interpersonal theory is the major alternative to Freud's drive theory, his failure to acknowledge Freud's thinking may have made his work unpalatable for those working within psychoanalysis.

Although there has been a tradition of publicly casting out detractors (e.g., Jung and Adler) from Freud's psychoanalytic inner circle, mainstream psychoanalysis' treatment of Sullivan's work has been more dismissive, eerily like Sullivan's treatment of Freud. An extraordinary example of this dismissive treatment by a psychoanalyst as a way of separating from Sullivan came from Karen Horney. During the early 1930s, Horney was initially a close colleague of Sullivan and member of the Zodiac group with Sullivan, Fromm, Clara Thompson, and others credited as the founders of social psychological or Neo-Freudian psychoanalytic theory. Yet later, at the height of a serious controversy with the American Psychoanalytic Association, Horney (1939) only mentions Sullivan's work in a footnote and a brief reference. She credited him along with others for suggesting that satisfaction and security as the basic foundation for human motivation (a concept Sullivan pioneered), but further stated that his theory was weakened by his failure to pay sufficient attention to the problem of anxiety. As we shall see throughout this book, perhaps the most central tenet of Sullivan's theory of personality was his unique and penetrating insights on the pervasive influence of anxiety in interpersonal living. The only conclusion for anyone familiar with Sullivan's work to reach was that Horney's statement was motivated by factors other than a careful assessment of Sullivan's thinking.

As mentioned before, another reason why people, including many who studied with Sullivan, may have been ambivalent in furthering his ideas, or had frankly turned away from his work, was that he held an attitude toward many psychoanalysts and psychiatrists that varied from disapproving to downright contemptuous. Perhaps Sullivan's own words, from *The Interpersonal Theory of Psychiatry (ITP),* best convey this assertion ...

I think that there is no other field of scientific endeavor in which the worker's preoccupations are as troublesome as in psychiatry. To illustrate this I will give three definitions of psychiatry. The first and broadest definition would run like this: it is all the confounding conglomerate of ideas and impressions, of magic, mysticism, and information, of conceits and vagaries, of conceptions and misconceptions, and of empty verbalisms. That is the broadest definition of psychiatry and, so far as I know, a good many people are very far advanced students of that field.

(Sullivan, 1953: 13)

While Sullivan next proposed his radical and rich definition of psychiatry as the study of interpersonal processes, including "the characteristic actions and operations in which the psychiatrist participates," it appears that he must first insult or devalue others' work. His style of criticizing psychiatry is reminiscent of a dynamism about which he writes eloquently under the topic "The Learning of Disparagement" ...

Learning by human examples is extremely important, as I have stressed; but if every example that seems to be worth emulating, learning something from, is reduced to no importance of worth, then who are the models going to be? I think that this is probably the most vicious of the inadequate, inappropriate, and ineffectual performances of parents of juveniles.

Sullivan (1953: 243)

Here we traverse the best and worst of Sullivan. His disparaging style was not limited to his lectures alone; one only need read the excellent book edited by Kvarnes and Parloff (1976), *A Harry Stack Sullivan Case Seminar,* to see how withering Sullivan could be to the seminar participants, all of whom were younger psychiatrists and potential proponents of Sullivan's work. If Sullivan's behavior in this seminar was any indication of how Sullivan usually conducted himself around other psychiatrists, it is a testament to those who have promoted and extended Sullivan's work such as David Rioch, Leon Salzman, and Robert Kvarnes for their ability to separate the rich Sullivan wheat from a very abrasive chaff. This is not to say that Sullivan has not had powerful supporters; it just appears that many of them may have been ambivalent about Sullivan, as evidenced by the lack of response to challenges about his work and the failure to insist that Sullivan should be acknowledged for his role in the development of ideas in psychoanalysis. Parenthetically, as word got around that I was researching a paper on why Sullivan had been forgotten at the Washington School of Psychiatry (Evans, 1992), a number of people volunteered war stories about Sullivan's capacity to raise psychiatrists' anxiety. I must add that I also heard an equal number of stories about Sullivan's real kindness toward patients and fellow psychiatrists. Additionally, when reading his clinical studies (e.g., Sullivan, 1956), one can only be impressed, by his uncanny ability to empathize with the most troubled individuals. This is further evidence of Sullivan's paradoxical nature. As Perry (1982: 73) stated ...

> Many of Sullivan's colleagues described him as being exclusively one or another of three kinds of characters: a withdrawn and cantankerous drunk; a somewhat pretentious high-stepper and sophisticate; the kindest, most considerate man who ever lived. Seldom did he show all three sides to the same person.

While Sullivan believed that humans are acutely tuned, by social anxiety, to threats to self esteem, he was largely blind to the enormously deleterious effects his rough treatment of his fellow professionals would have on the acceptance of his ideas. Clearly, Sullivan had very important ideas to convey, yet his disparagement of psychiatric trainees and colleagues undoubtedly made many enemies among those close to him.

The fourth and last speculation about why Sullivan has been forgotten involves a rumor that exists often in the shadow of any discussion of Sullivan's contributions, i.e., the conjecture that Sullivan was schizophrenic and homosexual. Leston Havens (1973) stated that Sullivan was "at least twice acutely psychotic himself." The major source for the idea that he was schizophrenic comes from Sullivan himself (Perry, 1982). Yet, Sullivan biographers, Chapman (1976) and Perry (1982) could find no solid evidence for this assertion. Perry thoroughly researched the hospital admission records in all likely New York state mental hospitals and interviewed people who knew the Sullivan family during the suspected period of Sullivan's purported psychosis but could find no evidence of a schizophrenic break.

Evidence for Sullivan's possible homosexuality is somewhat stronger. Chapman stated that he had spoken with people who knew that Sullivan had some homosexual experiences, although Chatelaine (1981) noted that Chapman was unwilling to state his sources publicly. Chapman also believed that the "clearly autobiographical" (Chapman's words) nature of Sullivan's writings proves his homosexuality, an odd interpretation at best. While Perry also found people who claimed to have "direct knowledge" (Perry's quotes) of Sullivan's homosexual experiences, she also stated that she heard of his sexual experiences with women as well. Whatever may be the truth regarding his sexuality, Sullivan was, by all accounts, an unmarried and lonely individual, who saw "homosexuality as a developmental mistake, dictated by the culture as substitutive behavior in those instances in which the person cannot do what is the simplest thing to do" (Sullivan, 1954: 225). A host of writings about Sullivan's homosexuality, starting with Allen (1995), and the role it may have played in his writings (Wake, 2006) emerged subsequent to the first edition of this book, which will be discussed later in the book.

A question infinitely more interesting than whether Sullivan was schizophrenic or homosexual is why psychoanalysts and others might discount Sullivan's work on the basis of these two, tentatively supported claims about his behavior. For example, one of the philosophical quotations often spoken by psychoanalysts as they regard their work is "the unexamined life is not worth living." This quote comes from Plato (1929), through Socrates, who lived in a culture in which the highest form of love, including physical love, was between men. Clearly, few, if any, scholars discount Plato's/Socrates' contributions to Western thought on the basis of their purported homosexuality. Also, an especially puzzling notion within psychoanalytic circles is that one's "personal psychopathology" would be a reason to discount intellectual contributions. For example, Chapman (1976) stated that Sullivan's "emotional problems ... prevented him from ... taking the attitude, 'There is the patient, whom I, a sounder person with special insights, shall treat.'" Sullivan's (1953) one genus hypothesis, "everyone is much more simply human than otherwise" suggested that the psychotherapist's personal problems in living, carefully transformed, might come in handy when formulating something about psychopathology in others. Clearly, Freud's major works, *The Interpretation of Dreams* (1900) and *Psychopathology of Everyday Life* (1901) are only two important of the many examples of Freud's courageous self-analysis and his recognition of the value of the psychoanalyst's understanding of his/her own psychopathology. Perhaps the most important difference from Sullivan's perspective was Freud's early notion that all sources of countertransference could be analyzed away, leading to a rather untenable position of the analyst as a fully conscious individual. Toward the end of his life, Freud (1937) took a humbler position in this regard, recognizing that analysis could be "interminable." Certainly, modern analysts, most notably Winnicott (1947) and Searles (1979), took a position closer to Sullivan, that countertransference is an inevitable part of psychotherapy and, in fact, the most useful tool in understanding the patient.

Why then might Sullivan's supposed deviances have been especially problematic for mainstream psychoanalysis? The answer may lie in Sullivan's idea that people's stereotypes and prejudices, however irrational, are terribly important interpersonal influences. It is clear that, whatever we may feel about someone personally, a scholar's ideas should rest on their own merits; anything less would simply be unfair and irrational. Two of Freud's formulations that have not held up to the scrutiny of time have been his ideas about schizophrenia and homosexuality (as well as his writings on women and rejection of the seduction/trauma hypothesis). For example, in the famous Schreber case, Freud (1911) stated that schizophrenics are untreatable by psychoanalytic methods (see Neiderland's, 1974, excellent research into Schreber's life and how his psychotic language symbolized actual interpersonal experience). Sullivan (1962) and his followers, most notably Fromm-Reichmann (1950), pointed out the serious limitations of Freud's ideas on schizophrenia by offering theoretical and clinical perspectives which led to successes in patient care.

Certainly, Freud's well-known position (1905, 1914) on homosexuality as a perversion arising from a narcissistic sexual identification with the father in response to castration anxiety has been roundly criticized and discarded by all but the most fervent Freudians. As Rieff (1959) pointed out, for all Freud's protestations about the scientific neutrality of psychoanalysis, he was a highly moral man and his ideas were not immune from the prevailing societal values of his time. Clearly, such values were present in his analysis of homosexuality. On the other hand, Sullivan (1953) demonstrated an unusual, sensitivity to, and sophistication about, the dilemmas of homosexual men. His ideas about homosexuality were highly advanced, especially for his time, and, as I will explain in Chapter 5, even for today.

At the time of his lectures in 1946–47 (Sullivan, 1953), homosexuality was considered by society, and the vast majority of the psychiatric community, as a sexual perversion, a view which was also psychoanalytic canon at the time. It is interesting to note that homosexuality was listed as a sexual deviance in the American Psychiatric. Association's *Diagnostic and Statistical Manual of Mental Disorders* until 1987 and World Health Organization's *International Classification of Disorders* only removed homosexuality in 1992. In contrast, Sullivan's (1953) remarkably advanced perspective was "to talk about homosexuality's being a problem really means about as much as to talk about humanity's being a problem."

One wonders if there is an element in mainstream psychoanalysis' treatment of Sullivan's implicit challenge to Freud's (and society's) values about homosexuality that is similar to Victorian society's outrage at Freud's open discussion of the importance of human sexuality and the costs of repressing this aspect of our humanity. Perhaps, psychoanalysts and psychiatrists have unconsciously found it difficult to accept, let alone honor, a fellow member who is seen as socially "deviant" (read socially unfashionable) at that given time, as clearly was the case with schizophrenia and homosexuality in significant parts of past (and present-day) society and psychiatry. I believe that Sullivan's theory would suggest the following interpretation about the problem of Sullivan's followership. Do we secretly feel subtle, unacknowledged, and irrational shame over allegiance to Sullivan, not because of Sullivan's actual character (which no one can know for sure), but because of the social anxiety engendered in us by the rumors about him and by our need to maintain interpersonal security? Leaving aside issues of a political nature to scholars of psychoanalytic history, what I suggest here is that there may be unacknowledged interpersonal forces at work, which have inhibited embracing the work of this very complex man.

In summary, it is my hope that the reader will find in this book that Harry Stack Sullivan was a visionary genius who pioneered an original and revolutionary way of conceptualizing human behavior. While the corpus of his writing is sparse, incomplete, and inadequately tested (and at times difficult to understand without significant elaboration), there is much evidence to suggest from modern developments in psychoanalysis, psychiatry, psychology, and social science that he was definitely on the right track. He was a problematic man who did not inspire an easy allegiance and was the subject of troublesome and embarrassing rumors. Yet, he was also a man of deep compassion and humanity, who actually believed that we were all simply more human than otherwise (unless you were a psychiatrist). He transcended his own personal problems and prejudices to formulate the interpersonal theory of psychiatry, which insisted on the essential interrelatedness of all people as the foundation of personality theory and social understanding. While Sullivan rarely used the word love in his writings, his work strongly implies that it is love between humans that ultimately liberates us.

# Chapter 2

# Harry Stack Sullivan, the Man

Harry Stack Sullivan is one of the least widely known of great men. Within his own profession, his name is legend ... Sullivan is not among the writing psychiatrists. He belongs rather to a bardic tradition ... his ideas have spread more rapidly than his fame. By a trained awareness of his own processes ('The wounded surgeon plies the steel,' said T. S. Eliot), the psychiatrist is qualified to recognize distortions in the patient's behavior, caused by unresolved past situations.

(Frankenberg quoted in Perry, 1982: 402)

As mentioned in Chapter 1, Harry Stack Sullivan's life was shrouded with mystery and controversy. There are whole periods of his life for which there are no accounts of his activities or whereabouts. Yet, as with Freud before him, it is clear from his writings that Sullivan draws on his own life experiences, especially interpersonal experience, as an important source for his theories about personality and human nature. While it is well beyond the scope of this book to write a detailed biography, a summary discussion of his early life experiences, his early professional training, and his later personal and professional life are in order. Readers interested in greater depth on this topic are referred to Helen Swick Perry's (1982) excellent book *Psychiatrist of America: The Life of Harry Stack Sullivan.* Perry's book is by far the most thoughtful and well-researched biography to date. Perry edited five of the seven books that comprise the Sullivan opus and therefore knew his writings intimately. Her book not only thoroughly chronicles Sullivan's life, but is an excellent example of a biography from the perspective of Sullivan's interpersonal theory.

Sullivan was born of Timothy Sullivan and Ella Stack Sullivan on February 21, 1892, on a cold winter day in Norwich, New York, a small rural farming community several hundred miles northwest of New York City. Both parents were of Irish descent, first-generation American immigrants fleeing the Irish potato famine. Their families came to Chenango County, New York within a year of each other, into a community that looked down upon Irish Americans. Ella Stack descended from a family of landed gentry both in Ireland and eventually in Chenango County. While there was always a

DOI: 10.4324/9781003305712-3

whisper of family failure because her father had been dismissed from seminary, by and large the Stack family was favorably regarded in the Irish-American community of Chenango County. She was the oldest daughter of her father, a schoolteacher and farm owner, and most of her siblings eventually went on to college in the United States and later established themselves in businesses or professions. Ella Stack did not go to college and was perilously close to being an old maid and the only unmarried child, when, at nearly 33 years of age, she married Timothy Sullivan, at 28, a man four-and-a-half years younger.

From all accounts, Timothy Sullivan had worked as a laborer at Stack farm or other nearby farm, which is likely how he met Ella Stack. As with many Irishmen of that era, Timothy's father left Ireland as an impoverished, landless farm worker to work on the railroads in North America. Although the Sullivan family worked diligently to save money to obtain land in the United States, when Timothy was seventeen his father was killed in a railroad construction accident, leaving behind a poor family of six children with no means of support. The older sons, Timothy included, were sent to work as laborers or servants on local farms to provide support their mother, Julia Sullivan, and the younger children. The sons were also expected by the mother to make good, which meant to purchase the farmland, the fulfillment of her dream. Only one son, Timothy, would ever do so. At the time of his marriage, Timothy worked in a hammer factory farm outside of town as an unskilled or semi-skilled laborer, without land of his own. Ella Stack married a man without money, prestige, or education, all qualities highly valued by the Stack family. Even though they faced considerable prejudice from without, Irish Americans had their social stratification, specifically the landowner, upper class "lace curtain Irish" as opposed to the landless, lower class "shanty Irish." According to the Stack family, Ella Stack had "married down" by taking Timothy Sullivan as her husband. This family tension would repeat a generational pattern, with a few exceptions, that began before the Stacks and Sullivans left Ireland and remained for generations afterward. As will be described further, the underlying Stack/Sullivan tension was a fertile ground for an enormously intelligent, perceptive, and sensitive young man to study intrafamily struggles and the social context in which they occur. It is no wonder that Sullivan experienced and described the power of social and cultural pulls more vividly than the relatively culturally insulated Freud.

Harry Stack Sullivan was Ella and Timothy Sullivan's third child. Their two previous children were born in the same house in the month of February, respectively, two and four years earlier and both had died in convulsions, probably due to diphtheria, before the Fall of their first year of life. Ella Stack Sullivan was 39 at the time of Harry Stack Sullivan's birth, despaired of dying childless, and now had another February baby. Fueled by the local old-time belief that winter babies did not have a good chance to live through the first summer, as well as her two losses bearing out the prediction, Ella Sullivan must have keenly experienced, and Harry Stack Sullivan must have been surrounded by, the maternal anxiety that would become the core concept of his developmental theory. Adding to her dread, they lived on Rexford Street, a bad part of town, in a neighborhood of lower social status and literally on the wrong side of the railroad tracks, near an abandoned, improperly drained canal ditch thought to be the source of "black diphtheria," which raged in epidemic proportions during the late 1880s. The confluence of being the only surviving child of a mother who had lost two previous children in similar circumstances and growing up in a feared social environment must have naturally led to Ella Stack Sullivan's overprotectiveness of Harry Stack Sullivan, which later marked his powerfully ambivalent feelings towards her and other women.

From the beginning of their marriage, there was considerable family struggle between Timothy Sullivan and Ella and the other Stacks. Ella Stack Sullivan deeply resented living on Rexford Street and, now with the birth of Harry, also feared it. Her brother Ed Stack was a prosperous businessman in nearby South Otselic, New York and there was considerable family pressure on Timothy to move his family there to take part in Ed's business. Yet, there was no Catholic church in South Otselic, an exclusively Protestant town apart from Ed Stack's family, who either did not go to church or attended the local Protestant services. A deeply religious man, Timothy Sullivan would not abide the move to South Otselic based on his commitment to Catholicism. In the midst of this period of disagreement, Timothy purchased, apparently precipitously and unilaterally, the Rexford Street house, taking out a large mortgage to do so. Shortly thereafter, another of the frequent shutdowns occurred in the hammer factory where Timothy Sullivan was employed, leaving the Sullivans in very tight financial straits. These events led to the next important chapter of young Harry Stack Sullivan's life.

When Harry Stack Sullivan was two-and-a-half years old, he moved from Norwich to the Stack family farm in Smyrna NY to be raised by his maternal grandmother, Mary Stack. While the actual events leading to this move are shrouded in mystery, it strongly appears that Sullivan's mother disappeared, amid rumors that she suffered a nervous breakdown and tried to harm herself and possibly young Harry. Whether she was put in the attic of the family farm or went to her brother Ed's or some other place for convalescence has never been determined. What is clear is that Harry Stack Sullivan, who heretofore had been raised exclusively and overprotectively by his mother, was now being raised by his Irish born, superstitious, strict grandmother who spoke predominately Gaelic. Events in the Sullivan family's life underwent further rapid change. Ella's father and Mary's husband, Michael Stack, died soon after Harry moved to the farm, leaving the Stack family farm without anyone to run it or to support Mary Stack. Timothy Sullivan was elected to run the farm for family and acceded to circumstance. He sold his Rexford Street house to Ella's brother Ed Stack and purchased the farm, which was deeded to him in a highly specific and humiliating way, suggesting that the Stack family believed he could not be trusted. An example of the West Irish concept of *cliamham isteach*, literally the son-in-law going in, Timothy Sullivan, shrouded by failure and isolated from his home and friends in Norwich, withdrew into himself and, for the next 36 years until his death, owned and farmed the Stack farm by which it was always to be known. For Ella Stack Sullivan, once she recovered, the move also represented a defeat, a move to the farm from which Ella Stack had married Timothy Sullivan to escape. It was an isolated farm outside Smyrna, New York, well away from the larger, more prosperous town of Norwich. Smyrna was geographically isolated and economically poor. Nativism of the Protestant majority was especially high and prejudice of school children toward an Irish Catholic boy would be worse than in the better-situated Norwich. The burning of a cross within the sight of the Stack farm in the 1920s by the anti-Catholic Ku Klux Klan bears witness to the social world of Harry Stack Sullivan's childhood. These life tragedies in childhood would provide fertile ground for his extensive and unique perspective on the role of cultural, interpersonal, and family dynamics on the development of personality and mental illness. His multiple family influences and misfortunes would lead him to emphasize "mothering" and other processes of social learning over the exclusive reliance on the mother-child relationship found in Object Relations and other psychoanalytic theories and to develop tremendous empathy and insight into severe mental illness. As Freud used his penetrating insight to pierce the veil of civility of the European Victorian era in his discovery of the origins of neurosis, so had Sullivan, using his painful family and community experiences in rural America to plumb the causes of psychosis and severe personality disorders.

During what he termed the Childhood Era (after Infancy and before the Juvenile Era) which coincides with the beginning of schooling, Sullivan was raised primarily in the company of adults, mainly women. His grandmother played the central caretaking role; his mother, who reappeared during this period, was a shadowy figure and his father was remote and even more uncommunicative than before. As his dear friend and colleague Clara Thompson (1949) stated at Sullivan's memorial service, his closest childhood friends were livestock on the farm. Sullivan often autobiographically referenced the importance of imaginary playmates and the freedom a lonely child without real playmates had from the group allegiances and assumptions which are so deeply engrained that they go otherwise unnoticed. His isolated farm existence was interrupted only rarely by occasional visits from an aunt, uncle, or cousin. His mother's direct role in his upbringing became less central than before her disappearance, yet her loss of status from the myriad failures that accompanied this period (e.g., as a woman dependent on her mother, herself as a mother, and the loss of her husband's status) must have had a tremendous influence on young Harry. It surely provided the lonely perceptive boy Sullivan with a wealth of experience to observe the workings of what he was later to call *self esteem*, one's sense of self as compared to one's sense of important others, and *security operations*, activities verbal and non-verbal that avoid or reduce anxiety that signals dangers to self esteem. A curious side note regarding his own self esteem experience, Sullivan intense hated of the color blue. He refused to wear blue clothes or even sit in a blue chair. He explained to friends that his aversion came from his mother's use of the color in his baby clothes, which she preserved and showed proudly to guests.

Sullivan's entrance into grade school marked a critical turn in fortune for him, as he was to find some important sources of self-esteem in his academic abilities and successes. To quote Sullivan (1953: 227) "This (the Juvenile Era) is the first developmental stage in which the limitations and peculiarities of the home as a socializing influence begin to be open to remedy." He attended a school where all grades through high school were physically in one building, the lower school (grades 1 through 6) on the first floor and upper school (grades 7 through 12) on the second. Unlike most of his peers, Sullivan already knew how to read when he entered school. He was soon noticed by the school principal Herbert Butts, who influenced and greatly enhanced Sullivan's interest in science, especially from geography trips in the fossil-rich area surrounding Smyrna.

Learning the scientific name of things was a passion throughout Sullivan's schooling. His interest in Latin and Greek derivations, along with complications of using in the brogue of his Gaelic-speaking grandmother, probably contributed to his curiosity about words and was seminal in the difficulty in expression for which he was often justly criticized throughout his later career. Often the teacher's pet, Sullivan's school years were not without significant problems. Living in the last house in the school district, a one-and-a-half mile walk from school, he was a loner who lacked experience in knowing how to be part of his peer group. The problem of being the brightest student, but an Irish Catholic boy to boot, gave rise to the envy and misunderstanding among his rural peers. As mentioned earlier, the community of Smryna was high in virulent anti-Catholic sentiment, which Sullivan (1938a) was to liken later in life to anti-Semitism. Perry (1982) quotes one of Sullivan's grade schoolteachers as saying of Sullivan, "He was just born too smart," and conjectures that the teacher did not think it fair for an Irish-Catholic student to be so superior. Ever the brilliant outsider, his school years gave Sullivan ample opportunity to explore the interpersonal themes of the Juvenile Era – the comparison of authority figures inside and outside the family, the learning of different values of different social groups, and the importance of the peer group's acquisition of the social skills of compromise and cooperation. Needless to say, it was also an excellent time to learn the powerful social forces of prejudice, envy, and ostracism.

While Sullivan drew much self esteem from his school academic experience and some relief from the encompassing familial worldview occasioned by his physical separateness from peers, his early grade social world was still influenced by peer isolation at school and complex family dynamics at home. At home, while Sullivan's grandmother continued to dominate his mother, diminishing her self-esteem, Ella became more involved with Sullivan during the school years. This odd, overindulgent, and verbal woman pushed him socially and intellectually to succeed in school, seeing young Harry destined for Stack family greatness. While Sullivan did achieve this greatness, he was most ambivalent about it. Clearly Sullivan's overprotective/abandoning, highly insecure mother had an enduring impact on his life. His own ambivalence regarding many stories of Stack superiority told by his mother to bolster her fragile sense of self is nowhere more perceptively revealed than by Perry's (1982) research into the names he used throughout his adult life. He was first known as Harry Francis Stack Sullivan (Francis being his confirmation name given at age 13), then as H. F. Sullivan, next as H. Stack Sullivan, a surgeon in Chicago, and finally as Harry Stack Sullivan, in which the Stack is variously spelled out or initialized in his signatures. In contrast to this hothouse of maternal expectation, Sullivan's relationship to his father was remote. His father was hardworking, withdrawn, and inarticulate, and attempts by his father to involve Sullivan in work on farm were undermined regularly by his mother with well-timed trips to the library. Sullivan did not get to know his father until after his mother died in 1926. In later life, Sullivan would come to share his father's hardworking and withdrawn tendencies.

In what Perry termed "the quiet miracle," Sullivan's life once again made a significant turn with the formation of his first peer friendship. This person, who Sullivan (1953) called in later theory the *chum*, marking the beginning of the *Pre-Adolescent Era*, was in real life Clarence Bellinger. Bellinger was a boy five years older than the eight-and-a-half-year-old Sullivan, lived on a more prosperous farm next to Sullivan, and like Sullivan was a bright only child who was doted on by his mother. In high school, they rode together in Bellinger's horse-drawn wagon to Smyrna, delivering milk to a cheese factory on the way to school. Fellow schoolmates probably despised and ostracized the twosome for many reasons – both for their intelligence and air of superiority when together, Sullivan for his Irish Catholicism, and Bellinger for his shortness, obesity, and privilege. Bellinger's family were also religious outcasts, because they did not go to the Protestant church regularly. Yet for Sullivan, his preadolescent chum must have been a godsend. Intellectually matched, equally isolated and ostracized, and special only sons with doting mothers, one can readily understand his interest in "*isophilic love*," i.e., being in love with someone like oneself. *Chumship* is a time when friends share openly their inner evaluations of their families and life in general. Sullivan and Bellinger must have had much to talk about.

Set apart from other adolescents their age by their attendance in high school, neither boy participated in friendships apart from their own, paralleling the exclusivity of relationship they had with their mothers. Sullivan and Bellinger had no known significant relationships with girls or young women in Smyrna, likely reflecting their over-merger with the sexual prohibition of their mothers. Sullivan was later to write penetratingly about the major role of *"not me"* anxiety about sexuality in the development of schizophrenia and other severe mental illnesses. Interestingly, given their rural Smyrna background, neither Sullivan nor Bellinger ever married, both became important psychiatrists (Bellinger became the Superintendent of Brooklyn State Hospital, a large psychiatric in New York state hospital system), both worked at St. Elizabeth's Hospital under the direction of the great William Alanson White, and both became psychiatric researchers, which was uncommon for psychiatrists during their time. Bellinger published his first paper in 1925, the same year as Sullivan's first paper and both wrote papers on the role of inadequate child training on mental illness. Despite these great similarities, after Bellinger graduated high school (two years ahead of Sullivan) and matriculated at Syracuse University Medical School, they never communicated again. Clearly, they had a significant falling out. In fact, Bellinger was said to be outwardly contemptuous of Sullivan to others throughout the rest of his life, while Sullivan was never known to speak of Bellinger. Sullivan mentioned poignantly in his discussions of the *Pre-Adolescent Era* about the vulnerability of the lonely preadolescent who could be easily misused by a post-puberty adolescent chum for chum's satisfaction.

Two other influences on Sullivan's boyhood years are important to mention. Aunt Margaret Stack, his mother's sister, took an active role with Sullivan's upbringing during his school years. She was an unmarried schoolteacher living in New York City, near Park Avenue. On her visits to Smyrna, she brought him many books unavailable to him in Smyrna on a broad array of interests and engaged him in lively intellectual discussions that served for him as an introduction to the larger world of ideas. Her visits would eventually help him make the significant transition from Smyrna to the outside world. Not insignificantly she provided money for his medical education. Will Sullivan, his father's cousin and one of the few successful men on the Sullivan side of the family, was a highly regarded attorney and later judge. Influenced by the numerous suicides and bizarre murders in Chenango County (one of which was the basis of Theodore Dreiser's famous 1925 novel An *American Tragedy*), Will Sullivan was a pioneer in applying psychological knowledge to the law during his years as a practicing attorney,. He used the insanity defense, though unsuccessfully, in several murder trials and was known as a fair and compassionate judge. His actions and ideas served as a backdrop for Harry Stack Sullivan's interest in human problems. Will Sullivan probably also contributed financially to Sullivan's education.

As a culmination to his success in high school, variously nurtured by his mother's neurotic ambition for Stack greatness, his Aunt Margaret's introduction to the intellectual world beyond Smyrna, his cousin Will Sullivan's compassion for the emotionally troubled, and his own budding intellect, Harry Stack Sullivan won the prestigious New York State Regents Scholarship to Cornell University. In doing so, he experienced a rare and special glory for a rural boy from Chenango County. Clearly, this event must have done much for his self-esteem, precariously based on academic achievement as it was. Unfortunately, his moment of glory was to be short-lived.

In 1908, at the age of 16 and without much to say goodbye to in Smyrna, Harry Stack Sullivan matriculated in the College of Arts and Sciences at Cornell University with dreams of becoming a physicist. Physically delayed in puberty and emotionally immature compared to his classmates, his academic performance in the first semester was good for his level of high school preparation, but he most definitely was not the smartest, nor the most academically successful, student. The role of good, but not best, student was new for him and much of his personal security hinged on school success. Additionally, problems with a lack of social and sexual maturity surfaced. In *The Interpersonal Theory of Psychiatry*, Sullivan's writing on the failure of the integration of lust dynamism reveals an understanding of obsessive preoccupation with fantasy women of a lonely, immature late adolescent that was likely drawn from his own experience. One of Sullivan's great contributions to personality theory and psychopathology was his cogent analysis of the grave dangers in adolescence of the failure to integrate the dynamisms of lust, interpersonal security, and intimacy, which is likely based on the cataclysmic events of his life which began at Cornell. His grades slipped dramatically in second semester and was involved with a group of boys who were illegally obtaining and selling chemicals through the mail. While all evidence suggests that his role in the scam was minor and tangential, he was the one caught and convicted of mail fraud, a serious crime. For both his academic difficulties and involvement in the crime, Sullivan was suspended from Cornell for a semester (a light punishment), but never returned. For the next two years, his whereabouts were unknown. While some speculation suggested that he was sent to jail or reform school, Sullivan did obliquely mention to Perry (1982) and other professional colleagues that he had experienced a schizophrenic state and implied that he had been hospitalized during this period. While she did find some circumstantial evidence that he may have been treated at Bellevue Hospital in New York City by the colleague of the son of his family doctor or A. A. Brill or both, Perry's (and Chatelaine's, 1981) research failed to find direct evidence for this claim. Additionally, David Rioch (1985: 142), a close colleague of Sullivan, suggested that, "The rapidity, efficiency and stability of his recovery from his debacle ... at Cornell in no way suggest a chronic psychotic condition (as gossip in professional circles has implied)." The most accurate statement of Sullivan's two years after Cornell is that he appeared to drop off the face of the earth, only to resurface in Chicago in 1911. The disgrace of the Cornell failure and criminal conviction must have been keenly felt in Smyrna, after which Sullivan's mother would walk away at the mention of his name, even after he graduated from medical school. Episodes of severe failure and disgrace are quite rare in the histories of many of the other makers of modern psychotherapy, with perhaps the exception of Erik Hamburg Erikson. Sullivan's ability to survive, and later make great use of, these failures was quite central in his development of interpersonal theory.

After Sullivan's two-year disappearance, he matriculated medical school at the Chicago College of Medicine and Surgery in the Fall of 1911. The Chicago College of Medicine and Surgery, founded by Valparaiso University to provide "high grade" medical education regardless of financial circumstances, did not require the bachelor's degree prerequisite, unlike medical training in the United States today. In all likelihood, given its proximity to Cook County Hospital and other noted Chicago clinics, the Chicago School provided an average medical education for its day, but under no circumstances should it be compared to the superior medical or academic training received by Freud and other psychoanalytic luminaries. In his records at the Chicago College, there was no mention of his attendance at Cornell, beginning perhaps the pattern of exclusion and falsification of applications and records that would continue for many years. He completed his formal course work in 1915, but was not awarded his medical degree until 1917. It is not known whether this delay was to allow him to pay back fees (not uncommon for the period) or to permit him to complete or make up courses, as Sullivan's grades at the Chicago College were uneven. Loyola University of Chicago acquired the Chicago College of Medicine at the end of Sullivan's medical training and he received the last medical diploma awarded by Valparaiso University.

Sullivan's early medical career was hardly illustrious. Initially, he took medical jobs that did not require the completion of medical training, first as an industrial surgeon for a steel mill and, in June 1916, as an enlistee in the Illinois National Guard, where he was assigned to an infirmary in San Antonio, Texas. By November 1916, he was released for physical disqualification, presumably because he broke his jaw in a riding accident. This explanation is somewhat suspect in that his release from the National Guard began another period of disappearance in 1916–17. On later application and documents, Sullivan noted as part of his professional training that he received 75 hours of psychoanalysis roughly during the period in question. Shortly thereafter, he apparently opened a private practice in Chicago under the name of H. Stack Sullivan, Surgeon. In 1918, he applied to the Army for an appointment to the Reserve Medical Corps. According to Perry's (1982) research, Sullivan's application contained numerous inaccuracies and falsifications, including false claims of prior hospital employment and even a wrong birthdate that made him appear older than he was. Be that as it may, he passed his examination for medical licensure and received a commission as first lieutenant in active duty until Armistice, after which he was appointed Captain in Officers Reserve Corps. Between 1919–20, he moved between Chicago and Washington, DC in a variety of medical jobs for the Division of Rehabilitation for Disabled Soldiers, Sailors and Marines, Federal Board of Vocational Education. He left the Federal Board in late 1920 and records lose track of him again until his appointment as a liaison officer for the Veterans Bureau at St. Elizabeth's Hospital in Washington, DC. in November 1921. At the age of 30, Sullivan's career as a psychiatrist was launched at long last.

The first year of Sullivan's psychiatric career was spent at St. Elizabeth's Hospital, a national institution famous for its sympathetic understanding and care of patients, under the direction of William Alanson White. White was a pioneer in the application of dynamic psychiatry to psychotic patients, who before St. Elizabeth's had worked New York psychiatric hospital close to Sullivan's boyhood home. Active in psychiatric research as well as clinical care, White co-founded the prestigious journal, Psychoanalytic Review, where Sullivan later published one of his first two papers (Sullivan, 1925) on schizophrenia. St. Elizabeth's was a hot bed of psychiatric innovation and research with thinkers such as White (1935) and Edward Kempf (1921), who modified (and discarded aspects of) psycho-analytic method for the treatment of schizophrenic and manic-depressive patients. Fascination with dynamic methods for treatment was high and White actively encouraged his staff's initiative and thoughtful experimentation.

Adding to this milieu of learning for a young psychiatrist, White had an ability to inspire confidence from his staff and apparently got to know much about Sullivan's earlier life. Sullivan felt that White rescued his medical career and helped establish him as an accepted professional. White's special sympathy and understanding for mental illness and crime must have certainly helped in this regard. White's (1933: 31) one genus postulate that, "The difference between the so-called insane person or the criminal on one hand and so-called normal or sane person on the other is only a difference in quantity, a difference in the strength or weakness and the balanced relationships of the various tendencies and stimuli with which he has to deal." is essentially same as Sullivan's one genus hypothesis (1940/1953: 16), "we are all much more simply human than otherwise, be we happy and successful, contended and detached, miserable or mentally disordered, or whatever." This central organizing principle of both men's approach to humanity must have been White's great personal, one could say therapeutic, contribution to the brilliant, but troubled Sullivan. Instead of hiding his troubled past, it became the data by which Sullivan came to formulate his theory and develop his approach to treatment.

While Sullivan also felt the influence of Kempf (who was no longer at St. Elizabeth's when Sullivan was there) on his theory, borrowing and expanding Kempf's concepts of "not I, not me, not myself" and "social esteem," it was William Alanson White who became Sullivan's professional and intellectual father. It is a mark of Sullivan as a man that in 1933 he would choose the name, the William Alanson White Psychiatric Foundation, as the governing body for the Washington School of Psychiatry and the journal *Psychiatry* and call the New York branch of the Washington School of Psychiatry, the William Alanson White Institute. Sullivan's well-known lectures, which became the only book published in his lifetime (*Conceptions of Modern Psychiatry*, 1940/1953), were the First William Alanson White Memorial Lectures. Sullivan (CMP: 177–78) gave White first honors for "maintaining the healthy eclecticism that has characterized American psychiatry and that has carried it far beyond psychiatry elsewhere in the world."

Apparently, White was less impressed with Harry Stack Sullivan. When Sullivan was no longer satisfied to be a liaison officer between the Veterans Bureau and St. Elizabeth's Hospital, he approached White about a full-time clinical position at St. Elizabeth's. White told Sullivan that there was no position available nor would there likely to be one in the immediate future. In response to a letter of reference request for Sullivan from Ross McClure Chapman for a position at Sheppard Pratt Hospital, White mildly questioned Sullivan's abilities, and gave a reference that was one of faint praise. Apparently, when the word got back to Sullivan, he began to question White's candor and honesty with him. Nonetheless, he maintained an active professional, if somewhat distant personal, relationship with White, acknowledging White's importance to him and staying connected to White's role as gatekeeper to a vast network of psychiatric communications.

In 1922, although White's letter of reference was less than inspiring, Ross Chapman, Medical Director of the Sheppard Pratt Hospital in Towson, a suburb of Baltimore MD, immediately hired Sullivan for his first position as a psychiatrist with direct clinical responsibility. In December 1922, Sullivan began the eight years at Sheppard Pratt, which led to the most important clinical work of his career. Sheppard Pratt Hospital, a private Quaker hospital with a provision for accepting indigent patients (an unusual policy for private hospitals in the United States then and now), afforded an excellent match for Sullivan's socially conscious awareness of the connection between social class and mental illness. Ross Chapman was a clinical innovator who was William Alanson White's first assistant at St. Elizabeth's before assuming the superintendent of Sheppard Pratt. In many ways, Chapman became as important an influence on Sullivan's development as a psychiatrist as White was.

Whereas White was an inspirational, sympathetic, though doubting "father," Chapman became the unprecedented champion of Sullivan's talents. A strong believer in the importance of the therapeutic milieu in the hospital and of specialized training for hospital nurses and attendants, he granted privileges to Sullivan regarding the design and conduct of his clinical unit that were unprecedented for their time (and perhaps remain so today). Chapman allowed Sullivan to establish a small ward for schizophrenic men set apart from the rest of the hospital that was staffed with hand-picked male attendants and excluded female nurses. Sullivan requested, and was given, recording equipment to assist him in his research on schizophrenic thought patterns. He carefully trained his attendants in his theories and gave them much autonomy to operate on their own with the patients. De-emphasizing the various social status roles of doctor, attendant, and patient as much as he could, Sullivan established a social treatment environment of people responding empathically to the troubles of others without prejudice of role differences. As Sullivan stated ...

the chosen employees ... ceased to regard (the patient) in more or less traditional ideology as "insane," but instead had stressed to them the many points of significant resemblance between the patient and the employee— we created a much more useful social situation; we found that intimacy between the patient and the employee blossomed unexpectedly, that things I cannot distinguish from genuine human friendship sprang up between patient and employee, that any signs of the alleged apathy of the schizophrenic faded, to put it mildly, and that the institutional recovery rate became high.

(1962: 223)

To clarify this passage, Sullivan (1953) believed strongly that intimacy was not essentially sexual, but was instead the desire for humans to be close and to receive validation of self-worth. Sullivan's quotation suggests the central distinction between the interpersonal (or object relation) theorist's belief that humankind is person oriented as opposed to pleasure oriented in Freud's drive theory (1905). Truly, Sullivan's one genus hypothesis and interpersonal orientation came to life on his Sheppard Pratt ward.

While Sullivan's statements appear idealistic, as would befit his American democratic philosophical leanings (see Mullahy, 1970 for his comparison of Sullivan to the famous American philosopher John Dewey), the results from Sullivan's treatment unit, what he called "social recoveries," made him famous as the man could successfully treat schizophrenics using psychodynamic methods. His series of articles on schizophrenia, the most important of which were collected for his book *Schizophrenia as a Human Process* (1962), describe his understanding of schizophrenia and suggested a novel approach to treatment. His work became widely known not only for its successful results, but also because he challenged a cherished psychoanalytic doctrine. According to Freud (1911) in his famous Schreber case, psychoanalytic treatment of schizophrenia was not possible, primarily because, unlike neurotics, the schizophrenic was unable to form a transference. Sullivan found the opposite, that schizophrenics form powerful, intense transferences that are often overwhelming for both the patient and the psychiatrist and that require significant modifications in psychoanalytic technique. His discoveries led to a busy schedule of paper presentations and article writing, which broadly disseminated his ideas on schizophrenia as well as his initial thinking on the role of social forces in the formation of personality and mental illness. His eight years at Sheppard Pratt were his most prolific as a writer. Sullivan came to Sheppard Pratt as an untried novice and left as a legend in the world of clinical psychiatry, as well as in social sciences where he was so well regarded that he was selected in the early 1930s to write both the "Mental Disorders" (1962) and "Psychiatry" (1964) sections of the *Encyclopedia of Social Sciences.* In his later years, Sullivan would despair that other psychiatric units did not replicate his results and that medical education failed to develop sufficient empathy for the patient to be useful for the schizophrenic problem. Putting Sullivan's work in historical context, it is important to remember, when evaluating Sullivan's successes at Sheppard Pratt, Salzman (1992) has suggested that many of the patients whom Sullivan considered schizophrenic would today be seen as borderline. The seminal papers about the borderline state (e.g., Deutsch, 1942; Kernberg, 1967, 1975; Knight, 1953; Stern, 1938) came well after Sullivan's writing on schizophrenia, so that the important modern distinction between schizophrenic and borderline states likely did not influence Sullivan's thinking.

While at Sheppard Pratt, Sullivan met the individual who would become one of his closest friends and professional colleagues and, directly and indirectly, one of his most important influences. When Sullivan first met her in Baltimore, Clara Thompson was a young psychiatrist working at the Phipps Clinic of the Johns Hopkins University School of Medicine under the direction of Adolf Meyer. From the beginning, Thompson and Sullivan shared an infinity for the psychiatric dilemmas of the "lonely ones," as they referred to their schizophrenic patients. They critiqued each other's emerging concepts and papers. Thompson introduced Sullivan to Adolf Meyer's (1957) psychobiology, which would validate Sullivan's emphasis on interpersonal and sociocultural events in the formation of the personality as well as the importance of symbols, meanings, and conscious integration in mental life. Sullivan would soon share Meyer's skepticism about the growing orthodoxy within psychoanalysis. Sullivan's influence on Thompson's thinking can be seen throughout her writings (Thompson, 1964). Perhaps his influence is in no place more powerfully demonstrated than in her brilliant challenge (Thompson, 1943) to Freud's concept of penis envy, which stated that the concept represents a symbol of women's underprivileged status in society rather than an innate, biologically determined wish to be a man or to have a penis. When Sullivan became interested in the work of Sandor Ferenczi in

1926 (especially his interests in so-called hopeless cases, in the role of culture in personality, in providing treatment for the poor, and in challenging Freud's belief in the detached, objective stance of the analyst), he convinced Thompson to travel to Budapest to be analyzed by Ferenczi in late 1927. In turn, Thompson became Sullivan's training analyst when she returned from Europe, on the basis of which he was later admitted to membership in the American Psychoanalytic Society. While very close during the Baltimore days, they never married, although Sullivan alluded to an event in which he agreed one evening with a young woman to marry; "the next morning ... they broke their necks to the first to telephone and break the engagement" (Perry, 1982: 202). Champions of the power of intimacy and the interpersonal, both Sullivan and Thompson remained devoted friends, though were unmarried throughout their lives.

The Sheppard Pratt years brought important losses and new attachments. Sullivan had gradually achieved rapprochement with his family again and visited often during his mother's illness in 1925–26. During one of these trips to Smyrna, he visited his closest cousin Leo Stack, who became ill while dining. A local doctor was called, pronouncing Leo as suffering from an attack of indigestion. Not satisfied with the doctor's diagnosis, Sullivan insistently urged Leo to see another doctor, which Leo and his wife politely ignored. Tragically, Leo Stack died that night of a massive heart attack. Leo's death was a marker event for Sullivan, beginning his lifelong skepticism with his medical colleagues. Shortly thereafter on February 25, 1926, Sullivan's mother died, ending his relationship with the woman whom he often said was a chronic invalid and complainer and formed "her personification of him as a clotheshorse on which to hang her illusions" (Perry, 1982: 223).

Later in 1926, Sullivan met Edward Sapir, a professor of cultural anthropology at the University of Chicago. Sapir introduced Sullivan to the Chicago School of Thought, including the work of Charles Cooley (1937, 1964, 1966) and, especially, George Herbert Mead (1934, 1952, 1956), whose concepts of mind, self, and society are building blocks from which Sullivan developed his interpersonal theory of personality. Sapir, a specialist in the language and life of Northwest Indians, was interested in the possibility of a collaboration between psychiatry and social sciences. Sapir arranged to meet Sullivan in Chicago where Sullivan was attending a professional meeting. As a result of this meeting, they became devoted friends and colleagues until Sapir's untimely death in 1939. In Sullivan, Sapir found a wise and compassionate confidante and broad and creative psychiatric thinker. Sullivan found a true adult male chum in Sapir as someone who deeply appreciated him and helped Sullivan gain greater assurance in the world of social sciences because of his relationship with a scholar possessing a first-rate intellectual mind.

Sullivan's access to the Chicago School of Sociology (containing departments of social anthropology, social psychology, and political science) began his famous interdisciplinary collaboration between psychiatry and the social sciences. The Chicago School's place in United States intellectual history is considerable. In addition to Cooley and Mead, the Chicago School listed as its contributors such great thinkers as philosopher and educator John Dewey, sociologist Robert E. Park, cultural anthropologist Ruth Benedict, and political psychologist Harold Lasswell, all of whom contributed significantly to Sullivan's thinking. Through Sapir within the Chicago School, Sullivan chose to spearhead this collaboration with W. I. Thomas, a contemporary of George Herbert Mead, who had significant political clout, and a prodigious scholarly reputation within the Chicago School and the academic field at large. Understanding the importance of obtaining funding to advance psychiatric research, a zealous Sullivan joined with Thomas, Harold Lasswell, and a somewhat reluctant William Alanson White to place psychiatry on the Social Science Research Council (SSRC). The SSRC was composed of seven disciplines that made recommendations to private foundations which comprised the major resource for funding research and sponsoring conferences. Driven by the belief in the critical role psychiatry research would play in addressing social issues, Sullivan personally funded much of the cost associated with this endeavor. In fact, his 1931 bankruptcy was largely traced to these expenses. Unfortunately, because the social sciences did not easily cede power to their medical brethren and the prevailing fashion within social science emphasized statistically oriented research as opposed to psychiatry's more case study approach, the proposal for psychiatry's inclusion on the SSRC was turned down. Undaunted, Sullivan shifted gears and quickly arranged an interdisciplinary conference demonstrating the importance of psychiatry and social science collaboration.

Together with Thomas and William Alanson White (heading the American Psychiatric Association's Committee on Relations with the Social Sciences), Sullivan organized the highly successful First and Second Colloquia on Personality Investigation in 1928 and 1929 (American Psychiatric Association, 1929; 1930), a meeting of over 20 top social science and psychiatry scholars. While White was the psychiatry chair of First Colloquium, Sullivan was clearly the driving force. Were it not for the 1929 Stock Market Crash and the Great Depression, which eliminated much foundation research money, perhaps Sullivan's dream for the fusion of science and psychiatry would have come to a more immediate realization. As a result of World War II, money for research in the United States came increasingly through government agencies and interdisciplinary research which Sullivan envisioned was funded. Psychiatrist Alfred Stanton and sociologist Leslie Schwartz's (1956) classic study of the mental hospital, conducted at Chestnut Lodge, was the first of numerous critical interdisciplinary research studies which revealed the power of the mental hospital social structure's influence on patient care and would redefine mental hospital practice (e.g., Caudill, 1958; Evans, 1976; Goffman, 1961; Levinson & Gallagher, 1964; Stotland & Kolber 1965). Dorothy Blitstein, a sociologist and his longtime friend, would state that "Harry Stack Sullivan was a social scientist whose specialty was psychiatry" (Perry, 1982: 258). Sullivan was the pioneer among the makers of psychodynamic psycho-therapy to integrate the findings of psychiatry and psychoanalysis with other disciplines and to insist on the importance of research, a rich tradition later furthered by Bowlby's (1969, 1973, 1980) integration of ethology, infant research, and psychoanalysis and recently by Stern's (1985) and Lichtenberg's (1983) integration of infant research and psychoanalysis.

As Sullivan turned his focus to the outside world of psychiatric research and social science collaboration, events in Baltimore transpired that made leaving Sheppard Pratt inevitable. Sheppard Pratt was in the process of building a new Clinical Center and Sullivan was quite active in its design. The centerpiece of Sullivan's design was a new reception (admissions) unit which was highly responsive to the patient's first 24 hours, and even first hour, of hospitalization, acknowledging that the patient's initial impression of the hospital was critical to the patient's later recovery. Additionally, this unit emphasized that intensive treatment of the first acute attack schizophrenic person who, properly treated, had greatest chance of recovery. While Sullivan's design suggestions were largely followed, he was not chosen to head the new reception center. His significant problems with budgetary casualness and his "inability to behave patiently toward the average indi-vidual" (Perry, 1982: 288), especially the nursing and maintenance staff, led the Board of Trustees to effectively censor Sullivan despite Chapman's active support for him. Additionally, with the illness and death of Champlin Robinson, president of the Board of Trustees who actively supported Sullivan and his research, the new Board president canceled Sullivan's action research plan to determine whether his techniques would work on a small number of patients, which then could be used for a larger number. Sullivan resigned from Sheppard Pratt in late 1930 with plans to join Sapir and Lasswell at the University of Chicago to collaborate on psychiatry and social science research. Unfortunately, the funding initially promised to Sullivan did not materialize, beginning a series of painful, but ultimately fortunate, profes-sional reversals.

At the same time Sullivan was battling to include psychiatry in social science research funding and to establish his action research and clinical design initiatives at Sheppard Pratt, he began a hard campaign to upgrade psychiatric education. In 1927–28, he proposed a new degree, Doctor of Mental Medicine, and a new approach to the training of psychiatric physi-cians, emphasizing greater empathy and understanding of the patient's ex-perience, which he thought nearly impossible to attain from current psychiatric education. With initial support from William Alanson White, he campaigned tirelessly for a major planning conference on standards for psychiatric education, similar to the Flexner report on medical education. Political maneuvers within the American Psychiatric Association (aPa) led White to withdraw from the planning committee, leaving Sullivan alone on a committee of psychiatrists with a dissimilar orientation. White's defection led to Sullivan's resignation from the committee and a serious break in his relationship with White. Unfortunately, no report on psychiatric education was developed by this committee and even today there is nothing comparable in psychiatric training to the Flexner report. Additionally, on advice of his colleagues, he withdrew his book, *Personal Psychopathology* (Sullivan, 1972), from publication consideration on the grounds that it was too premature a statement of his theories.

Over these years from 1927–30, Sullivan experienced a series of resounding professional defeats and disappointments, which led him to move away from Sheppard Pratt, William Alanson White, the aPa, and social science funding associations. His response was to take the central responsibility himself for what Perry (1982: 301) termed the "blueprint for much of his life's work," the founding of his own psychiatric educational institute and of an inter-personally oriented journal. In 1933, he founded the William Alanson White Foundation, the governance body for what would become the Washington School of Psychiatry (with its New York branch now called the William Alanson White Institute) and the journal *Psychiatry*. There was no small irony in naming the Foundation after William Alanson White, by which Sullivan honored White, but also in assisting in obtaining funding. While the founding of the White Institute was the most impressive of his many rises from adversity, Sullivan's problems had not yet ended with his resignation from Sheppard Pratt.

In December 1930, Sullivan arrived in New York City to start a private practice and to collaborate with Sapir and Lasswell, who both had moved from the University of Chicago to Yale University in New Haven, Connecticut. As Rioch (1985) notes, Sullivan's concept of private practice was to study prodromal states that precede schizophrenia, especially compulsive-obsessive syndrome, which could only be studied in an outpatient setting. With limited funds and much debt, he rented an expensive, well-appointed apartment. With him moved James Inscoe Sullivan, his adoptive son, whom Sullivan took in as a vagrant at age 15 while at Sheppard Pratt. Jimmie Sullivan became his devoted and meticulous secretary, lifelong companion, and only heir. From 1930 until 1936, Harry Stack Sullivan worked in New York City, planning on patients that never came in sufficient numbers (he turned down a large number of referrals of schizophrenic clients because it did not fit his research plan), living in extravagant surroundings, and paying himself for psychiatric research and travel.

In 1931, his father died, with whom Sullivan had achieved some small intimacy, unlike with his mother. Yet, Timothy Sullivan died with more debt than his farm was worth, because of expenses from his illness and outstanding taxes, and Harry Stack Sullivan had to shoulder those debts, including his father's burial expenses. His severe money problems, caused by circumstance, generosity to patients and supervisees, professional ambition, and extreme financial impracticality, became insurmountable and he filed for bankruptcy in 1932. Much of his large debt included loans, some quite large, from friends and colleagues, including Clara Thompson, A. A. Brill, and Ernest Hadley (with whom he formed the William Alanson White Foundation). While he defaulted on many people, including the later publishers of *Psychiatry*, it is interesting that many of the same people remained committed to him and his plans with financial and personal support throughout his life. On the other hand, his bankruptcy, especially his failure to repay close associates, did not little to stop Sullivan's "reputation as incorrigibly eccentric" (Perry, 1982: 325).

In the midst of his katabasis during the early New York days, Sullivan began a resurgence that would propel him into the main of his life's work. He traveled weekly to New Haven to participate in Sapir's seminar on culture and personality. Sullivan, along with Clara Thompson, Karen Horney, Erich Fromm, and William Silverberg (who had briefly taken Sullivan's ward at Sheppard Pratt), formed the famous Zodiac Group, a regular meeting on Monday evenings in a local bar of friends sharing social and professional interests. This informal collaboration gave rise to the branch of psychoanalysis that has been called the social psychological theorists and the neo-Freudians (Greenberg & Mitchell, 1983). Horney (1939, 1967) and Thompson (1943) worked out powerful new conceptualizations regarding gender, personality, and psychoanalysis; Fromm (1941, 1947, 1955), the only trained social scientist in the group, explored the role of the political state and personality; and Sullivan (1940/1953, 1953) continued his development of an interpersonal theory of personality. In addition, the group included well-known artists such as poet Lloyd Frankenberg and artist John Vassos. Through this connection, Sullivan saw quite a few (many non-paying) clients who were artists and writers, including photographer, Margaret Bourke White. Working with an often highly articulate outpatient population allowed Sullivan to focus on the treatment of pre-schizophrenic and related disorders, broadening his context for both his understanding of psychopathology and of personality, especially how fortunate social circumstances and inner resilience mitigated against severe psychopathology (Sullivan, 1956). From a psychotherapy perspective, deviating from the growing psychoanalytic canon of unending analysis (see Freud, 1937), Sullivan did not want to see clients indefinitely, but instead focused on circumventing anxiety long enough to help the client discover a more satisfying life.

In 1933 in Washington, DC, Sullivan, along with Edward Sapir, Harold Lasswell, and Ernest Hadley, founded William Alanson White Foundation (WAW Foundation). The WAW Foundation was the beginning of a dream that Sullivan had that would allow Sapir, Lasswell, and himself to obtain funding to support their collaborative research together for life, unfettered by financial need and institutional pressure. The Foundation was to include research, psychiatric education, and publication branches with its goals of: 1. most important, funding collaborative social science and psychiatry research with Sapir and Lasswell; 2. establishing an interdisciplinary school for training in a wide range of specialties and 3. beginning an eclectic journal, which emphasized the interpersonal dimensions of psychiatry. While Sullivan was the driving force from the beginning, Ernest Hadley was centrally involved in the development of the WAW Foundation, carrying with Sullivan the major burden of administration and fund raising. After 1939, the WAW Foundation would be mainly be the result of Sullivan's and Hadley's work. Throughout their collaboration, Hadley significantly supported Sullivan's financial needs, even when they were unrealistic. Yet, Hadley's orientation to psychiatry was not same as the other three. Specifically, Sullivan and Hadley had early differences in their respective emphases on psychiatry versus psychoanalysis. Even their approach to private patients differed, with Hadley interested clinical practice with government officials, the power elite of Washington, DC, and Sullivan favoring the creative, artistic, and unusual patients as a source of data for his theories on a wide range of social problems. Their differences would later surface in a divisive way, affecting the direction of the Foundation.

The research component, and the opportunity to work with Sapir and Lasswell, was Sullivan's first priority. He had already begun to collaborate with Sapir and Lasswell in New Haven, in Sapir's seminar on culture and personality (the manuscript of Sullivan's (1972) *Personal Psychopathology* was part of required reading) and with numerous discussions with Lasswell on personality and politics. It is interesting to note that Erik Erikson came to Yale University's Institute of Human Relations in 1936. His main work *Childhood and Society* (1950) appears highly influenced by Sullivan and Sapir's thinking, although he cited only one footnote for Sullivan and none for Sapir. Sapir became seriously ill in 1937, which set off frantic efforts to get funds to support Sapir and family, as Sullivan and Lasswell believed Sapir's survival depended on not returning to Yale. The increased necessity for an endowment through the Foundation to support Sapir became an ill-fated, unsuccessful, and deeply frustrating attempt to raise money through a not very skillful fund-raiser hired by Lasswell, which led to a parting of the ways between Lasswell and Sullivan. When Sapir died in 1939, he left a legacy of important influence on both Sullivan and Lasswell, but also caused the dissolution of the research triad. Sullivan characteristically immersed himself in a new project studying Black American adolescents in Memphis, Tennessee and Greenville, Mississippi with Charles Johnson (1941). In late 1939, six months after Sapir's death, Sullivan moved to Bethesda, Maryland near Washington, DC for the last decade of his life, leaving behind his financially precarious New York lifestyle and his dream for a mid-life research chumship with his dear friend Edward Sapir. Sullivan's vision of a high-level inter-disciplinary research program would not materialize until after his death in the form of David Rioch's Neuropsychiatry Davison of the Walter Reed Army Institute of Research.

The Bethesda years were the most productive and successful ten years of Sullivan's professional career and life. He was afforded some financial security because Dexter Bullard, Director of Chestnut Lodge, provided Sullivan with a steady consultantship. Bullard was one of several successful psychiatrists, who recognized Sullivan's brilliance as a clinician, theoretician, and teacher and who saw to it that Sullivan was provided for financially. Chestnut Lodge, a mental hospital with sensibilities similar to Sheppard Pratt, was the site of Sullivan's regular staff consultation and student clinical seminars (see Kvarnes & Parloff, 1976). Through Chestnut Lodge, Sullivan met and influenced important Washington clinicians who became the core members of the Washington School of Psychiatry and contributors to interpersonal theory, such as Frieda Fromm-Reichmann (1950), Edith Weigert (1970), Mabel Blake Cohen (1952, 1959), and David Rioch (1985) as well as important students such as Otto Will (1961), Margaret Rioch (1960, 1970), Leon Salzman (1966, 1980), Robert Kvarnes (Kvarnes & Parloff, 1976), and Don D. Jackson (1968). Soon upon arriving in Bethesda, Sullivan also undertook an ambitious psychiatric consultantship, establishing psychiatric standards for the Selective Service. In 1942, disagreements with new Director of the Selective Service General Lewis Hershey, who was opposed to psychiatry, led Sullivan to resign. Sullivan's model for screening of draftees was later adopted and used for many years. When, some years later, General Hershey was asked if there was a problem between himself and Sullivan, he replied, "No problem. We both wanted to run the Selective Service, and there was room for only one of us" (Rioch, 1985: 149).

As part of the White Foundation's plans for a journal, Sullivan and Hadley originally attempted to purchase the *Psychoanalytic Review* from Smith Ely Jelliffe, William Alanson White's co-editor, after White's death in 1937. When they could not agree on a price, Sullivan decided to start their own journal. The advantages of this decision would soon become apparent. Sullivan was especially insistent that the name of the journal should not include the word psychoanalytic to reflect interdisciplinary and eclectic origins, in which psychoanalysis was seen as a contributing, but not pre-eminent, discipline. While this philosophy and decision would lead to problems in the future, the journal *Psychiatry* auspiciously began in 1938 with papers by Sapir, Lasswell, Hadley, and Sullivan, among others. The journal rose to eminence during Sullivan's Bethesda years. *Psychiatry* was an unusual publication with an interdisciplinary focus, which explored the boundaries between psychiatry, psychoanalysis, social science, and biology. Additionally, *Psychiatry* provided room for the conceptual and the empirical, the operational and the speculative. It was a journal, which in the words of Margaret Rioch (1989), "kept the questions open." Above all, as reflected in its two subtitles, "The Journal of the Biology and Pathology of Interpersonal Relations" and in 1948 "The Journal for the Operational Statement of Interpersonal Relations," *Psychiatry* embraced Sullivan's interpersonal orientation in the broadest sense, both in terms of presenting his conceptions, but also encouraged the ideas of others, even quite disparate ones. In many ways, Sullivan was surprisingly open-minded for both his time and for psychoanalysis in general. As Marianne Horney Eckardt (1978) noted, Freud was both a scientist and an autocrat, stressing progressive modification of his theory based on empirical evidence, yet not giving his followers a similar freedom. In Sullivan's era, American psychoanalytic circles were beginning to strongly replicate Freud's autocratic style. For example, when Erich Fromm (1941) published his controversial book, *Escape from Freedom*, he was roundly denounced in psychoanalytic circles. Sullivan responded to this condemnation with a 1943 edition of *Psychiatry* containing eight reviews of Fromm's book, including three by psychiatrists/psychoanalysts, two by famous anthropologists (Ruth Benedict and Ashley Montague), and one each by a philosopher, a sociologist, and a theologian.

*Psychiatry* became the most important source for disseminating Sullivan's thinking, in the form of his many articles, unsigned editorials, and, especially, the only book he published in his lifetime. In 1939, Sullivan gave five public lectures, titled the First William Alanson White Memorial Lectures, outlining his views on personality, psychopathology, and psychotherapy. In 1940, the lectures were published as *Conceptions of Modern Psychiatry* (1940/1953), a monograph taking the entire edition of *Psychiatry*. This monograph was in such demand that Psychiatry published two subsequent bound reprintings in 1943 and 1947, with an added commentary by Patrick Mullahy. *Conceptions of Modern Psychiatry* was reviewed in *New York Times Sunday Book Review* on August 3, 1947 by noted poet, and Sullivan admirer, Lloyd Frankenberg. Aided by Frankenberg's review, the second printing was a remarkable success totally over 13,000 copies sold in five years, an unheard-of sales number for an essentially privately published book.

As with all of Sullivan's projects, *Psychiatry* would not be without controversy. For example, Perry cites letters between Karl Menninger and Ernest Hadley regarding an article by Erich Fromm (1939) in *Psychiatry*. Menninger warned Hadley that Fromm was not paying close enough adherence to Freud's ideas to merit publication and that the psychoanalytic community in New York was taking a dim view of the publication of material so disparate from Freud's ideas. Menninger wrote to Hadley, "As a Freudian, I should think that you would want the more egregious errors [in the article] corrected. I have heard a great deal of criticism of the article from those whose opinions I know you respect" (Perry, 1982: 381). Hadley, who was very involved in the psychoanalytic community, attempted to placate Menninger by suggesting that Menninger write a reply letter for *Psychiatry*. When Sullivan got wind of what can easily construed as a threat to Hadley and *Psychiatry*, he wrote to Menninger, inviting Menninger to submit articles clarifying Freud's position and making it clear that he had no intention of allowing censorship by the psychoanalytic elite. While Sullivan's lack of circumspection may have compensated for only by his unwillingness to be swayed by expectations of autocratic adherence to Freudian doctrine, this disagreement began the time when many psychoanalysts would come to see Sullivan and other interpersonal theorists as radical and dangerous. These early rumblings about the editorial policy of *Psychiatry* would take on greater intensity in the training philosophy of the Washington School of Psychiatry. Be that as it may, over the years, *Psychiatry* would do a commendable job of providing an outlet high quality, non-doctrinaire, eclectic, and interdisciplinary scholarly writing from an interpersonal perspective. Perhaps most importantly, *Psychiatry* would come to reflect Sullivan's deeply felt belief the psychiatry should not emphasize the psychopathology, but instead focus on the study of interpersonal living and its difficulties.

Sullivan's second great contribution during the Bethesda years was the formation of the Washington School of Psychiatry, which emerged into a multi-disciplinary, theoretically eclectic post-graduate school emphasizing training from an interpersonal perspective. The Washington School of Psychiatry began as a psychoanalytic institute with a curriculum relatively indistinguishable from other analytic institutes, which was offered under the auspices of the Washington-Baltimore Psychoanalytic Society. The growing schisms between psychiatry and psychoanalysis and within schools of psychoanalysis disturbed Sullivan, who saw both psychiatry and psychoanalysis as emerging fields that were incomplete and needed research and cross-fertilization from other disciplines, especially the social sciences and biology. Additionally, as he felt from his Sheppard Pratt days, training in psychiatry and psychoanalysis often lacked teaching empathy for the patient's actual experience, substituting instead theoretical doctrine for close listening and a deep understanding of a person's actual circumstances. Guntrip's (1975: 145) reflection would later state Sullivan's position well, "Theory ... is a useful servant, but a bad master, liable to produce orthodox defenders of every variety of faith." Gradually, the curriculum at the Washington School increasingly began to reflect the interpersonal thinking of Sullivan and his colleagues, such as Freida Fromm-Reichmann, Clara Thompson, Erich Fromm, David Rioch, and cultural anthropologist Ruth Benedict. Under Sullivan's (and later continued under David Rioch's) direction, the Washington School of Psychiatry instigated an energetic curriculum revision in 1943 that differentiated itself from standard psychoanalytic training. In addition to Sullivan's lectures on interpersonal theory and psychotherapy, courses on sociology, social psychology, cultural anthropology, biology, and philosophy became part of the curriculum. While the American

Psychoanalytic Association was closing ranks by prohibiting non-physicians from becoming psychoanalysts, the Washington School of Psychiatry responded to the post-war need for more well-trained mental health professionals by developing a Certificate in Applied Psychiatry Program for psychologists, social workers, and ministers, which was essentially its same program for psychiatrists. By 1948, over 400 students were registered for courses at the Washington School, over 80 of whom were in intensive training in psychiatry and psychoanalysis. The Washington School dropped the word psychoanalysis from the title of its certificate program, instead calling it Intensive Personality Study (Rioch, 1948, 1949, 1950).

By 1943, Sullivan was joined at the Washington School by David Rioch, a noted psychiatric research scientist and neuroanatomist. Rioch (e.g., 1938, 1940), who did groundbreaking research at Harvard University on specific brain-behavior mechanisms, provided the Sullivan and the Washington School's training program with a first-rate thinker on the neurobiological underpinnings of personality and on comparative psychology. After serving as Director of the Washington School during Sullivan's last years and after his death, Rioch would go on to direct the famous interdisciplinary Neuropsychiatry Division of the Walter Reed Army Institute of Research, the training ground for several Nobel laureates, many American psychiatry department chairs(at one time 40%), and many important scholars of human behavior. Rioch (1985) credited Sullivan for the vision of the interdisciplinary behavioral research program, a vision that would later come to fruition at the Walter Reed Army Institute of Research.

In addition to the Washington School, Sullivan began a parallel training program in New York City, through the William Alanson White Foundation. The faculty core consisted of Clara Thompson and Erich Fromm, who both lived in New York and Sullivan and Freida Fromm-Reichmann, who traveled from Washington on a weekly basis. Soon David Rioch joined the visiting Washington contingent as well as Ruth Benedict from Chicago. By 1943 the Washington School and its New York branch were no longer affiliated with Washington-Baltimore Psychoanalytic Institute, although many faculty members taught at both the Washington School and the Psychoanalytic Institute. The New York branch, which separated in 1946 from the Washington School, became quite successful and today still stands as the renown William Alanson White Institute, which provides training in psychoanalysis and psychodynamic psychotherapy. It should be noted that Sullivan's supportiveness and openness to strong female leadership (e.g., Thompson, Fromm-Reichmann, Edith Weigert, and Mabel Blake Cohen) have contributed to favorable training environment for women found at the Washington School and the White Institute over the years unlike what was found in psychoanalytic institutes.

While the Washington School of Psychiatry was undergoing its transformation, important happenings to and between two of the other major

Zodiac group members, Horney and Fromm, were part of the environment that fueled Sullivan's and the Washington School's individuation from the psychoanalytic community. In 1941, Horney was disqualified as a training and teaching analyst by the New York Psychoanalytic Society for "disturbing the students" (Perry, 1982: 386). Clara Thompson and others walked out of the meeting where this action was decided and soon developed the Association for the Advancement of Psychoanalysis, a rival psychoanalytic training society with Horney as its Dean. In December 1941, the American Psychoanalytic Association expressed concern that certain local psycho-analytic groups, e.g., the Washington-Baltimore Psychoanalytic Institute, were becoming dominated by some other authority than Freud, i.e., Sullivan. A resolution was passed to separate the Washington School of Psychiatry from training institute of Washington-Baltimore Psychoanalytic Society. By 1943, Horney dropped Fromm from her training program, because he was a lay (non-medical) analyst in order to a maintain cordial relationship with the American Psychoanalytic Association, in spite of Freud's (1926) own questions about the sagacity of training only medical analysts. The devel-oping problem of professional schisms was addressed by Sullivan (1943) in a *Psychiatry* article exploring the roots of professional divisiveness and calling for the different groups to find a way to work together. Later the American Psychoanalytic Association would place the new Washington Psychoanalytic Society on probation until it denied any association with Sullivan and his radical ideas. By 1945, each psychiatrist/ psychoanalyst in Washington was forced to take sides on the growing rift, ending the highly productive working relationship between Sullivan and Hadley. At the height of this animosity, the Washington Psychoanalytic Society did not accept books, including first editions of Freud, if the nameplate indicated that the book came jointly from the Washington School of Psychiatry. It is interesting to note that in 1939 Sullivan achieved an important dream when he was appointed as Full Professor and Chairman of a new Psychiatry Department at Georgetown University Medical School. His name was withdrawn by Georgetown University for his insistence on including psychoanalytic methods in the psychiatry training program, in opposition to the university's Catholic orientation, which opposed Freud and psychoanalysis.

While Sullivan's efforts with *Psychiatry* and the Washington School of Psychiatry moved ahead with great success, he became seriously ill in 1945 with bacterial endocarditis and was bedridden for many weeks. He was under much medical pressure to retire due to his seriously weakened heart and to refrain from any strenuous activity. Rather than devote his life to academic work of low stress and tension, Sullivan took up the invitation of Brock Chisholm, the Canadian psychiatrist who was soon to become the first head of the World Health Organization, to serve as a consultant to the post-World War II International Congress on Mental Health. Always concerned about what psychiatry could do to alter social situations for the prevention of psychiatric disorder, Sullivan's collaboration with Chisholm set the course for the last years of his life, applying the principles of psychiatry (and interpersonal psychiatry was especially well suited) to the problem of world peace. Sullivan was quite interested in child-rearing practices that would assist in raising children with values for peace. Despite his weakened state of health, Sullivan agreed to participate in three meetings through UNESCO during the summer of 1948, the last summer of Sullivan's life. The first meeting was the UNESCO Tensions Project, held in Paris. Sullivan was one of seven social science specialists to attend this meeting. Each participant shared his views on the causes of international aggression through extended paper and all worked together to develop a Common Statement on the problem. The papers and Common Statement were later published as Cantril's (1950) famous *Tensions That Cause War*, which included Sullivan's (1964: 293–331) most comprehensive statement of the importance of psychiatry in world peace. Next, Sullivan participated in the International Preparatory Commission London Conference as part of UNESCO's plan to organize network of local groups throughout the world for the promotion of mental health. The World Federation for Mental Health arose from these meetings. One of Sullivan's proudest accomplishments was his contribution to adopt the use consensus decision making for the upcoming International Congress on Mental Health. Here Sullivan came full circle by invoking the Quaker ideals which he first learned at Sheppard Pratt. Sullivan's last meeting of that summer was the UNESCO Seminar on Childhood Education Towards World-Mindedness in Podebrady, Czechoslovakia which lasted five weeks. Together with friend Ruth Benedict, Sullivan was among the forty participants from fifteen countries who explored ways that children could be raised to overcome group insecurity and destructive nationalism.

Sullivan returned to Bethesda excited with the new ideas he encountered, but was extremely tired which was bad for his health. His optimism was high from the meetings and he was full of future plans and ideas. Within a short time after Sullivan returned, both Ruth Benedict and Ross Chapman died within one week of each other. In December, Sullivan attended a Christmas party with White Foundation colleagues and was reported to look frail, but full of good cheer. He expressed worry about the stress of his trip to Europe for meetings of the World Federation for Mental Health.

On January 14, 1949, on his mother's birthday and about one month short of his 57th birthday, Sullivan died in a hotel room in Paris, France, heading home from the frustrating UNESCO meeting in Amsterdam. He died after ordering breakfast and was found with his pills scattered on the floor. Several Paris newspapers suggested suicide and one suggested the possibility of homicide. Chatelaine (1981: 480) strongly suspected that Sullivan planned to commit suicide based on a letter to Jimmie Sullivan which stated, "I probably will not return, but remember this and do not forget it. I will be controversial, there is no way to avoid it." Yet, Rioch (1985) reported that both Sullivan and Chisholm expressed concern to Otto Will that Sullivan might not survive the stresses of this trip. Perry's (1982) thorough research found that his autopsy report stated that he died of a meningeal hemorrhage, a cause of death consistent with his existing medical problems, and that an additional autopsy by a toxicologist, because of suspicion of suicide, revealed no overdose. Sullivan was cremated, per his request, and his ashes returned to the United States. A Captain in the U.S. Army Medical Corps in World War I, he was buried at Arlington U.S. Cemetery as befitted his military service. Sullivan wrote his own epitaph in 1947 urging his psychiatric colleagues to work toward "enduring peace and social progress."

Begin;

and let it be said of you,
if there is any more history,
that you labored nobly
in the measure of man
in the XX century
of the scientific Western world.

                              (1947b: 245)

Sullivan's death left behind much work to be done. His powerful ideas could be found to some degree in his many journal articles and in the privately published *Conceptions of Modern Psychiatry*, but his writings were not nearly a complete statement of his thinking nor were his most developed ideas readily available. Fortunately, through the William Alanson White Foundation, a group of Sullivan's colleagues, Mabel Blake Cohen, David Rioch, Janet Rioch, and Clara Thompson, as well as later Dexter Bullard, Sr., Otto Will, and Donald Burnham, with Helen Swick Perry as Editorial Consultant, formed the Committee on the Publication of Sullivan's writings. From 1953 through 1972 in collaboration with W. W. Norton & Co. publishers, the Sullivan Committee published three books based on Sullivan's notes and tape recordings, one on interpersonal theory, *The Interpersonal Theory of Psychiatry* (1953); one on interpersonal psychotherapy, *The Psychiatric Interview* (1954); and one on psychopathology, *Clinical Studies in Psychiatry* (1956). *Conceptions of Modern Psychiatry* (1953) was republished as part of the Norton series as well as two collections of his most important published articles, one on schizophrenia, *Schizophrenia as a Human Process* (1962) and another on psychiatry and social sciences, *The Fusion of Psychiatry and Social Science* (1964). In 1972, Sullivan's first book of his earliest formulations, written during his Sheppard Pratt days, would finally be published as *Personal Psychopathology*. Later, Kvarnes and Parloff (1976) published a transcription of tapes of a continuing clinical teaching seminar with Sullivan for psychiatric residents, thus completing the cycle by providing a view of Sullivan as a clinical supervisor. Without this remarkable effort, sustained over a twenty-three-year period, much of Sullivan's most important contributions would have been lost. We are deeply indebted to the Sullivan Committee for preserving this great intellectual treasure.

Uniquely American, a second-generation immigrant of humble beginnings, who crossed class lines, Sullivan provided a unique perspective on humankind that emphasized interpersonal events in the formation of personality and psychopathology and suggested a novel form of treatment for very challenging clinical problems. He left as his legacy the famous Washington School of Psychiatry, the journal *Psychiatry*, and extraordinary and extensive clinical and research traditions. Most of all, Harry Stack Sullivan has left us with a point of view on what it means to be fully human that remains alive and vibrant gmany years after his physical death.

# The Interpersonal Theory of Psychiatry

# Chapter 3

# Basic Concepts

Personality is made manifest in interpersonal situations, and not otherwise.
(Sullivan, 1938b: 32)

Perhaps Harry Stack Sullivan's most important, fundamental, and neglected contribution was his extraordinary theory of personality, which may be more properly put as his vision of humankind. Whereas great thinkers like Freud, Jung, and Kraepelin oriented their penetrating insights on the functioning of the individual, Sullivan offered a systematic conception of humankind in our social world or context. So central was the interpersonal and social world of humankind that, in his later years, Sullivan (1964) wrote a highly controversial and disturbing paper entitled "The illusion of personal individuality." For Sullivan, psychiatry, and all that derived from it such as theories of personality and treatment, was redefined as the science of interpersonal living, quite radically different from previous psychoanalytic conceptualizations (see Greenberg & Mitchell, 1983). It is the purpose of the next four chapters to give an overview of the main concepts of Sullivan's interpersonal theory. I will often use the term "interpersonal theory" in place of the usual term of "personality theory" to remind the reader that, from Sullivan's perspective, everything about the person must be placed in an interpersonal context. To develop a deeper understanding of Sullivan's interpersonal theory, the reader is strongly encouraged to read Sullivan's primary sources – *Conceptions of Modern Psychiatry* (1940/53), *Personal Psychopathology* (1972), and, most importantly, *The Interpersonal Theory of Psychiatry* (1953).

Sullivan's conception of psychiatry as the science of interpersonal living clearly challenged the two prevailing alternative perspectives – Kraepelin's (1918, 1968) descriptive psychiatry, perhaps the oldest trend in modern psychiatry, and Freud's more individual-based psychoanalysis. Like other areas of medicine, Kraepelin's tradition focused on the careful description of symptoms within a clinical syndrome, looking for points of divergence and convergence with other syndromes. Within this model, psychiatric research explores symptom patterns from which clinical syndromes are discovered, differentiated, or merged, resulting in an end point of a clear, definable

DOI: 10.4324/9781003305712-5

taxonomy of mental disorders. Kraepelin's underlying assumption was that mental illness is more purely biological and genetic and that the mentally ill can be clearly differentiated from normals. Descriptive or biological psychiatry, as it is referred to today, has grown in influence and popularity, as evidenced by the wide and largely unchallenged use of the *Diagnostic and Statistical Manual of Mental Disorders, 5th Ed.* (DSM-5, American Psychiatric Association, 2013). While this orientation to psychiatry has produced some important advances, e.g., in the areas of bipolar disorder (formerly manic-depressive disorder), Sullivan's critique of the problems of the Kraepelinian model remains relevant to the present day (see *Schizophrenia as a Human Process*, 1962). For similar modern critiques of Kraepelinian psychiatry, the reader is encouraged to read seminal thinkers such as Szasz (1961) and Laing (1965, 1967). As will be discussed in Chapter 7, more recently these critiques include Frances (2014), one of the authors of the DSM-4; the British Psychological Association's (see Johnstone & Boyle, 2018a) radical paradigmatic shift from traditional diagnosis to classification of behavior and experience; and, a direct extension of Sullivan's work, Pincus, Hopwood & Wright's Contemporary Integrative Interpersonal Theory (see Pincus, 2005; Wright et al., 2020).

Sullivan did not deny the importance of, and actually encouraged, research on biological substrates of psychiatry as evidenced by his close working relationship with neuroanatomist David Rioch, the many biopsychiatric articles in *Psychiatry*, and the inclusion of neurobiology in the training programs at the Washington School of Psychiatry. His basic critique of Kraepelinian psychiatry was that powerful interpersonal, social and cultural forces play the determining role in creating ineffective patterns of interpersonal living, which are often mistaken for disease. Additionally, Sullivan believed that social and cultural forces were critically important even when people demonstrated clear biological disorders. As important as physical differences are, Sullivan believed that people's need for social order and conformity, and the anxiety toward others who appeared markedly different, were potent social influences that could turn a troubled individual into a social outcast. Modern social psychology research (see Fiske & Taylor, 1991; Hogg & Abrams, 1988; Miller, 1982) has more than amply demonstrated the devastating impact of stereotyping and prejudice on individuals, especially stereotypes regarding race and gender (see Steele, 2011). What Sullivan most feared from descriptive psychiatry was its failure to look beyond symptoms and view the whole person in his or her psychosocial context. Additionally, descriptive psychiatry's limited focus on symptoms failed to reveal what the person had in common with everyone else, as well as special strengths and abilities which could be used to compensate for biopsychosocial trouble.

While Sullivan differed with Freud in numerous and subtle ways which will be discussed throughout this book, it is important to note Sullivan's most central distinction was his insistence on the development of a scientifically accurate and robust theory must not focus on "me," but "on the basis of common humanity" (1954: 4). While Freud recognized the reality of the interpersonal dimension in his powerfully important clinical concept of transference (Freud, 1910a) and somewhat in his concept of the superego (Freud, 1917, 1923a), his theory did not follow these concepts to their logical conclusion. Freud's emphasis on the individual's internal psychological mechanisms gave rise to the intra-psychic approach. For Sullivan, that which is truly intra-psychic is purely private and essentially unknowable. Once a person discusses, or even anticipates discussing, an "internal" experience, it is no longer private or internal, but becomes an interpersonal event, affected by social forces. For Sullivan, speculations about people's unconscious fantasies are, at best, inferences which are terribly hard to prove or, at worst, wild and potentially harmful speculations. Sullivan believed that there was more than enough to learn from the patient's description of his or her own experience and perception of the world without resorting to conjecture about unconscious fantasy. Sullivan's emphasis was not on the individual and the workings of internal psychic mechanisms, but the individual in his or her interpersonal world and the dynamisms of energy transformations between persons. While Clara Thompson (1964) suggested that Sullivan's theory was an important complement to and extension of, but was not fundamentally different than, Freud's psychoanalytic theory, Greenberg and Mitchell (1983) suggested that Freud and Sullivan were the primary examples of the two fundamentally different trends in understanding object relations in psychoanalytic theory. Rychlak (1973), a philosopher and psychologist, suggested that the meta-assumptions of Freud and Sullivan were essentially different from the perspective of the philosophy of science underlying their perspective theories. Both Rychlak and Havens (1976) suggested that the meta-scientific assumptions of Sullivan's relational approach share more in common with modern quantum theory and relativism than the Newtonian mechanical underpinnings of Freud's drive theory.

## What Is Psychiatry?

In the beginning of *The Interpersonal Theory of Psychiatry*, Sullivan revealed fundamental difficulty in the development of any theory of personality and its pathology. As Sullivan observed, everyone has his or her own conception of human living (i.e., our personal "theories of personality") which is experienced and strongly held as intuitively correct. This deeply personal conception of "reality" is central to bringing coherence to the personal and non-personal world around us and to who we are in that world. Naturally, on one hand, our conceptions are bound by our particular socio-cultural experiences, while, on the other hand, we tend to see the world through the very personal experience we call "me" which Sullivan referred to, tongue in cheek, as "our most valuable possession" (1953: 4).

In his concept of the *self-system*, Sullivan suggested that we form protective illusions to ward off uncertainty and inconsistency, to simplify the enormous complexity of the world, and especially to avoid social disapproval and disappointment. The work of cognitive psychologists Kahneman and Tversky (Kahneman et al., 1982; Kahneman, 2011) amply demonstrated the use of mental shortcuts, called heuristics, in complex decision making. Social psychologists Taylor (1989) and Janoff-Bulman (1992) cite research demonstrating the power and importance of these illusions in determining mental health and mental disorder. Thus, psychiatric scientists attempting to form an objective, accurate view of mental disorder and normal functioning are hampered by the very nature of their decision-making processes under high complexity. Similar to Heisenberg's (1958) principle of indeterminacy (which in sub-atomic physics the measurement of a phenomenon with the same level of phenomenon alters the phenomena measured), the psychiatrist observer participates in and alters every interaction that he or she observes. Unlike Heisenberg's measurement of electrons, whose properties are well known, the properties of the psychiatrist's decision making is far more puzzling.

This fact of interpersonal science led Sullivan to the conclusion that explaining human living was extremely complex ...

I think that there is no other field of scientific endeavor in which the worker's preoccupations are as troublesome as in psychiatry. To illustrate this I will give three definitions of psychiatry. The first and broadest definition would run like this: it is all the confounding conglomerate of ideas and impressions, of magic, mysticism, and information, of conceits and vagaries, of conceptions and misconceptions, and of empty verbalisms. That is the broadest definition of psychiatry and, so far as I know, a good many people are very far advanced students of that field.

Now there is a second definition ... and this is a polite definition of psychiatry in the prescientific era. This second definition sets up psychiatry as an art, namely, the art of observing and perhaps influencing the course of mental disorders.

The third definition of psychiatry, which is relevant here, may be approached by considering it as an expanding science concerned with the kinds of events or processes in which the psychiatrist participates while being an observant psychiatrist ... The actions and operations from which psychiatric information is derived are events in interpersonal fields which include the psychiatrist ... not events that he looks at from atop ivory towers ... (and) are those that are accompanied by conceptual schematizations or intelligent formulations which are communicable ... (and) which are precise and explicit ... with nothing significant left equivocal or ambiguous.

(1953: 13–14)

As such for Sullivan, psychiatry must focus on developing frames of reference, which are guides to exploration, as opposed to developing premature, immutable laws about the human condition. Sullivan tried to take extra pain in defining his frame of reference in clear language, relatively unencumbered with psychiatric jargon (although his own arcane mode of expression made this goal occasionally difficult for him). Sullivan took a modest position regarding what could be known in psychiatry, but insisted on scientific integrity, with measurable, reliable, and consensually validated concepts. For Sullivan, it was simply not enough to think something is so; it must be conclusively shown to be so. As noted by Greenberg and Mitchell (1983), Sullivan's cautiousness demonstrated deep respect for the complexity and uniqueness of the experience of others ...

> There is an essential inaccessibility about any personality other than one's own ... There is always an ample residuum that escape analysis and communication ... No one can hope to fully understand another. One is very fortunate indeed if he approaches an understanding of himself.
>
> (1972: 5)

As a result, Sullivan's concepts presented in the interpersonal theory of psychiatry served to guide his exploration of the vast intricacy of human behavior and interpersonal relationships.

A special aspect of Sullivan's reflections on the philosophy of science underlying psychodynamic theory was his deep concern about the misuse of psychiatric jargon. Sullivan cautioned that such jargon could lead to a guild-like encapsulation of believers from non-believers and argued that psychiatrists should use words of common usage that can be broadly understood. For Sullivan, language in psychiatry was best used as a way to understand, and integrate with, others, the essence of his concept of *syntaxic experience*. He was openly critical of Freud's and his followers' use of overly complex, hard to validate, and jargon-ridden concepts, constantly warning that inference and metaphor could be mistaken for actual experience. A relative lack of jargon marks the interpersonal approach, as compared to other psychoanalytic approaches (of course, with an occasional wild exception). While Sullivan may not have fully achieved his goal in his writings and lectures, one of his most important contributions was his observation, furthered by the writings of Fromm-Reichmann (1950), about the high potential for psychiatric jargon to be used in defensive and divisive ways. Ironically, as mentioned in Chapter 1, the lack of an array of jargon in interpersonal theory, so often found in other psychoanalytic schools, may have contributed to difficulties in developing an enduring group of disciples.

## Basic Theoretical Concepts

In *The Interpersonal Theory of Psychiatry*, Sullivan provided core definitions and postulates, which underlay his approach to understanding human living. As mentioned above, Sullivan's central definition and most distinguishing contribution is a revision of *psychiatry as the science of interpersonal living*, that personality could not be separated from the interpersonal world in which the person lives. The interpersonal theory is a significant critique and reworking of Freud's psychoanalytic approach and major departure from Kraepelin's descriptive psychiatry, both of which focus on the individual.

Perhaps Sullivan's most elegant postulate was his *one genus hypothesis* in which he states, "everyone is much more simply human than otherwise" (1953: 32) or, "we are all much more simply human than otherwise, be we happy and successful, contended and detached, miserable or mentally disordered, or whatever" (1940/1953: 16). While the one genus hypothesis has a seemingly maudlin ring to it, on closer examination it becomes clear that Sullivan meant that we are more alike Jack the Ripper, the pederast, and the hopeless schizophrenic, as well as Albert Schweitzer, Mother Teresa, and Gandhi, than otherwise. For Sullivan, understanding what is common to all humanity, the basic biological, psychological, and social principles of living, was more crucial than the relatively insignificant differences between people. For example, though vastly different from our experience, a baseball hurtling at us at 100 miles per hour or one softly lobbed to us are both understood by the physicist as similar events, describable by physical laws of motion and expressed in a common equation. The search for verifiable, underlying laws, which explain seemingly diverse experiences and events represents one of the elements of what Kuhn (1962) called a paradigm shift from the pre-scientific to the scientific phase. Sullivan's struggle to understand his common humanity with the patient provided both scientific accuracy and a highly empathic stance for listening to his patient's troubles.

Another important element of Sullivan's theory is the concept of *experience*, which is …

> anything lived, undergone or the like. Experience is the inner component of events in which a living organism participates in as such—that is, as an organized entity. The limiting characteristics of experience depend on the kind of organism, as well as on the kind of event experienced. Experience is not the same as the event in which the organism participates.
>
> (1953: 26–27)

For Sullivan, our experiences are our basic data of the world and the point of contact between outer reality and the inner world. We may have our experience in an utterly private mode, not communicable to others, or we may be able to readily engage in language transactions in which we make our needs known to others and theirs to us. The flow of sensation, i.e., experiences, from our inner and outer worlds of needs and the resulting energy transformations, rapidly becomes organized into ever more complex cognitions, an inner bundle of interpreted experience which Sullivan called a *percept*. Sullivan also suggested that experiences were organized and developed into three, increasing more complex, modes of representation – the *prototaxic*, the *parataxic*, and the *syntaxic* modes.

As Mullahy (1948) has elaborated, the *prototaxic* mode is the earliest and most primitive, described as the infant's limited awareness of himself or herself as separate from the environment. The newborn infant "knows" only in the moment, and barely senses or *prehends* earlier and later states. The overall experience is a flowing, undifferentiated, and cosmic sense of the world. As experiences and percepts accumulate in the very young infant and actions become attached to relatively reliable consequences, the sense of undifferentiated wholeness is broken and the infant begins to develop experience in the *parataxic* mode. Experiences become associated with consequences as the infant develops *recall*, memories of prior consequences attached to certain experiences, and *foresight*, the anticipation of certain consequences associated with experiences and actions taken to modify these experiences. As Sullivan noted, "The comparatively great influence of foresight is one of the striking characteristics of human living in contrast to all other living" (1953: 39).

Yet, in the parataxic mode, these experiences are linked by association, not by logic. The infant does not make logical distinctions and differentiations, but experiences things "naturally" occurring together. For the infant in the parataxic mode, crying magically brings milk. As certain events in the inner and outer world become consistently associated with certain experiences and consequences of these experiences, through recall and foresight these events become *signs and signals* for the satisfactions, frustrations, security, or insecurity that follows. Attached to each sign therefore is a particular *meaning* for the infant, which develops into the person's own experience of the foresight and recall of needs and their consequences. Since all satisfactions and security for the infant require *interpersonal cooperation*, signs and their meanings are representations of interpersonal transaction as well. As these experiences become represented through language, signs, signals, and meanings can be spoken and the child can begin to *consensually validate* his or her experience with the experiences of others, that is, develop common understanding about the signs, signals, and meaning of experience. Communicative behavior (both speech and gesture) and its potential for greater logical differentiation and precision become the primary ways of knowing, which Sullivan called experience in the *syntaxic* mode, the third and most advanced mode of experience. Developmental movement from mode to mode is not assured for all experiences; indeed, Sullivan stated that "any experience that can be discussed—that is any experience in the parataxic or syntaxic mode is always interpenetrated by elements of the ... past" (1953: 38–39) and that experience in all three modes are present by later childhood into adulthood. Sullivan's attempts at conceptualizing a model of cognitive development are unique among the early psychoanalysts and, as Youniss (1980) pointed out, paralleled the theoretical formulations of Piaget (1965) and other cognitive developmental theorists.

Perhaps the major psychoanalytic critique of Sullivan's theory, with Jacobson (1955) and Kernberg (1976) being the most representative, has been that Sullivan is overly sociological or behavioral, without concern for the deep, inner human experience such as fantasies and wishes. This criticism is either the result of not carefully reading Sullivan's work, or having done so, fails to grasp his meaning. His basic concepts of *experience* and *meaning* showed his deep respect for the importance of inner life. Sullivan (1962: 34) cautioned, though, to remember that the psychiatrist "knows" the inner experience of the patient through the "verbal report of subjective appearances (phenomena)," a verbal report which is influenced by the patient's experience of the psychiatrist, including real experience and transference (i.e., *parataxic distortions*). As mentioned above, Sullivan noted that truly private experience cannot be communicated, is immutable, and cannot be included in psychiatric inquiry. Sullivan valued the physicist P. W. Bridgman's (1945) principle of operationalism as the basis for scientific psychiatry and took the position that, while public and private modes of human interaction exist, psychiatry could only study the public modes. While, as his critics state, this position is similar to Skinner and other radical behaviorists (see Ferster & Skinner, 1957; Skinner, 1953), Sullivan believed that many "internal" states, people's inner experiences and meanings, could be shared with the psychiatrist and that carefully drawn, valid inferences could be made, if the psychiatrist would take pains to listen carefully. It is important to remember again that *human experience*, not social behavior, was the organizing principle for Sullivan's interpersonal theory. On the other hand, Sullivan was especially critical of clinical psychiatric theorizing that was based on presumed processes taking place inside the person, which was not verifiable to either the psychiatrist or the patient ...

> The unconscious ... is quite clearly that which cannot be experienced directly, which fills all the gaps in the mental life. In that rather broad sense, the postulate of the unconscious has ... nothing the matter with it. As soon as you begin to rearrange the furniture in something that cannot be directly experienced, you are engaged in a work that requires more than parlor magic and you are apt to be embarrassed by some skeptic.
>
> (Sullivan, 1962: 204)

As Greenberg and Mitchell (1983) pointed out, the sharpest contrast between Sullivan's interpersonal model and British object relations theory (BORT) is evident in the BORT's use of language regarding internal objects, structures, and processes that presumed experiential referents. In particular Melanie Klein (Klein, 1964, 1975; Klein & Riviere, 1964) and her followers (Heimann, 1952a, 1952b; Riviere, 1936a, 1936b; Segal, 1964) elaborated a theory utilizing a world of inner unconscious fantasy within the infant, which is most inimical to Sullivan's position. For Sullivan, the infant's experience, through close observation, could at best be roughly inferred and certainly not with the precision and meaning subscribed to by Klein and her followers. Additionally, Sullivan's criticism of psychoanalysis's tendency to rely on interpretative, inferential constructs over those based directly on the patient's experience was that such an approach was fundamentally anti-empathic, leading to inaccurate theory and poor clinical practice.

Like all psychodynamic theorists, Sullivan addressed the question of human motivation, most particularly in his postulates regarding reduction of tensions. Much like Freud's (1905) pleasure principle, Sullivan believed that humans experienced the alternation of states of *euphoria* and *tension*. He stated that euphoria is the experience of a state of well-being arising from the reduction or elimination of tensions regarding human biological and psychosocial requirements of living. Quite unlike Freud's pleasure principle in which euphoria came as the result of gratifying psychosexual (oral, anal, phallic, and genital) needs, Sullivan defined two distinct categories of tensions, *tension of needs* and *tension of anxiety*.

Sullivan's concept of the *tension of needs* referred to the experienced component of various specific biological requirements. While the tension of needs is conceptually close to Freud's psychosexual needs found in his theory of the libido (Freud, 1905, 1911, 1915, 1923b), Sullivan explored the concept more deeply and included such tensions as hunger, thirst, warmth, dermal physiochemical regulation (e.g., removal of urine and feces from the skin), and oxygen requirements, as well as general biological requirements such as the need to sleep and the need for touch and human contact. Sullivan's tension of needs was either in experienced through specific *zones of interaction* or experienced in *general*. Sullivan's concept of zones of interaction was different from the developmental sequential character of Freud's theory, which required that the psychosexual needs must be satisfied in moderation (not too much, not too little) and in correct order, otherwise consequences specific to that psychosexual phase would hinder further psychic development. Instead of focusing on the satisfaction of specific physiological needs, Sullivan made the innovative observation that all of the infant's needs require interpersonal cooperation because of the utter dependency of the human infant. Therefore, the critical element in interpersonal theory was that the reduction (satisfaction) of the tension of needs could not be considered independently from the interactions between people. Sullivan thought that, as the person matured and developed through the various epochs of development, the tensions of need, and the energy transformations used to integrate with others to satisfy these tensions, underwent change and required increasingly more complex forms of interpersonal cooperation. For Sullivan, the quality of the interpersonal cooperation required in meeting physical needs, as well as the characteristic way that purely interpersonal needs were met, were the essential determinants of human development, rather than Freud's speculations about the overarching importance of the satisfaction of specific psychosexual needs in and of themselves.

The critical process of the linking of satisfaction of zonal and general needs to interactions with others is expressed in Sullivan's (1953: 39) *theorem of tenderness*, "The observed activity of the infant arising from the tension of needs induces tension in the mothering one, which tension is experienced as tenderness and as an impulsion to activities toward the relief of the infant's needs." The child then experiences the mother's behavior towards the relief of his or her needs, not only as a zonal satisfaction, but also as a tender act. The relaxing effect of the satisfaction of the need is associated with the tenderness of the mother creating a general *need for tenderness* as well. The need for tenderness, as well as the need for contact (such as touch and later emotional contact), are "the very genuine beginnings of purely interpersonal or human needs" (1953: 40). Sullivan further noted the consequences of the failure the mothering one to attend to the infant's repeated expression of the tension of needs, a state which he called *apathy*. While he remarked on the physical dangers of long episodes of uninterrupted crying and the immediate organism-preserving qualities of apathy, Sullivan was also aware of Ribble's (1938) research on the life-threatening effects of chronic apathy arising from serious disturbances in maternal cooperation. Spitz's (1945, 1946) hospitalism studies dramatically further confirmed infants' need for maternal care and tenderness beyond meeting physical requirements.

Sullivan's second tension, *tension of anxiety*, is perhaps the most unique and central motivational postulate within his interpersonal theory and clinical practice. This concept had no parallel in Freud's drive theory and marked the beginning of the relational model in psychodynamic theory (see Greenberg & Mitchell, 1983). Sullivan put forth the following definition ...

*The tension of anxiety, when in the mothering one, induces anxiety in the infant*. The rationale for this induction—that is, *how* anxiety in the mother induces anxiety in the infant-is thoroughly obscure. This gap ... has given rise to some beautifully plausible and perhaps correct explanations. I bridge the gap simply by referring to it as a manifestation of an indefinite-that is, not yet defined—interpersonal process to which I apply the term *empathy*.

Now, in discussing anxiety, I have come to something that has nothing to do with the physiochemical needs of the living young. The tension called anxiety primarily appertains to the infant's, as also in the mother's, communal existence with a *personal* environment, in utter contra-distinction to the physiochemical environment.

(1953: 41–42)

In this definition, Sullivan posited a distinct interpersonal tension, which could only be relaxed, i.e., have euphoria restored, through the removal of anxiety, which in turn leads to the experience of **interpersonal security**. Along side of the infant's need for satisfaction (reduction of tension of needs), the infant also has the need for interpersonal security. The tension of anxiety appears as part of the person's psychological "apparatus," but does not operate like a zonal tension. Unlike zonal tensions of need which have easily foreseeable actions to relieve them, and which therefore become differentiated quickly into parataxic, and later into syntaxic, experience, early experiences of the tension of anxiety are overwhelming, because the infant cannot readily locate the source of his or her anxiety. As such, infant experiences of anxiety remain in the more primitive prototaxic mode and are only gradually and poorly differentiated later in life. As Sullivan stated, "the infant has no capacity for action toward the relief of anxiety" (1953: 43), leading to an underlying deep-rooted sense of helplessness or power-lessness. Just as tenderness in the mother increases the feelings of well-being in the child, which in turn induces further tenderness in the mother, the induction of anxiety from the mothering one to the child establishes a similar, but disintegrative, feedback loop of ever-increasing anxiety in the interpersonal field. Too much anxiety would lead to **somnolent detachment** in the infant, a process like apathy, but more interpersonally focused, a process crucial in the development of dissociative patterns later in life. Greenspan's (Greenspan & Shanker, 2007) research on infants' gaze aver-sion to avoid the intolerable anxiety of psychotic mothers empirically es-tablished the impact of impaired early maternal-child bonding on later severe mental disorder.

The need for interpersonal security, i.e., the absence of the tension of anxiety, was especially critical from Sullivan's perspective. As will be dis-cussed later, significant early experience with anxiety exerts a distorting effect on development and personality. Not only does frequent or prolonged anx-iety profoundly disturb the infant's sense of interpersonal security and ex-pectations for positive interpersonal cooperation, but his or her cognitive development is impaired as well. When anxiety becomes attached to zonal needs such as hunger and eliminative process or with general needs such as a need for closeness and tenderness, the development of normal processes of need resolution become disturbed or impaired. As such, Sullivan frequently remarked that significant early experiences of anxiety could establish patterns of interaction in opposition to the infant's other needs. Throughout his dis-cussion of the tension of anxiety, theorem of tenderness, and the need for interpersonal security, Sullivan put forth the implication that interpersonal relatedness, as a need independent from the satisfaction of needs, was present at birth and was essential for the survival of the infant. In Scotland, without the knowledge of Sullivan's work, W. R. D. Fairbairn (1952, 1963) arrived at essentially the same conclusion, though using quite different language to express his ideas.

### Tension of Anxiety and Attachment Theory

However powerfully Sullivan demonstrated the impact of the tension of anxiety, his definition of anxiety was, and remains, undeveloped and un-satisfying from a theoretical perspective. In his failure to grasp the core of Sullivan's tension of anxiety, Bowlby (1958) somewhat inaccurately criticized Sullivan's theoretical inconsistency in failing to distinguish physiological needs from the primary need for contact and human relatedness. Perhaps the greatest critic of his formulations concerning anxiety was Sullivan himself. In the Preface to the 1940 Second Edition of the *Conceptions of Modern Psychiatry*, Sullivan (1940/47: ix) stated, "The theory of anxiety, its bearing on personality development, and its crucial importance in observing and influencing interpersonal relations, is not adequately stated." Later, in the most advanced statement of his thought before he died, Sullivan (1953: 8) remarked, "In discussing the concept of anxiety, I am not attempting to give you the last word; it may, within ten years, be demonstrated that this concept is wholly inadequate, and a better one will take its place."

As with Freud, Erikson, Spitz (1965) and other psychoanalytic theorists, Sullivan discussed the motivational goal of the need for satisfaction and the signal for its frustration – fear – quite clearly. Sullivan's confusion became pronounced when he attempted to describe his second, more purely inter-personal motivational component, the *tension of anxiety*. As Fairbairn (1952) theorized and later Bowlby (1969, 1973, 1979, 1980, 1988) demon-strated empirically, the goal of the second component of human motivation was the maintenance of the primary need for contact and human related-ness, a need that Bowlby aptly called **attachment**. While it is beyond the scope of this book to give a full discourse on Bowlby's work (See Holmes (1993) excellent book on Bowlby's attachment theory in the *Makers of Modern Psychotherapy* series), a brief discussion of attachment theory fills an important gap in Sullivan's interpersonal theory. As an interesting his-torical note, Bowlby's (1958, 1960, 1961) first papers formulating the out-line for attachment theory appeared within ten years of the publication of Sullivan's last statement about the inadequacy of his formulations on anxiety, just as Sullivan predicted.

Seeing the difficulties inherent in Freud's drive theory, Bowlby, like Sullivan, looked beyond the speculations of psychoanalysis and searched for a scientific base for psychodynamic theory. To complement his psychoanalytic understanding, Bowlby found that the field of ethology, the scientific study of animal behavior in natural conditions with special attention to the animal's interaction with its whole environment, provided an excellent methodology for studying attachment. Influenced by the works of Lorenz (1952), Tinbergen (1950), and later Hinde (1982), Bowlby tested his ideas about the central importance of attachment, initially in the mother-infant psychological bond, as a motivation in its own right and not as a secondary elaboration of the meeting of oral needs in the infant. Particularly based on Lorenz's observations of bonding in geese and Harlow's (1962, 1971) monkey studies, as well as Bowlby's own observational study of human infants (e.g., Bowlby et al., 1952), Bowlby formulated an empirical grounding for his belief in the importance of attachment as a primary motivation for humans, other primates, and other animals. He saw attachment as a central foundation for the development of the human personality.

Bowlby found that attachment behavior is essential to the survival of many species and is not a learned behavior that can be extinguished, but rather is deeply embedded in the biopsychosocial makeup of these species. Attachments could be either *secure attachments*, experienced as feelings of safety and security, or *insecure attachments*, experienced as fears of abandonment and rejection, intense dependency, irritability, and vigilance. *Attachment behavior* is defined by Bowlby as behavior that seeks to attain or retain proximity or closeness with a significant and preferred other. The attachment motivation and behavior (perhaps translated into Sullivan's language as the "tension of attachment"?) is organized into an *attachment behavioral system* (perhaps "the dynamism of attachment"?) which regulates attachment needs and encodes representations of the self, significant others, and the interrelationships of their patterns of attachment. Thwarting the need for attachment has powerful consequences. As van der Kolk (1987: 40) stated, based on extensive examination of both human and animal research, "In most mammalian species, dependency on adult caregivers is so strong that separation from the mother alone, even without external danger, causes distress in infants." Bowlby named this intense distress reaction the *separation protest*, a characteristic set of responses, also called the separation cry or the protest-despair response (see van der Kolk, 1987), which included behaviors such as crying, screaming, clinging, kicking, or biting designed to induce the caretaker to provide proximity, safety, and nurturance. If the separation protest fails to bring desired attachment, the characteristic despair response of "low-keyedness," depression, and, eventually, interpersonal detachment becomes evident, much as Sullivan discussed in his concept of somnolent detachment. Repeated successful interactions between the mother and infant attending to the attachment needs of the infant are necessary for the development of a *secure base* (Ainsworth, 1982; Bowlby, 1988). If the secure base is not achieved, then environmental exploration necessary for psychological maturation is inhibited and separation anxiety becomes a prominent and disabling aspect of the personality.

Though better organized and more systematic, Bowlby's and Ainsworth's conceptualizations of attachment were in many ways parallel to, and certainly expanded, Sullivan's interpersonal concepts of the tension of anxiety, interpersonal security, tenderness, need for closeness, empathy, somnolent detachment, and security operations. Upon a more careful reading, Sullivan was much closer to attachment theory than Bowlby gave him credit for. Much of both the trouble and the advantage of Sullivan's formulations arose from his theoretical orientation toward the experience of the person. Sullivan organized his thinking about the personal relatedness dimension of human motivation around the infant's experience of disturbance in the relational field with the mothering one (anxiety in the mothering one evoking anxiety in the infant), as opposed to Bowlby's emphasis on the concept of attachment as a more purely proximal event. The later research and theory of Ainsworth (1982, 1989), considered the co-founder of attachment theory, focused especially on the important roles of empathic attunement and maternal responsiveness. She empirically validated Sullivan's concept of empathy and his emphasis on the extraordinary acuteness and subtlety of infant-caretaker interaction in determining the later quality of interpersonal connectedness. i.e., the attachment bond.

On the other hand, Bowlby's critique of Sullivan for failing to discriminate physiological needs from the primary need for contact and human relatedness is inaccurate, likely a misreading of, or failure to understand, Sullivan's core concepts. As stated earlier, Sullivan carefully distinguished the *tension of needs*, which is physiological, from the *tension of anxiety*, which Sullivan explicitly stated was purely interpersonal and social. In fact, both Bowlby's and Sullivan's separation of physical and relatedness needs should be re-thought in light of van der Kolk's (1987: 39–40) findings, "Primate research demonstrates that social attachment is not only a psychological event; it is related to the development of core neurobiological functions in the primate brain." Indeed, in their research summary of the neurobiology of infant attachment and fear, Landers and Sullivan (2012) make it clear that the attachment neurobiological circuit in the brain has a twin function of keeping infants proximate to the caregiver as well as shaping long-term emotional and cognitive development. Cozolino (2014) provides a comprehensive review of how attachment schemas enhance or detract from the development of a biochemical environment in the brain conducive to providing healthy emotional regulation, growth, and even immunological functioning. He notes that negative early parent-child attachment patterns are found in individuals with greater physical and psychological illness throughout life.

Since the publication of the original edition of this book, the study and research of attachment in field of child development has exploded beyond Bowlby's and Ainsworth's original studies (see Cassidy & Shaver, 2016) and established itself as perhaps the most important single determinant of child development (see Marvin et al., 2016; Sroufe, 2016). Research has firmly established disordered attachment as powerful predictors of childhood, adolescent, and adult psychopathology (see Atkinson & Zucker, 1997). The compelling nonhuman primate research following the cohort of monkeys from Harlow's original colony has established the intergenerational transmission of attachment difficulties in nonhumans as well as the capacity to correct them (Suomi, 2005). Further, based on their comprehensive review of the human attachment literature, Van IJzendoorn and Bakermans-Kranenburg (1997: 163) concluded "intergenerational transmission of attachment should be considered as an established fact." In particular, the expansion of Ainsworth's original internal working model of attachment called *disorganized attachment*, has opened the door to fresh perspectives on understanding, diagnosis, and intervention for children with dysregulated and disorganized parent-child relationships (see Solomon & George, 2011).

These findings from attachment theory and research have opened the door to important interventions for children and their problematic parents. In particular, the Circle of Security® Intervention (Marvin et al., 2002; Powell et al., 2013) was developed to change damaging attachment interaction patterns in high-risk parent-child relations through parent education and psychotherapy intervention. Research has shown that the three models using Circle of Security® Intervention to be effective for children and their caregivers in highly troubled family situations that previously defied treatment intervention (Woodhouse et al., 2018; Yaholkoski et al., 2016). Further, understanding the impact of attachment problems in infancy and childhood has led to important advances in individual adult psychotherapy (see Fonagy 2018; Slade, 2016), especially with complex psychological difficulties such as borderline personality disorder (Bateman & Fonagy, 2004). Not surprisingly, attachment-focused couples' psychotherapy has been found to be useful in assisting dysfunctional attachment in couples' relationships (Diamond et al., 2016; Shaver et al., 2019). Spieker and Crittenden (2018) discussed the value of applying attachment theory to forensic settings, especially in child protection, while Solomon and George (1999) and Byrne et al. (2005) have discussed the importance of attachment theory in child custody, parenting plan assessments and forensic decision-making.

To further add to the contributions from the study of attachment, several useful psychological assessment methods have been developed (Solomon & George, 2016). Originally a laboratory-based procedure to evoke and mimic stressful situations for children and caretakers, Ainsworth's Strange Situation Procedure (SSP: Ainsworth, 1969) was intended to reveal patterns of caregiver-child attachment and has been adopted as the gold standard for attachment assessment in a variety of intervention situations. While the SSP is an observation procedure that yields valuable information, becoming proficient to administer the procedure requires considerable training, and scoring behavioral interactions is complex. Adapting attachment theory to measurement of adult attachment, George et al. (1985) developed the Adult Attachment Interview (AAI), an hour-long interview that measures inner attachment working models in adults. The AAI has been shown to be reliable and valid for its intended purposes (Bakermans-Kranenburg & Van IJzendoorn, 1993) and has held up well to further research (Hesse, 2016). One disadvantage of the AAI, like the SSP, is that learning the scoring of AAI takes considerable time and effort and the scoring of AAI itself by experienced assessors is also very time-consuming. As a way of obtaining similar information in a less time-consuming format useful in standard psychological assessment, George developed the Adult Attachment Projective Picture System (AAP: George & West, 2001, 2012), a projective instrument with eight pictures designed to provide a valid assessment of adult attachment states of mind and characteristic defensive processes not available in other available psychological assessment methods.

However, Sullivan and Bowlby and Ainsworth may have differed in the language or emphases of their respective theories, it is clear that together they shared a deep respect for the value of empirical scientific inquiry in understanding interpersonal patterns and for the fundamental interpersonal relatedness of humans. Bowlby and Ainsworth's attachment theory achieved in excellent theoretical organization and empirical verification what Sullivan had hoped to accomplish in his theory of anxiety – that humans are by their nature highly attuned to stimuli that signal possibly dangerous disruptions in interpersonal relationships and are programmed to respond with anxiety. One area of difference between Bowlby and Ainsworth's attachment theory and Sullivan's interpersonal theory is how "experience near" each are. While attachment theory primarily focuses on the transactions between child and caretaker and the cognitive schema of the internal working model, Sullivan's concepts of anxiety and empathy attempt to capture the following: both the description of the child's/person's experience of the impact of separation, of anxious or destruction parenting types or of relationship betrayal. In addition, he describes relational patterns similar to cognitive schema of the internal working model. As such, it seems to this author proper to consider the two theories of human relatedness complementary.

## Dynamism

Before considering Sullivan's theory of development, an additional core idea essential to his thinking must be considered, his concept of the *dynamism*. Sullivan (1953: 103–104) defined a *dynamism* as a "relatively enduring pattern of energy transformations which recurrently characterize an organism in its duration as a living organism" and defined a *pattern* as "an envelope of relatively insignificant particular differences." Sullivan emphasized that the common principles of interpersonal behavior were more critical than the relatively insignificant, particular differences between people. In the concept of the *dynamism*, Sullivan stressed that, while human behavior was a process of ever-unfolding flux and change within the interpersonal field, i.e., dynamic, it became organized into habitual "relatively enduring patterns" toward characteristic satisfaction of needs and the avoidance of distress. For Sullivan, all significant variations or patterns occurred between species and that, within our specie, humans were simply more human than otherwise.

Sullivan's dynamisms were either *zonal dynamisms* directed at satisfaction of needs, or *interpersonal dynamisms* directed toward attachment, anxiety avoidance, and interpersonal cooperation. Sullivan defined human experience in terms of process and function, rather than concrete mechanisms to "avoid too close an association of known function to an unknown structure" (1972: 17–18n). He opposed using mechanistic concepts, which lent themselves to a reification of energy transformations and to the reduction of the pattern of processes into hypothetical structures. Sullivan directly criticized Freud's (1923a) structural theory of the id, ego, and superego, because Freud's concepts were mechanistic and inferential metaphors which could too easily be mistaken for actual processes. It can be said that Sullivan used the term *dynamism* somewhat loosely both to describe small patterns of interpersonal transaction or to refer to a vast organization of experience and behavior, such as the lust dynamism, oral dynamism, or self dynamism. On the other hand, Rychlak (1973) suggested that Sullivan concepts like the dynamism represented a paradigmatic shift from Freud's drive theory, much akin to the shift from mechanistic, structural Newtonian physics to the modern physics of relativity theory, quantum theory and indeterminacy.

## Developmental Theory

Another of Sullivan's essential postulates was the importance of the **developmental approach**. For Sullivan, the understanding of the normal human developmental processes which continue throughout our lives was fundamental for interpersonal theory. Given the opportunity to develop in a sane social environment, Sullivan viewed humans as oriented ultimately to becoming more fully human, empathic, secure, and inclusive with the capability of living in relative harmony with our social brethren throughout the world. This developmental approach, with its emphasis on the underlying process of interpersonal living, vehemently argued against Kraepelin's (1918) descriptive psychiatry's narrowly construed focus on naming and categorizing common symptoms and syndromes with no basis in human development. Sullivan further challenged Freud's (1920, 1930) more pessimistic ideas about the presence of an innate, core aggressive and destructive drive. While Sullivan followed Freud's similar emphasis on the importance of child developmental in shaping personality, he greatly broadened Freud's psychosexual theory with its exclusive reliance on sexual and aggressive drives

(Freud, 1905, 1920). Sullivan brought the child into the great interpersonal drama of the family and the larger society and more clearly explicated the critical influence of interpersonal learning and education on human development. Sullivan's human became a learning, thinking, person-seeking being, rather than Freud's drive-ridden, pleasure-seeking human. Additionally, Sullivan took a less deterministic perspective than Freud by commenting repeatedly throughout his discussion of human development about impact of fortune and misfortune in a person's life course. Like Dr. Jonathan Hullah in Robertson Davies' (1995) novel *The Cunning Man*, whose emblem was the caduceus under the Greek symbol for *anangke*, Sullivan took seriously the role of fate and accorded a proper place for bad luck, capriciousness, and the unknown as well as luck and good fortune.

Sullivan's interpersonal developmental approach stressed the essential need for interpersonal relatedness, the utter dependency that infants and young children has on their parents and family, and the role of learning in human development. Sullivan did not ignore biological aspects of the infant, but rather emphasized the interpersonal nature of all infant experience, including how biological processes such as eating, drinking, eliminating of waste, and even breathing were affected by caretaking. While retaining the advantages of a broad psychodynamic orientation, Sullivan's developmental theory also added the processes of human learning shared with Skinner's analysis of behavior and Bandura's social learning theory (see Rychlak, 1973), and, as Youniss (1980) had noted, included a cognitive development orientation similar to Piaget.

Like Freud's (1905) psychoanalytic developmental theory and Piaget's cognitive developmental theory, Sullivan's development approach is organized around specific *epochs of development*. Each epoch has its own distinctive developmental tasks and successful movement to the next epoch is largely dependent on negotiating the tasks of the prior epoch. Sullivan outlined in detail six pre-adult developmental epochs – Infancy, Childhood, the Juvenile Era, Preadolescence, Early Adolescence, and Late Adolescence, as well as early work on understanding Adulthood. Sullivan defined *Infancy* as the period from birth until the development of articulate speech. *Childhood* begins with the appearance of the need for playmates, both adult and child, and is the first step in developing interpersonal communication through language. The *Juvenile Era* commences with the child's entrance into school and continues until when the child finds a *chum*. Most importantly, this was the first developmental stage in where family limitations and peculiarities were open to substantial modification. In *Preadolescence*, the need for *chumship*, an intimate relationship with a compeer, a person of comparable age and status, is the central developmental event. *Early Adolescence* begins with puberty and genital sexuality, the psychologically strong interest in members of opposite sex, and involves resolving the complex interplay between the *dynamisms of lust, security, and intimacy*. In *Late Adolescence*, the person begins to integrate the partially developed aspects of the personality into an age-appropriate, early adult identity. The task of **Adulthood** is to establish a relationship of love with another person, someone who becomes as important as oneself. For Sullivan, while this adult intimacy is "not the primary business of life, but is, perhaps the principle source of satisfactions in life" (1953: 34). It is worth noting that Sullivan's early, though incomplete, writings on *adulthood* were novel in psychoanalytic theory and presaged the later adult development of Levinson (1978).

The next three chapters of this section on Sullivan's interpersonal theory will be devoted to a detailed overview and critique of Sullivan's epochs of development. While the author will present the main ideas, it is important to note that the scope of this book cannot do full justice to Sullivan's ambitious and complex thinking. While reading Sullivan can be frustrating, it is hoped that the reader will use this chapter as a map to the treasure trove of Sullivan's many ideas, concepts, and unique perspectives on human interpersonal development.

# Chapter 4

# Infancy

## The Beginning of Interpersonal Living

> We shall now consider the infant's success or misfortune in bringing about the appearance, approach, or cooperation of the good mother in the satisfaction of a need.
>
> (Sullivan, 1953: 92)

Much of Sullivan's developmental theory is based on his thoughts about the role of *infancy* in the formation of the person. Eight of the twenty-two chapters of *The Interpersonal Theory of Psychiatry*, constituting over one-third of the total pages of the book, are devoted to Sullivan's ideas about *infancy*, the first developmental epoch. Sullivan's acute interest in this earliest phase of human development is curious, in that Sullivan did not marry nor did he have children of his own. In fact, as mentioned in Chapter 2, he was an only child with no friends in the main of his own for much of the time covered by his developmental epochs (except for an important, but troubled friendship in pre- and early adolescence with Clarence Bellinger). Unlike Klein, Bowlby, Winnicott, Erikson, and Mahler, he never worked clinically with children. Even Freud, Fairbairn, and Kohut, the great psychoanalytic theorists who worked with adults, were married and had children. At best, Sullivan occasionally observed the children of his adult colleagues and friends, although it is unlikely that he spent much time observing the behavior of infants. On the surface, Sullivan's considerable lack of direct background experience gives us pause in considering his plausibility as a theorist of infant and child behavior.

As Stern (1985) has pointed out, there are significant problems with using the data from the "clinical" infant, retrospective reports of infancy obtained clinical work, as opposed to data from the observed infant, i.e., actual observations of infant behavior. Yet, Sullivan appears to have made extraordinary use of his limited contacts with children, retrospective accounts of childhood from his patients, his pediatric rotation in medical school, his voluminous reading, and his ability to carefully and conscientiously reflect on the human condition. As we have seen in the previous chapter and will see further, many of Sullivan's observations about child development have

DOI: 10.4324/9781003305712-6

considerable accuracy based on the convergence of his work with later child development research findings, especially in light of his foretelling of theoretically and scientifically robust attachment theory. His ideas of child development far outweigh the contributions of Freudian psychoanalytic theory. Sullivan's interpersonal theory is a testament to his exceptional powers of observation and reflection, gathered from his experience as one of life's outsiders.

Sullivan's detailed illumination of infancy was the cornerstone of his developmental theory. Many of his initial postulates mentioned above, e.g., tension and euphoria, the tension of need and anxiety, theorem of tenderness, and modes of experience, organized his thinking about the infant's biopsychosocial underpinnings. Unlike other psychoanalysts, Sullivan entered the infant world through a compelling description of infant's first post-natal experience – the danger of anoxia. Sullivan observed that the infant's reaction to anoxia, upon his or her umbilical separation from the mother, was an intense response of fear akin to what could easily be called terror and rage. For Sullivan, this first tension of fear arising from "unsatisfied, extremely aggravated needs" (1953: 57), and the terror and rage behavior it provoked, revealed the tremendous energy of young infants, which are clearly designed to call forth an interpersonal response from caretakers. The infant's first biologically separate act in the extrauterine world was to cry out, evoking help from those upon whom he or she depends. Sullivan further elaborated on the four ways in which the tension of fear could be altered – removal or destruction of, escape or avoidance from, neutralizing, or ignoring – the fearful situation. On one form or another for the infant, the removal of the tension of fear by the first three operations can only be achieved by interpersonal cooperation of the caretaker. Ignoring the fearful or anxiety-provoking situation, through apathy or somnolent detachment, occurs when the call for interpersonal cooperation necessary for reducing the tension of need or tension of anxiety is not attended to or is malevolently attended to. Early in his conceptualizations about maternal responsiveness, Sullivan straightforwardly addressed the reality of ***malevolence*** in childrearing, which he distinguished from non-responsiveness to the infant's immediate needs or from the anxiety-provoking presence of the anxious mother. He used the word *malevolence* to refer to the infant's experience of a disintegrating, destructive interpersonal presence, i.e., where the interpersonal response of the mothering one was the opposite of tender cooperation, but where the mothering "instead hurt or otherwise provoked fear in the infant" (1953: 115). While we shall address later some of the consequences of transactions with malevolent parenting, it is important to note that, early in his interpersonal theory, Sullivan made a link between malevolent mothering and somnolent detachment, the complex dynamism of ignoring a fear.

For Sullivan, anxiety was an especially complex threat for the infant. The infant cannot destroy, remove, avoid, or neutralize the source of anxiety, (the mothering one) and crying is ineffectual, or worse, brings the infant in greater proximity to anxious, anxiety-provoking, or malevolent mothering. The operation of ignoring, in response to prolonged severe anxiety, leads to the attenuation of tension of needs or anxiety through *somnolent detachment*, literally interpersonal detachment by falling asleep. The infant's over-reliance on the last strategy, which Sullivan believed was a very complex operation, became a central aspect of his theory of severe *problems in living*, i.e., his term for psychopathology. While a necessary short-term response, the interruptive power of anxiety can eventually become a chronic dangerous response for interpersonal and biological regulation and maturation. Greenspan's (1983) observational research on infants of psychotic mothers has provided evidence for Sullivan's perspective. Greenspan's work revealed a high frequency of disturbed interpersonal behaviors such gaze aversion (interpersonal avoidance) and apathetic, interpersonal detachment in infants of psychotic mothers, which he reasoned were sources of interpersonal disturbance predisposing these children to later severe psychopathology (DeGangi et al., 2000). Greenspan and Shanker (2007) further demonstrated the crucial importance of the development of facial affective signaling and pattern recognition and joint attention as essential capabilities necessary for cognitive and language development.

Sullivan observed that the infant, with appropriate cooperation of the mothering one, has the capacity to deal with the external world of stimulation directly opposed Freud's (1911) original and Mahler's (Mahler, 1968; Mahler et al., 1975) later formulations of a period of "normal autism." While the infant enters the world in the prototaxic mode of experience, Sullivan, along with Bowlby, Fairbairn, and Winnicott, strongly believed that, from birth, the infant is "built" for interpersonal relatedness and requires a supportive "facilitating environment" to mature (see Winnicott, 1965). Based on their review of infant research as it bore upon psychoanalytic theory, Lichtenberg (1981, 1983) and Stern (1985) concluded that Mahler's concept of normal autism should be discarded. Additionally, Sullivan's observations that rage behavior is a fear-induced reaction to the failure to bring forth adequate interpersonal cooperation in the presence of significant physical and interpersonal needs was closer to Bowlby's empirically demonstrated concept of separation protest than to Freud's (1920) or Klein's (1975) conceptualizations of a primary aggressive drive existing independent of environmental stimulation. Learning theorists Dollard and Miller's (Dollard et al., 1939) research on psychoanalytic concepts demonstrated that aggression was a response to frustration, not a primary drive as suggested by Freud.

As stated above, Sullivan described the infant entering the world in the prototaxic mode, experiencing two kinds of tensions – *tension of needs*, requiring satisfaction and relief from physical and interpersonal needs, and the *tension of anxiety*, requiring interpersonal security. Because of the utterly dependent state of infancy, the satisfaction of needs and interpersonal security for the infant could only occur through interpersonal cooperation with the caretaker, called the *"mothering one"* in Sullivan's theory. As such Sullivan was always concerned with relations with others, especially the dyad of the child and the mothering one. As Winnicott (1965) so elegantly stated, "there is no such thing as an infant' meaning, of course, that wherever one finds an infant one finds maternal care, and without maternal care there would be no infant."

Sullivan's use of the term *"mothering one,"* as distinguished from the term "mother" found throughout the writings of other psychoanalytic theorists, emphasized again the importance he placed on process and function. The young infant experiences *mothering*: it is only much later that the person "mother" is differentiated out of prototaxic experience. The infant experienced mothering through what Sullivan called **zones of interaction**, the point of contact between the infant's inner world of tensions and the interpersonal environment. Different from Freud's focus on the specific tension, e.g., need for oral gratification, Sullivan's concept of zones of interaction stressed the importance of the quality of interpersonal cooperation, which is inseparable from the infant's need satisfaction. Like Freud, Sullivan believed in the central importance of the very young infant of the oral zone, though Sullivan expanded Freud's emphasis on sucking to eat to include breathing and communicating distress (crying) and pleasure (cooing). Unlike Freud, Sullivan discussed the significance of other zones of interaction with the infant as well in terms of the quality of interpersonal cooperation in regulating the infant's body temperature, providing the "removal of noxious physical circumstances" (1953: 62) such as urine and feces from the skin, burping, untangling the bound infant from his bedclothes, and the like.

Sullivan emphasized that communication of needs by the infant brings satisfaction or disappointment (sometimes grave disappointment) of these needs and additionally the experiences of either tenderness or anxiety (or possibly even malevolence) from the mothering one. When the infant repeatedly experiences the satisfying and tender mothering one, the infant develops successful patterns of cooperation in the oral zone and experiences his or her needs as bringing durable, favorable change in his or her state of being. Sullivan expressed his preference for concepts which emphasized process and function in describing feeding, an interaction in the oral zone, rather than simply oral gratification. He stated that, when the infant experienced hunger, the infant soon learned that crying (the biologically built-in response to fear) frequently brought the tender, satisfying, **nipple-in-lips situation**. In the process, these cooperative interactions between the infant and the mothering one establishes the experiences of *foresight* and *recall* within the infant, beginning the differentiation into the *parataxic mode*. Through the ever-growing capacities of recall and foresight, the infant eventually comes to anticipate (*prehend*) that his or her experience of need will bring about a durable change in the unpleasant experience. Hunger soon brings, through foresight and recall, a prehension of satisfactory interpersonal cooperation as well. The infant begins to notice *signs* – patterns in experience of events which are differentiated from the general flux of experience and which occur in the recall and foresight of particular satisfactions or distress. Sullivan stressed that signs, and behavior conditioned by signs, were part of the infant's *experience*, not "outside objective reality." Sullivan believed strongly that it was more important for the mothering one to understand what the infant's actions and thoughts were actually **intended** for, in terms of the infant's actual experience, rather than what the mothering one speculated them to mean. Ainsworth's research (Ainsworth et al., 1978) on empathic attunement and maternal responsiveness confirmed the importance Sullivan placed on maternal empathy.

Further differentiation in the infant's emerging cognitive world occurs when the infant experiences that crying-when-hungry frequently, but not invariably, produces the correct (satisfying) nipple-in-lips situation. The infant comes to learn that, simply because he or she experiences hunger and cries for the good nipple-in-lips, the environment (mothering one) does not necessarily supply it. The adult necessary for satisfaction (a parent with milk-producing nipples) may be absent, the nipples of a satisfactory adult may not produce milk, and the like. As a result, the infant may experience a good, but unsatisfactory, nipple-in-lips (e.g., a bottle provided by the father) or the wrong nipple-in-lips (a breast without milk). Additionally, the infant may experience what Sullivan drolly called the *evil nipple-in-lips*, which was the nipple of an anxious mother. This nipple was preceded by the aura of extremely disagreeable tension of anxiety, which the infant would struggle to avoid, even if the infant were hungry. Experience with the unsatisfactory, wrong, or evil nipple-in-lips leads to differentiated zonal experience, to the identification of differences, and to the generalizations of good and bad. As the infant matures and develops, zonal and general dynamisms, the characteristic way the individuals interact with the interpersonal environment, are established. Sullivan talked about the development of oral dynamisms, which are patterns of integrating tendencies like hunger that lead to resolution or disintegration of oral needs, determined by the needs of the infant, the socialization of the infant and the quality of interpersonal cooperation. When experiences of anxiety occur with sufficient frequency in meeting of zonal needs, disintegration of interpersonal situations, complex relationships, and primitive modes of experience predominate. The accretion of bad experiences with a particular zone of interaction will lead to serious difficulty in developing straightforward, satisfactory dynamisms.

### Personality and Personification

After setting down the nature of early infant-caretaker cooperative patterns, Sullivan next introduced his concept of *personality*, "the relatively enduring pattern of interpersonal situations which characterize a human life" (1953: 110–111). Through the recall and foresight of experiences with others, the infant develops the capacity to differentiate dynamisms, which lead to satisfaction and integration of needs through interpersonal cooperation, from anxiety and fear-driven dynamisms which lead to apathy, detachment, and disintegration of interpersonal cooperation. While the infant-mothering one's interpersonal interaction initially involves meeting zonal needs of the infant, general and broader interpersonal dynamisms rapidly develop through the infant's fundamental experiences of tenderness, unsatisfactoriness, or malevolence with the mothering one. Sullivan noted that these interpersonal dynamisms contained both a behavioral component, predispositions towards action, and an "intrapsychic," cognitive component, the representation of interpersonal relatedness. In keeping with his strong emphasis on cognitive-emotional development, Sullivan reasoned that the infant formed an increasingly complex elaboration of experience in recall and foresight of interpersonal events, which he called *personification*.

*Personification*, a central organization within Sullivan's view of the overall personality, is the essential way the infant comes to interpret the interpersonal world, through the formulation of a set of internal assumptions, ideas, emotions, and fantasies about people and the self based on actual interpersonal experience. The first personification is of the *good mother*, formed early in infancy, which is the infant's recall and foresight about the pattern of recurrent interactions with the mothering one in which she satisfactorily responds to the infant's needs. i.e., situations have been resolved with satisfaction. As Sullivan (1953: 111) stated, "Thus the infant's personification of the good mother ... symbolizes the integration, maintenance, and resolution of the situations that are necessary for the infant's appropriate and adequate action in the satisfaction of his needs."

Sullivan (1953: 112) strongly emphasized that, "this personification is not the 'real' mother-a particular living being considered as an entity ... (but) an elaborate organization of the infant's experience." Sullivan defined the initial sense in which personification occurs as a cognitive-emotional representation of learned experiences of transactional relatedness, i.e., the representation of the transactions of interpersonal cooperation and of the concurrent experiences of interpersonal security. From Sullivan's perspective, this earliest form of personification was not yet differentiated into an object (the "real" mother) or a subject (the self). Carson (1982) cited empirical research on the functioning of human memory and how complex schemas of interpersonal perception are formed by past interpersonal experience which confirms the remarkable accuracy of Sullivan's concept of personification. Ainsworth's (1979) concept of the *internal working model of attachment* is very close conceptually to Sullivan's concept of personifications, which has been shown to have substantial support in the research literature on neurobiology of attachment (Bretherton & Munholland, 2016), infant development (Sherman et al., 2015), child and adolescent development (Thompson, 2016), and psychopathology in adulthood (Stovall-McClough & Dozier, 2016).

As experience with the mother increased, Sullivan (1953: 122) believed that "the infant is bound to have two personifications of any mothering person," i.e., the infant develops personifications of the *good mother* and the *bad mother*. From Sullivan's perspective these two concepts are actually representations of good and bad *mothering*, i.e., representations of the flow of experience where the distinction between self and other is a primitive and vaguely differentiated sense of satisfying, unsatisfying, or seriously anxiety-ridden interpersonal transaction. From Sullivan's perspective, though not "autistic," the prototaxic differentiation between inside and outside, you and me, self and other was in no sense the infant's earliest representation. What the infant first experiences is the quality of relatedness, out of which experiences of self and other later arise. As Greenberg and Mitchell (1983: 97) pointed out, personifications are the "infant's earliest organization of experience ... based on the distinction between anxious states (bad mother) and nonanxious states (good mother)."

Because of the transactional nature of human living, the development of personifications is a crucial element in the development of the personality. While the infant is "built" for interpersonal relatedness, the impact of the facilitating environment is especially critical during the highly dependent state of early infancy. Sullivan expressed numerous times and in many ways that humans are far more socially dependent and interconnected than our prevailing Western conceptions of autonomy would indicate. Basic attitudes about interpersonal connection, what Stern (1985) referred to as the domain of core-relatedness, are formed in a generally "unconscious" way; that is to say, they are so much an implicit part of the developing person's worldview that this core sense of relatedness operates largely outside the person's awareness. Virtually identical to Erikson's (1950) later description of the first psychosocial task of trust versus mistrust, Sullivan insisted that the infant must form a sense of secure interpersonal connectedness or serious problems would ensue. Without the relatively consistent experience of interpersonal security, similar to what Ainsworth (1982) and Bowlby (1988) called the *secure base*, the infant is placed in a dangerous situation where he or she cannot form consistent, reliable representations of interpersonal cooperation. Instead, the infant develops what Sullivan called malevolent personifications ...

> the malevolent person may behave toward the infant in ways quite other than giving tender cooperation in satisfying the infant's manifest needs; she may instead hurt and otherwise provoke fear in the infant. Since malevolent behavior is also apt to be accompanied by anxiety and to induce anxiety in the infant, the infant's prehensions ... come to be organized as the experience of the bad mother.
>
> (1953: 115–116)

The impact of anxiety in infancy is crucial in that, if experiences of anxiety become associated with need states, the development of the necessary personification of interpersonal cooperation for the resolution of needs, i.e., the good mother, is hindered. Greenspan's (1983) previously mentioned research on gaze aversion in infants of severely emotionally disturbed mothers provided an excellent illustration of the effects of anxiety on development of personification. These infants turn their heads and crane away with their bodies to avoid the unpleasant visual contact with their mother's faces. Greenspan found that, once this pattern of gaze aversion was established, it was very difficult to get the infants to establish contact with any adult, thus cutting off the possibility of positive, nurturing experiences with maternal surrogates. Literally, consistent, early experiences of severe anxiety with the mothering one led the infants to anticipate the facilitating environment as malevolent, virtually assuring them of serious psychopathology in later life.

Sullivan's good mother and bad mother personifications appeared superficially similar to the psychoanalytic concept of inner objects, which were the basis for understanding intrapsychic experience in classical psychoanalytic and object relation theories. Where Sullivan parted company with these psychoanalysts was his emphasis on the transactional relatedness in the development of personifications of the good and bad mothering one. Unlike psychoanalysts like Melanie Klein (1964, 1975), he did not stress the importance of intrapsychic life and did not see the infant as having inner representations of the good and bad mother as a well-differentiated other person. He attended to the experiential sense of transactional or core relatedness in which self and other is experienced but could only vaguely be described. To Sullivan, the infant did not experience complex interactions between self and the object world of good and bad mothers as suggested by the work of Klein and Edith Jacobson (1964). For Sullivan, the infant experiences described by Klein and Jacobson resided primarily in the mind of the psychoanalyst.

## The Development of the Self

After establishing the concepts of personification of the good mother and bad mother, i.e., how the infant developed cognitive-emotional representations of transactional relatedness, Sullivan next addressed the development of the infant's sense of himself or herself as a person. From his conceptualizations about the good and bad mother emerged the first psychodynamic theory of the development of the *self*, or in Sullivan's terms, the *self-dynamism*. Heavily influenced by social psychologist George Herbert Mead (1934, 1952, 1956), while Sullivan defined personality as the entire interpersonal functioning of the person, his concept of the *self* concerned the representation of those experiences about what one takes oneself to be. The process by which one develops this sense of self comes through interpersonal interaction. As Sullivan stated (1940/1953: 22), "The self may be said to be made up of reflected appraisals of others." For Sullivan, the infant's sense of self begins first by learning about "my body." As the infant's sensory systems become more differentiated and acute and his or her capacity for foresight and recall increases, the infant begins experiential "differentiation that is based on sentience from more than one zone" (1953: 136). Sucking a thumb requires the infant to coordinate the thumb to the mouth – "the thumb feels sucked" (1953: 136), but no milk comes forth. The thumb feels different than the nipple. The infant experiences a variety of different zonal sensations, including his or her tactile exploration of his or her own body as well as tactile contacts with others. Stern's (1985) review of infant research found strong support for multizonal sensory experience in the development of internal representations or schemas that become linked to an infant's emergent sense of self.

While, through these multizonal interactions, the infant learns a sense of her or his own body, the interpersonal component is inextricably tied to this learning as well. As the infant's sensory apparatus matures, his or her increased visual and auditory acuity allows the infant to better differentiate himself or herself from the external world, which also includes an increasing ability to discriminate and read *signs* and *signals*. The infant especially visually discriminates various facial gestures and auditorily differentiates sounds and phonemes, which interpersonally become as signs of integration and disintegration of interpersonal situations. Sullivan accurately observed that infants have a particularly acute early capacity for the learning of facial gestures and the learning of phonemes, which he hypothesized occurred in mid-infancy, at about the age of 6 to 8 months. Much infant research, e.g., Haith (1980) indicating the babies attend more closely to faces that speak and Field et al. (1982) reporting that infants can reliably imitate adult facial gestures, have provided empirical support for Sullivan's observations but found that the processes of facial gesture and auditory discrimination occurs much earlier than Sullivan suggested. Nelson's (2001) review of the infant facial recognition literature supported the view that infants unambiguously recognize faces within the first six months of life and that the neural systems involved face recognition also become activated during this period.

Sullivan stated that the infant learns that, through the generalization of experiences with needs satisfaction and interpersonal cooperation, the anticipation of the personifications of the good mother and bad mother becomes linked to the infant's increasing sense of his or her body. Through that seamless flow of behavior, interpersonal reaction (consequences), and cognitive encoding of these sequences, i.e., learning, a second kind of personification arises from this linkage of experience of the personifications good and bad mother to the increasing sense of body. Sullivan called this personification the *sense of self*, found within the dynamism of the self-system. Sullivan's **self-system** was the anti-anxiety dynamism which led operationally

to the maintenance of interpersonal security and the avoidance of interpersonal situations likely to produce anxiety. As Barnett (1980) pointed out,
Sullivan's concept of the self contained both operational and representational
aspects of the self-system, which, in keeping with the concept of the dynamism, indicated the functional and operational aspects of the self, and the
personification of the self, which referred to the content or inner representations of the self. Because Sullivan's concept of the self personification is
intricately tied to the processes of human learning, it is necessary to first
discuss his thoughts about learning.

An aspect novel to psychoanalytic theory and likely the introduction of
this now central concept in psychology, Sullivan's postulates of the self-
system and the personifications of the self was the way he conceptualized how
this process took place. Rather than rely on the psychoanalytic concepts of
introjection or incorporation which he openly criticized as "a rather reckless
oversimplification, if not also a great magic verbal gesture the meaning of
which cannot be made explicit" (1953: 166), he leaned heavily on the concept
of *learning through experience*. Influenced heavily by experimental psychologist and learning theorist Charles Spearman (1923, 1930) and educator and
philosopher John Dewey (1922, 1929), Sullivan devoted considerable space
in *The Interpersonal Theory of Personality* to his formulations about learning,
indeed an entire chapter titled "Learning: The Organization of Experience."
Sullivan believed that experience is not organized through obtuse, noetic
processes, such as psychoanalytic concepts of internalization, incorporation,
and introjection, but through demonstrable, knowable processes. For
Sullivan, these experiences developed through the process of human learning,
"undoubtedly a field which requires multidisciplinary thinking" (1953: 150).
In this chapter, Sullivan described numerous processes of learning, including
trial and success, reward and punishment, trial and error by human example,
and the complex process of intellectual learning he referred to as education. It
is of historical note that Sullivan's formulations presaged, and were later
empirically supported by, important discoveries in the field of the psychology
of learning, such as the works of Ferster and Skinner (1957) on schedules of
reinforcement, Bandura (1977) on imitation and social learning, and Piaget
on cognitive development (see Flavell, 1963).

Perhaps the most important aspect of his discussion of learning and the
development of the self was Sullivan's postulate of three basic and specific
processes by which the infant learns about the self through interpersonal
cooperation – *reward*, *gradient of anxiety*, and *severe anxiety*. As the maturing
infant is increasingly expected by the mothering one to behave cooperatively
with her or him, educative experiences of reward and gradient of anxiety are
provided by the mothering one to socialize the infant. Sullivan pointed out
the importance of tenderness as a *reward* for what the mothering one regards
as good behavior. Consequently, the "reward "of tenderness can be withheld
or withdrawn. Instead, mildly forbidding visual and auditory gestures, such

as a frown or a sharp tone, can be indications of disapproval of certain of the infant's behaviors. Sullivan called this process the *gradient of anxiety*. Learning of socially appropriate behavior, from the mothering one's viewpoint, proceeds by this rewarding application of tender approval and the mildly punishing withdrawal of this approval. The infant learns that smiling and cooing, the production of babbling, and greedy acceptance of the breast brings forth tenderness. The infant further learns biting the breast, throwing toys, and kicking while having diapers changed occasions disapproving visual and verbal gestures. It is through this interpersonal interaction that the sense of self is formed, according to Sullivan, as stated in his formulation that the self is made up of reflected appraisals of others.

Next, Sullivan carefully elaborated on an extremely important, special example of learning through gradients of anxiety which he called *severe anxiety*, the infant's experience of intense insecurity in response to anxiety or malevolence in the mothering one. If infant exploratory behaviors such as touching the genitals or anus or playing with feces evoked this intense or even cruel reaction from the mothering, the infant would experience an abrupt transition to a state of very severe anxiety, a highly dysphoric experience from which there is no escape. The extreme insecurity of this interpersonal situation arrests cognitive processes of recall and foresight, making it impossible to either learn from or avoid the experience. Sullivan (1953: 160) noted that severe anxiety "has a little bit the effect of a blow to the head, in that later one is not clear at all as to just what was going on." Such an experience is by no means educational as practically prohibits clear understanding of the immediate situation. While memory of the event does occur, it would be hazy and of the nature of an uncanny taboo. This set of Sullivan's constructs was perhaps the earliest clear explanation in psychoanalysis and developmental psychology of the experience of severe attachment separation later described by Ainsworth and others.

Based heavily on his work with schizophrenics, Sullivan strongly believed that severe anxiety, and the resulting uncanny experiences and uncanny taboos that it created in the infant, produced "useless confusion" (1953: 152) and interrupted cognitive processes, thereby rendering any educative purpose effectively fruitless. Additionally, while mild gradients of anxiety are useful in social learning, severe anxiety interferes with the infant's attempts to meet of zonal needs and learn about his or her body. Severe anxiety can be associated erroneously with a zone of interaction, which later could lead to associations of uncanny emotion and disrupted behavior with important functions. For example, in the case of severe anxiety associated with the anal zone can create severe disturbance in the infant regarding the elimination of waste products that can carry into adulthood. Severe anxiety associated with the oral zone can lead to eating disturbances. In in the case of severe anxiety associated with the genitals, the development of a healthy dynamism of lust can be severely hindered. Most importantly, repeated experiences with severe anxiety impairs both the development of cooperative, non-anxious personifications of others and wreaks havoc with the development of the self. Because the infant cannot differentiate the causes of the experience of severe anxiety or take appropriate preventative action, the infant develops an underlying and pervasive sense of powerlessness.

Additionally, Sullivan described a related process that he saw of great importance in childhood, the precursors of which can appear in infancy. In a way idiosyncratic to the rest of psychoanalytic theory, he used the term *sublimation* to describe "the long-circuiting of the resolution of situations, chiefly those pertaining to zonal needs-a long circuiting which proves to be socially acceptable" (ITP: 153). Sullivan stressed, not the defensive nature of sublimation, but its function, which is to meet zonal needs in the face of powerful anxiety and prohibition of the mothering one. Although sublimation has a component of meeting needs in a socially acceptable way, it can also have very unfortunate consequences for the developing person, an aspect quite different from the thrust of Freud's use of the term.

### Good-Me, Bad-Me, and Not-Me

Having established these three aspects of learning through interpersonal cooperation, Sullivan described "the initial personification of three phases of what presently will be *me*, that which is invariably connected with the sentience of *my body*" (ITP: 161). These three personifications of "me" were what Sullivan termed *good-me*, *bad-me*, and *not-me*.

First, Sullivan discussed the self-personification called the *good-me*. In essence, the infant anticipates and connects his or her behavior and inner experience of need states with the affective state of the mothering one. The *good me* is the internal organization and cognitive representation of the infant's experience in which the infant's behavior meets with the reward, approval, and tenderness of the mothering one, leading the infant to feel comfortable and secure through this empathic link. When my mother tenderly smiles at me when I babble, all is well in the world. The self-personification called the *bad-me* is essentially the inner representation of the interpersonal experience of the gradient of anxiety with the mothering one. While not overwhelming to the infant, the mothering one's disapproval, communicated through facial gestures and words and tones, creates worry about the loss of tenderness, the shadow of the loss of attachment. The mothering one is not attuned to the infant's internal experience of his or her needs, but instead responds to the infant from her feelings about the social appropriateness of the child's behavior. For example, good children do not throw toys, bad children do; no matter that the infant enjoys (initially) the experience of throwing toys. The infant prehends the loss of tenderness (and attachment) with the mothering one and learns to reorganize his or her behavior to achieve behaviors which the mothering one will experience as,

and reply with tenderness to, the *good me*. Sullivan emphasized the importance of realizing that gradients of anxiety leading to bad-me personification
were mild enough not to interfere with the infant's cognitive state, so that
the infant can in effect act on the environment to deter the experience of
mounting anxiety.

Before describing Sullivan's last personification, it is important to note
here an interesting and significant concurrence between Sullivan's concepts of
the *good me* and *bad me* and research on the development of self-esteem. It is
important to keep in mind that concept of self-esteem is an essential part of
the lexicon in mental health, but that it was originally brought into the mental
health literature by Sullivan. Classic studies by Coopersmith (1967) and
Baumrind (1978) established a connection between parenting styles and
children's self-esteem. Coopersmith found the children with high self-esteem
had parents who clearly communicated acceptance of the children (leading to
feelings in the child that he or she belonged in the family), communicated
well-defined limits and high expectations for performance (leading the child
to recognize expectations for socially appropriate behavior and parental
confidence in him or her to meet these expectations), and communicated
respect and allowance for the child's individual differences (leading the child
to feel that he or she had latitude to express his or her unique self within
general boundaries). Not surprisingly, parents with high self-esteem children
were themselves higher in self-esteem and in experienced confidence.

In her studies of competence in children, Baumrind discovered family
patterns similar to those described by Coopersmith. Baumrind (1978: 275)
found that authoritative parents, who "balanced much warmth with high
control, and high demands with clear communication of what was required
of the child," tended to have children who were more interpersonally
trusting, contented, and competent. Authoritarian parents, who were more
self-centered and detached, but controlling and who valued obedience over
reasoning, tended to have children that were more withdrawn, dis-
contented, and mistrustful. Permissive parents, who were warm, but lax in
discipline, and made only weak demands for socially appropriate maturity,
tended to have children who had difficulties interacting with peers, were
dependent and demanding, and displayed immature social behavior.
Sullivan's realization of the importance of the place of gradients of anxiety
in the socialization of children, within the context of a generally tender and
encouraging attitude, for the development of positive self-esteem and
competence has received more empirical support than do proponents of
unconditional positive regard and unconditional love, such as Carl Rogers
(1961). A comprehensive review of the literature on parenting and self-
esteem by Collins et al. (2000) drew attention to the complexity of parental
influences on child development of self-esteem, while also confirming the
substantial research supporting the relationship between modes of parenting and later self-esteem in their children.

While Sullivan's concepts of the good-me and bad-me personifications are roughly similar to the concept of good and bad self-presentations found in Klein's and others' British object relations theory, there are no significant parallels to Sullivan's concept of *not-me*. The *not-me* personification arises from interpersonal experiences of severe anxiety. Sullivan stated that not-me experiences are rarely encountered directly in ordinary experience except perhaps in a very bad nightmare or in a severe schizophrenic episode. The "not-me" can be indirectly observed through phenomenon of dissociated behavior in which people do and say things of which they are unaware of themselves but is observable to others. Because dissociated behavior operates automatically and unwittingly to avoid the possibility of severe distress, it is not available to the educational effects of learning and is organized at the most primitive levels (prototaxic and parataxic) of cognitive experience.

In essence, when the infant engages in certain behavior that interacts with prohibitive aspects of the mothering one's personality, the infant can unwittingly arouse intense anxiety or malevolence in the mothering one. In turn, the infant is empathically exposed to severe, overwhelming anxiety from which he or she cannot escape. Drawing the mothering one closer with the infant's cries, an attempt to call the good mother, can only bring the very anxious or malevolent mother proximally closer, increasing the infant's anxiety, or causing the anxious mother to leave, creating unwanted separation. The bad or malevolent mother cannot be avoided, nor can the good mother be called. This situation for Sullivan "is the closest approach to absolute tension that one can imagine" (1953: 45). In fact, Sullivan commented throughout his writings that this level of tension is so severe that people will do practically anything they can rather than face with the hint of it.

Additionally, Sullivan inferred that the experience of not-me was part of everyone's developmental experience. What distinguished the "normal" person from the schizophrenic in Sullivan's thinking is that schizophrenics experienced frequent not-me experiences in their development, associated often with particular zones of interaction. The development of a self-system heavily laden with not-me personifications and dissociative adaptive processes is especially problematic in that the self-system becomes a dynamism of avoidance of interpersonal living, that is, its purpose is to avoid painful or overwhelming human experiences. While the self-system is necessary to ward off painful interpersonal experiences, Sullivan further commented that over time the person avoided signs that represented the possibility of bad me and not-me experiences derived from interactions in the past, which were not actual experiences in the here and now. As a result, the self-system was, in Sullivan's words, conservative, that is, slow to change, even in more optimal facilitating environments. An avoidant self-dynamism tended to cut the infant, and later the child and adult, off from the very experiences that could modify troubled personifications and problematic interpersonal relations.

Social psychological research on the powerful impact of face saving in social interaction (see Jones et al., 1971) can be viewed as considerable empirical confirmation of Sullivan's notions of the self-system and security operations. Additionally, Fairbairn's concept of the closed system in the schizoid situation expressed a very similar idea, leading him to tersely state that psychotherapy for the deeply disturbed client was a cure by the hair of the tail of the dog that bit him.

In his concept of not-me personification, Sullivan eloquently revealed theoretical thinking that has been confirmed, as we shall explore further in Chapter 7, by a wide variety of research on trauma, dissociation and dissociative behavior. What Sullivan provided was a theoretical rationale for understanding the internal representation of overwhelming experiences, at the heart (of darkness) of which unveiled our essential interpersonal relatedness by divining experientially the cost of losing the security of our primary attachments. Putnam's (1997, 2003) work on dissociative disorders and child abuse and dissociation and states of mind in normal functioning and psychopathology (Putnam, 2016) provides substantial evidence for the power and ubiquity of not-me states.

Throughout the next two chapters on the rest of Sullivan's developmental epochs, Sullivan will use the concepts of the self, self-system, personification, and learning by experience as the cornerstones of human development as the infant learns language and enters into an increasingly more elaborate interpersonal world. The infant, soon to be a child, will face the complex demands of interpersonal living with more or less positive personifications of self and other, which will enhance or inhibit future learning.

# Chapter 5

# Developmental Epochs of Childhood and the Juvenile Era

## The Expansion of the Interpersonal World

We are largely a product of acculturation: our security depends on others, for our self-system is developed exclusively from communicated values which we have picked up from others; and the satisfactions of our most difficult needs ... also involve other people.

(Sullivan, 1956: 106)

This chapter on Sullivan's interpersonal theory of psychiatry will focus on his next two *epochs of development* – the periods including childhood through the juvenile era. As we move away from the more specific interactions between the infant and the mothering one, we shall see how Sullivan cast his developmental epochs as times of changing patterns of socialization and of learning increasingly complex patterns of interpersonal cooperation. Naturally, the developing person will also modify or change his or her *personifications of self and others*, the internal representations of the interpersonal world. As Carson (1982) pointed out, Sullivan's concept of personification suggested that these representations of self and other will begin to take the form of several internal "generalized others" (not all of whom will be the source of difficulty) with reciprocal complementary "selves." The role of the self in personality theory has received considerable empirical support (e.g., Gergen, 1971; McAdams et al., 2021).

As compared to other psychoanalytic theories, Sullivan's concept of the epochs of development emphasized the relative plasticity in personality development, during which current interpersonal circumstances became important influences, as well as the past. Balancing his more skeptical view of the conservative tendency of the self-system, i.e., maintaining, no matter how problematic, the prevailing self and other representations and resulting interpersonal dynamisms, Sullivan stressed the importance of how the processes of learning can increasingly activate more effective patterns of interpersonal cooperation influenced personality development. Sullivan saw developmental epochs as more or less culturally determined age periods where important interpersonal tasks were mastered more or less well. With the possible exception of the effects of massively anxiety-ridden interpersonal

DOI: 10.4324/9781003305712-7

relations in infancy, he did not believe in the concept of critical periods of development in which certain maturation must be met by a certain age or an immutable distorting influence would ensue. As noted by Kagan (1984), intercultural research on critical periods in human child development largely has not held up the concept of specific age-related developmental periods, but instead has indicated a greater influence of developmental task learning on personality development. Foretelling competency-based theories of human motivation like Robert White (1959) and David McClelland (1961), Sullivan strongly believed that the human animal found learning and mastery to be innately rewarding. Like John Dewey's (1922, 1926) pragmatic and optimistic social theory, Sullivan's developmental theory subtly expressed an underlying belief in the possibility of personality change in even highly damaged individuals, given the intervention of fortunate interpersonal circumstances.

## Childhood

For Sullivan, the developmental epoch of *childhood* marked the expansion of the interpersonal world, including relationships with other children and adults, and was the first step in the development of the critical operation of interpersonal communication through language. While the child was primarily concerned with his or her relationship with parents, the focus of their interpersonal cooperation changed. Sullivan pointed out that the quality of interpersonal cooperation in childhood shifted from the mother's empathic attunement to and tenderness toward the infant's biological and security needs to the growing necessity for the child to meet parents' demands for socialization and for parents to empathically understand what they can reasonably expect from the child. This shift in development is perhaps best captured in Sullivan's *theorem of reciprocal emotion* ...

> Integration of an interpersonal situation is a reciprocal process in which (1) complementary needs are resolved, or aggravated; (2) reciprocal patterns of activity are developed, or disintegrated; and (3) foresight of satisfaction, or rebuff, of similar needs is facilitated.
>
> (1953: 198)

Sullivan began his discussion of childhood with his thoughts about the transition between infancy and childhood. The central elements of this transition were the increasing socialization of the infant by his or her parents and the acquisition of language with its critical role in interpersonal cooperation and the elaboration of personifications. Again, Sullivan emphasized the processes of learning, with an expanded focus of social learning and socialization. Sullivan stated that the frequency, consistency, and especially "*sanity of* the educational efforts" (1953: 173) of the parents' socialization of the infant were crucial. Sullivan further modified his concept of empathy with the concept of *sanity of educational efforts*, the ability of parents to set expectations for their child according to the child's developmental ability and readiness to meet these expectations. The parents' expectations of and reactions to (or, in the language of modern social psychology, 'attributions about') the child's natural needs-oriented behavior exerted considerable influence on the child's social maturation and development of a positive sense of self. Sullivan's thinking was very much in line with the current social psychological research confirming the powerful influence of social attribution (see Malle, 2011; Shaver, 2016). Sullivan cogently described situations where the failure of the parents to apply sane education would lead to inevitable failure of the child to meet with parental expectations, resulting in anxiety-ridden, bad-me or not-me self personifications. Examples given by Sullivan included parents ascribing willfulness to a one-year-old, seeing the increasingly autonomous child as less maturationally able than his or her demonstrated abilities, or responding to the body exploration of the child as an immoral sexual act to be prevented by tying the child's hands, all of which were particularly problematic to the infant's development into childhood.

Additionally, for Sullivan, the nascent parataxic sense of self and other begun in infancy underwent a significant change during the childhood era with the maturation of the child's cognitive capacity. Sullivan postulated that the child started to better identify distinct persons in outer reality, through the symbolic representation of language. The beginning of language fused personifications of good and bad mother(ing) into personifications of interpersonal cooperation with a specific other. The person called mother brought with her both good and bad experiences of interpersonal cooperation, fusing the experiences of the good and bad mothering once previously separated in the early infant's cognitions. Sullivan believed that the resulting fused personifications, while still parataxic, were considerably more differentiated into what he variously referred to as "illusory two-group patterns" or "me-you" patterns. He stressed that fundamentally there could be no sense of self in isolation from others. Personifications in childhood (and throughout life) remained representations of transactional interpersonal relatedness, only the sense of self and other became further differentiated. As Greenberg and Mitchell (1983) noted, Sullivan's concept of personifications were representations of relational integration based on actual interpersonal experience and were conceptually different from Klein's autistic, intrapsychic ideas and Kohut's universal need-oriented, self-object configurations. Based on infant studies (see Stern, 1985) indicating the infants clear ability to differentiate the mother from others by way of sight, sound, and smell, Sullivan may have overemphasized the role of language in the development of differentiating personifications. Even so, Sullivan's observations on the role of language in developing increasing differentiation of the sense of otherness are still cogent.

## Covert Processes: Sullivan's "Unconscious"

Sullivan believed that, when the child met with *parental insanity*, the child was faced with excessive complexity in experience. This complexity arose from parental attributions about the child which were grossly out of line with what expectations were reasonable for the child to meet and what needs the child could reasonably forgo, In essence, the child was landed with the difficulty of having to respond to parental prohibition and anxiety, while continuing to have the needs that motivated the child initially. In Sullivan's words, "the tension of anxiety acts in direct vector opposition to needs" (1953: 176). While the child's capacity for foresight and recall were developing at a rapid pace, the child still lacked both an extensive cognitive capacity to reason through such conflict and the sufficient autonomous interpersonal security to make decisions in opposition to parental anxiety and forbidding. For Sullivan, this situation led to the development of *covert processes* in interpersonal relations. Commenting on the problems of positing a nebulous, non-verifiable internal process such as Freud's concept of the unconscious, Sullivan stated that covert processes could be observed by examining the phenomenon of *delayed behavior*. Delayed or interrupted behavior indicated to Sullivan that late infant or child engaged in symbolic operations which sought to meet needs outside overt interpersonal relations toward a more direct satisfaction of needs. For example, while the child never explored certain forbidden body areas in the presence of parents, one could observe the child engaging in the forbidden behavior in private, interrupting the behavior when the parent appeared, and later continuing the behavior when the parent left.

Sullivan believed these operations were covert from self and parental others, if, as was likely, the child was unaware of these shifts and delays in behavior. Because covert processes were essentially private, once established they were not easily changed by later parental education. Additionally, since covert processes were involved to a considerable degree with the avoidance of anxiety, they were part of the self-system and were represented in *bad-me* personifications. As the child grew older and learned increasingly through social experience that certain interpersonal situations were forbidden, the child's covert processes would be themselves accompanied with anxiety and could become excluded from the child's referential processes and repertoire of behavior. These covert processes eventually lead to the later development of the more complex dynamisms of *security operations* and *sublimation*. When important needs of the child were excessively prohibited, that is, accompanied with severe punishment or excessive parental anxiety, such that adequate security operations and sublimations could not be developed, then the experience of these needs would become dissociated as part of the *not-me* personification.

Sullivan's concepts of overt and covert processes in interpersonal relations invite comparison to Freud's concept of the unconscious. In many ways, Sullivan appeared to describe a similar set of ideas to Freud's (1900, 1915b) concept of the unconscious, its relation to the collision of the primary drives' (the id) with constraints of social reality (the superego), and the elaboration of compromise formations (the ego) (Freud, 1923a). On closer inspection, Sullivan's concept of covert processes and Freud's unconscious have critical differences. Freud's concept included both the "mental contents" of an inferred intrapsychic structure called the *unconscious* and the processes by which aspects of experience became unconscious. As Greenberg and Mitchell (1983) stated, the presence of internalized reality within the unconscious representing the interpersonal component of these processes was of little importance to Freud; instead he believed that the contents of the unconscious were unconscious phantasies of "hallucinated" need satisfactions. As previously stated, Sullivan was seriously opposed to the idea of the unconscious as a "place" in the mind with knowable contents. He also warned that reified, inferential explanatory concepts, which could not be objectively demonstrated, could be very misleading and that unconscious processes were essentially unknowable in a direct sense. At best, covert processes could only be roughly inferred by observing later delayed or substituted behavior, which indicated that something had gone on in the mind of the child or adult that was outside of his or her awareness. Additionally, for Sullivan, social reality was the critical factor in the causation of these covert mental processes. Even though self and other personifications and the resulting security operations operated outside current interpersonal reality like Freud's unconscious phantasies, the motivations underlying these operations were oriented toward meeting social needs, the maintenance of interpersonal security, as opposed to Freud's conception of drive-based gratification of libidinal needs. As Sullivan (1950b: 302) stated, "everything that can be found in the human mind has been put there by interpersonal relations, excepting only the capabilities to receive and elaborate the relevant experiences. This statement is intended to be the antithesis of any doctrine of human instincts."

## Security Operations, Sublimation, and Regression

As mentioned above, the developmental epoch of childhood occasioned a distinct shift in parent-child relations toward increased socialization, requiring that the child restricted personal needs in order to adapt to the demands of adult world. Sullivan paid special attention to the effects of this change, as well as the effects of language, on the development of the personification of the self and others, the representational component of interpersonal cooperation. Under the pressure of socialization by the parents and other adults, the child learned to forgo immediate felt needs in order to avoid social disapproval and the activations of bad-me personifications. Because the child's need for interpersonal attachment remained so powerful, the avoidance of the experience of anxiety which signaled the impending withdrawal of tenderness from the parent continued to be an enormously powerful motivation. This central fact of early interpersonal life led Sullivan (1953: 190) to formulate the *theorem of escape*, "the self-system from its nature-its communal environmental factors, organization, and functional activity-tends to escape influence by experience which is incongruous with its current organization and functional activity." Once established, self-system operations were difficult to modify, even if the child was forced to relinquish important needs to maintain good-me personification. Therefore, the power of anxiety and its inner experienced component, the self personification of bad-me, led the child to adapt to social expectation of the parents, even in the unfortunate circumstances where the cost to the child was the distortion of the experience of inner need.

As Sullivan stated, *security operations* were psychological and behavioral maneuvers organized primarily to reduce anxiety by escaping the insecurity of experiencing the self as bad-me. The childhood era, with its increased opportunity for frustration arising from socialization, was a time of accelerated development of the self-system. Cognitively, the avoidant operation of the self-system derived from a primitively prehended sense of danger to attachment, consisting largely of felt, empathic attunement to forbidding gestures, disapproval, and other gradients of anxiety. These more primitive cognitive operations conflicted with the development of a more advanced comprehension of interpersonal situations, occasioned from the rapid expansion of the capacity for recall and foresight. In situations where learning by anxiety predominated, the child could never fully grasp the interpersonal situation, i.e., whether or not the child's needs were reasonable or the parental disapproval and anxiety was unreasonable. Because of this more primitive quality of learning by anxiety, aspects of the self-system may not be readily open to later educative influences, as later education is hampered by the imperfect observation and definite inventions which comprised the self-system. One such common invention of the self-system was what Sullivan called "an extravagant, superior formulation of the self" (1940/1953: 121), an observation quite similar to Kohut's (1971, 1977) much later formulation of the grandiose self.

As Safran and Segal (1990) have pointed out, the concept of security operations is similar to the psychoanalytic concept of defense mechanisms (see A. Freud, 1936), but with two important differences. First, Sullivan's orientation in the concept of security operations was distinctly interpersonal, as opposed to the intrapsychic formulation of defense mechanisms in Freudian theory. Security operations are learned through experience of anxiety, reflecting Sullivan's belief in the innate tendency toward interpersonal relatedness, while Freud's defense mechanisms arise from the innate struggle between libido and superego, revealing his belief in the opposition of the individual and society. Secondly, Sullivan's concept of security operations eschews reified, hypothetical constructs like the id and the ego, emphasizing observable interpersonal processes, particularly the process of selective inattention. Numerous research reviews (Dixon, 1981; Erdelyi, 1990, 1985; Shevrin & Dickman, 1980; Singer, 1990) lent considerable empirical support for the role of selective inattention in what has usually been called by Freudian thinkers as the defense of denial. While the concept of selective inattention has lost much of its popularity in recent years, studies of dissociation (see Putnam, 2016) in terms of psychopathology and neurocognitive explanations of attentional process (e.g., Driver, 2001) reveal the importance of this psychological concept.

The operation of the self-system can be illustrated by the phobic preoccupation found in obsessive-compulsive rituals of childhood such as "you step on a crack; you break your mother's back." Children who carefully sidestep cracks gain comfort by avoiding being the bad child who is angry at his or her mother or wishes her harm, i.e., avoiding a bad-me experience of self. In fact, children who do not step on cracks are very good children, superior in all ways to their careless mates. While naturally the ritual has nothing to do with harming or not harming mother or having superior goodness, the tendency of the self-system to endure over time can be seen by the sense of taboo found during much later periods in life. Too many areas of bad-me personifications and too much of the child's behavior involved in security operations inhibits free learning and open mastery necessary for healthy development of the personality. As Wilfred Bion (1976), a great believer of the importance of learning by experience, said, "True learning is quite difficult, because in learning something we know we have to admit to ourselves that, in some manner or another, what we knew previously about this subject is wrong. And people hate to be wrong."

Sullivan believed that *parental sanity* during this period of development provided the child with an important platform for later healthy interpersonal development. As illustrated in the earlier discussion of the supportive research of Coopersmith and Baumrind, Sullivan stated that the child who could successfully meet reasonable parental expectations for socialization, yet have his or her own needs acknowledged and supported, explored, and learned about the world with a sense of confidence, resulting in high self-esteem. The alternation between encouragement the child's exploration on one hand and caretaker support and security on the other in healthy development of attachment is captured well in the Circle of Security Attachment Model (Marvin et al., 2002). Kohut's (1971) ideas about the process of transmuting internalization appear to this author to be a restatement of Sullivan's ideas about the impact of parental sanity on the development of the self, albeit in far more turgid language.

Where this kind of healthy interpersonal cooperation did not exist, Sullivan (1953: 200) maintained that the child would develop a sense of "disgust" with his or her needs and "a still further elaboration of the part of experience of being disgusted in what is called the emotion of *shame*." In addition, when the child's needs were in continual conflict with parental expectation, the child would experience considerable confusion and increasing doubt about his needs, when they opposed the "superior reality" of parental expectation. Should this pattern of doubt become exacerbated, the child could develop a sense of shame about his or her needs. It is interesting to note that Erikson's (1950) psychosocial theory described the second task of development as the period of autonomy versus shame and doubt for the same period Sullivan called the childhood era. The role of shame has been extensively explored as a powerful mechanism in psychopathology and an essential aspect of treatment (Nathanson, 2014). This dynamism is especially difficult within families since early life experiences of parental shame can be transmitted intergenerationally to their children (DeYoung, 2015).

Sullivan next addressed the process by which the children resolved situations where their needs conflicted with parental socialization. As the child became older, primitive covert operations could work no longer as a primary mode of resolving this conflict. The child's growing cognitive capacity for foresight and recall, enhanced by the development of language, contributed to emerging self-awareness (especially good-me and bad-me). With increased recall, even need-driven, delayed behavior became tinged with anxiety, requiring a new security operation to meet the demands of prohibited needs. Sullivan (1953: 193) postulated a new dynamism, central to childhood, which he called **sublimation**, "the unwitting substitution, for a behavior pattern which encounters anxiety or collides with the self-system, of a socially more appropriate activity pattern which satisfies part of the motivational system that caused trouble." Because socialization of the child requires the restriction of immediate personal needs, processes that allow for partial satisfaction of needs without the excessive anxiety were particularly important in childhood. Sullivan emphasized that, to be successful, the dynamism of sublimation must be unwitting. A consequence of learning to live in an "essentially irrational culture," the child developed an automatic ability, outside of awareness, "of giving up immediate, direct, and complete satisfaction of a need and of utilizing some partially satisfying, socially approved pattern" (1953: 196). Interestingly, Sullivan stressed that, for sublimation to work well, "symbol processes occurring in sleep (to) take care of the rest of the unsatisfied need" (1953: 193) were important. Clearly, Sullivan's concept of sublimation was a reworking Freud's (1923a) ideas about compromise formation in dreams and behavior, a concept which escaped the problems of instinct theory and emphasized the interrelationship between interpersonal experience and inner life.

Following his discussion of sublimation, Sullivan described what he believed to happen in the unfortunate circumstances where the child's dynamism of sublimation was insufficient to meet even partial satisfaction and where excessive anxiety arising from intense parental disapproval or malevolence could not be avoided. He called this situation the **disintegration of behavioral patterns**, in which "the whole of living is rather disorganized" (1953: 196), which was closely related to the child's experience of not-me personification in infancy. In place of more complex and mature behavior patterns, the child undergoes **regression**, during which earlier and less well-organized patterns of behavior re-emerge. Sullivan emphasized that regression was neither a mysterious nor uncommon process, nor was it a sign of severe psychopathology. He believed that regression was likely experienced daily during childhood. Because the interpersonal and emotional pressures, socialization was particularly intense during childhood. More complex behaviors were not well established and could give way rather easily to earlier, less mature patterns. Sullivan believed that regression could be found during all later developmental stages, especially under the influence of fatigue and interpersonal complexity, without it being especially psychopathological. Naturally, repeated and frequent disintegrations of behavioral patterns and regressions at any developmental stage revealed difficult interpersonal situations which further indicated and reinforced problematic self-system dynamisms.

## Language and Communication

As alluded to above, Sullivan believed that the child's growing capacity for language was a major instrument of socialization and was the other major influence on the developing personality. As Sullivan (1953: 189) stated, "great energy (is) devoted by the more mature people around the very young child to equip him with this most important of human tools, language." This parental education effectively began a shift in the child's primary mode of interpersonal learning from empathic control to consensually validated language, which in turn occasioned the shift from the *parataxic* mode to the *syntaxic* mode of experience. Sullivan focused his thinking about language on the process of interpersonal communication, which included both speech and gesture. As the child used language to consensually validate his or her inner experience with the experience of others, he or she moved beyond prehension to *comprehension of interpersonal situations*. Beginning in childhood, Sullivan (1953: 187) believed that symbolic behavior, "activity influenced by the organization into signs of previous experience in terms of satisfaction, or ... avoiding or minimizing anxiety," became the almost exclusive human mental activity. The child made use increasingly of symbols to comprehend meanings and anticipate patterns of interpersonal cooperation between the self and others, leading to a conscious integration of mental and interpersonal life. Learning language by example and imitation and by reward and indifference differentiated early prototaxic (private and unsocialized) experience to parataxic, associational linguistic activity into the social realm of mutually validated syntaxic experience. As mentioned in the beginning of this section on childhood, Sullivan thought that learning of language was responsible for the fusion of personifications, leading to a more differentiated sense of the transactional patterns between self and other.

Additionally, Sullivan discussed how language was used by the child to deal with certain requirements of socialization placed on him or her by parents. He noted especially the impact of fear on the child's verbal behavior, specifically fear of parental punishment by the infliction of pain, and the child's attitude toward his or her relationship with the parental stronger authority. In a culture that used infliction of pain as a socialization tool, a practice which Sullivan believed irrational, the child soon discovered the high value placed on obedience in the definition of the good-me. Yet, the child also found that the impulse to act on some prohibited needs was too strong to avoid the pain of parental punishment and attendant parental anxiety, even though this punishment could be readily foreseen. As sublimation could not occur in these instances, the child's growing capacity for foresight allowed the child to make discriminations of situations of parental authority. Under these circumstances, Sullivan suggested that the child developed capacity to conceal thoughts and actions in order deceive authority, i.e., act in ways to prevent parental punishment and anxiety. The necessity to conceal and deceive was closely tied to the child's learning, what Sullivan referred to as, the *magical use of language*. Many a child learned that lying about a transgression or uttering verbalisms such as saying sorry could forestall punishment or at least diminish the degree of punishment.

While highly useful in the immediate situation, frequent lying could become ultimately an ineffective pattern of social cooperation. Another linguistic technique to avoid punishment was what Sullivan defined as a *verbalism*, "a plausible series of words ... regardless of its actual, remarkable irrelevancy, which has the power to spare one anxiety or punishment" (1953: 208), which he used roughly parallel to the psychoanalytic concept of rationalization. The other problematic pattern that served the need to conceal was what Sullivan called *"as if performances"*. With "as if" performances, the child acted like or sounded like adults as a way of concealing other behavior (dramatizations) or pretending to do something to evoke tenderness (personae). These sub-personifications were similar to Winnicott's (1960) concept of the development of the *false self*, which both Sullivan and Winnicott saw as injurious to a confident and healthy sense of self. In particular, Sullivan saw "as if" performance as the underlying root of preoccupations used to mentally and behaviorally ward off perceived punishment and anxiety that later developed into obsessional states.

Sullivan's detailed analysis of concealment and deceit was especially interesting in light of his own criminal behavior at Cornell and of his early tendency toward deception about his professional background discussed in Chapter 2. Sullivan apparently developed a deep understanding about the dynamics and consequences of deception and concealment based on reflections of his own behavior. He was fortunate indeed to have come under the compassionate influence of William Alanson White. As noted earlier, White was himself an enlightened thinker about the relationship between mental illness and criminal behavior, although one wonders, whether White knew in some way about Sullivan's early problems at Cornell and deception in representing his professional background and, if so, what role this knowledge played in White's later lack of support for Sullivan. Whatever may be the case, Sullivan did transform his early adult history of considerable deception and concealment into considerable professional integrity and an unfortunately ruthless and disparaging attitude toward self-deception in other psychiatrists.

## Anger, Resentment, and Malevolent Transformation

Sullivan concluded his chapters on the childhood epoch with a discussion about the operation of anger in the interpersonal world of the child. He rejected outright psychoanalytic ideas about a primary aggressive drive and innate sadism, but instead chose to emphasize the social function of anger and its mutation, under unfortunate circumstances, into the patterns of resentment and malevolent transformation. In essence, Sullivan saw these phenomena as patterns of learned behavior, with the latter two patterns resulting from irrational cultural assumptions about the value of the use of pain in punishment in child rearing. As mentioned in Chapter 4, Sullivan observed that rage was behavior found first in early infancy, arising from the failure to bring forth adequate interpersonal cooperation in the presence of significant physical and security needs. In childhood, anger, the felt component of rage behavior, was experienced when the child encountered the pain of punishment and parental disapproval and anxiety. The child soon came to see the special usefulness of behavioral expressions of anger as modified forms of rage behavior in interpersonal situations, such as temper tantrums. On the other hand, many children would find that their expressions of anger would evoke considerable punishment from parents as well. The powerful influence of parental anger in enforcing interpersonal cooperation was undeniable to the child and through imitation came to be utilized by the child as well. Sullivan saw behavioral expressions of anger beginning in childhood as a primary way of discharging the tension of anxiety due to conflicts with parents. Frederickson (2014) expanded this understanding of the function of anger as a discharge of anxiety rather than a genuine expression of feeling. Sullivan further stated, that, if parental authority was especially repressive toward the child's anger, the child learned that his or her anger would only serve to aggravate his or her situation with parents. The child learned to conceal his or her expression of anger, which in turn was felt as *resentment*. Often, the child would meet with parental punishment and anxiety about any displays of resentment, causing the child to conceal his or her resentment as well. Eventually, even the child's experience resentment became covert, which Sullivan postulated could led to psychosomatic disorders, especially disorders of digestion.

The consequences of an extreme example of parents' repressive use of authority were what Sullivan termed *malevolent transformation*. Sullivan tackled the knotty problem of parental cruelty and aggressiveness in childhood and viciousness in later life with characteristic insight. As noted in his discussion of malevolence in the mothering one, Sullivan looked unflinchingly at the effects of parental cruelty. He reasoned that, when the child of cruel, malevolent parents experienced and expressed his or her need for tenderness, the child received anxiety or pain back from the parent. Malevolent (and certainly highly insecure) parents took advantage of their position of superior authority to ridicule, ignore, lie to, and hurt the child. Initially the child felt anxious, laughed at, and ashamed. The child would soon come to anticipate that his or her need for tenderness will bring anxiety and pain. Eventually, as security operations acted to reduce this extreme distress, the child perceived his or her need for tenderness as a weakness and helplessness that could be preyed upon by the multitude of potential enemies who populated his or her interpersonal world and inner personifications. In turn, the child would treat those around him or her who showed benevolence with contempt and those who wanted tenderness as prey to be used and exploited. The childhood or juvenile bully is an excellent example of malevolent transformation. Naturally, the malevolent individual was soon mistrusted by those around him or her, leading the malevolent individual to develop more sophisticated ways of exploitation which seem initially innocent, but were ploys for his or her manipulative designs. For Sullivan, if established, the malevolent transformation became the core organization of the self-system and was extremely resistant to change, because it served critical protective function for extremely brittle self-esteem and it operated to isolate the individual from others to the greatest degree possible.

Dodge's (Dodge, 1986; Dodge et al., 1986; Dodge & Frame, 1982; Richard & Dodge, 1982) research on hostile attribution biases in aggressive boys provided support for Sullivan's ideas about the effects of the kinds of personifications found in malevolent transformation. As Mullahy (1970) pointed out, Sullivan thought that the development of malevolent transformation was the greatest disaster that could occur in childhood in large part because of its resistance to treatment. Sullivan's concept is similar to Kernberg's (1976) concept of malignant narcissism which he saw as the root of serious antisocial behavior and as untreatable. Contemporary conceptualization and research on psychopathy and antisocial behavior by Robert Hare (Hare, 1993; Hare & Neumann, 2008) captures well the interpersonal nature of Sullivan's concept of malevolent transformation, including traits such as conning and manipulative relationships with others, callous disregard for others, lack of empathy, shallow emotions, pathological lying, egocentrism, irresponsibility, and promiscuity. Much like Sullivan and Kernberg predicted, research has found that individuals with primary psychopathy are quite largely resistant to treatment in terms of reducing their criminal and violent behaviors, clearly the most important outcomes from a societal perspective (Harris & Rice, 2006; Ogloff & Wood, 2010).

In conclusion, Sullivan believed that the person's ability to meet important needs, balanced with the capacity to delay, refine, or forgo immediate satisfaction to adapt to the reasonable demands of others, while using language to bridge the gap between self and other, set down a cornerstone in childhood for later cooperative social living and healthy personality development. The children's ability and good fortune in navigating this first epoch of intense socialization laid the groundwork for them to confidently enter the new and vastly more complex interpersonal world of the school, with new adult and especially peer relations. Unfortunately, other patterns such "as if" performances, resentment, and malevolent transformation could have long term, debilitating consequences on social development. Child development research cited by Seligman (1995a) on the development of the optimistic personality has strongly confirmed Sullivan's ideas that delay of gratification (see also Mischel, 1974; Mischel & Patterson, 1976; Patterson & Mischel, 1976; Tobin & Graziano, 2010) and social adaptability are critical for later adult mental health. With the interpersonal foundation of either confidence and autonomy, insecurity and self-doubt, or frank malevolence, the child now enters the Juvenile Era, which unlike Freud's concept of latency, was for Sullivan a most active period of human development.

## The Juvenile Era

One of Sullivan's most novel and valuable contributions to psychodynamic theory was his formulation of the *Juvenile Era*, "the years between entrance to and the time when one actually finds a chum-the first landmark which ends the juvenile era, if it ever does end" (1953: 227). The juvenile era through preadolescence roughly coincided with the period of Freud's (1905) psychosexual stages of development which he called latency. Sullivan made it eminently clear that the juvenile era was anything but latent ...

> the importance of the juvenile era can scarcely be exaggerated, since it is the actual time of becoming social ... This is the first developmental stage in which the limitations and peculiarities of the home as a socializing influence begin to be open to change. (E)verything that has gone on before becomes reasonably open to influence; this is true even in the organization of the self-system
>
> (1953: 226–227)

Sullivan believed that the juvenile world introduced a vastly broader scope of socializing influences than those found in the childhood era. These new social influences not only provided the juvenile with an opportunity to evaluate the sanity of his or her parents' expectations, through comparisons with teachers and other juveniles' parents, but more importantly opened the juvenile to world of peer relationships. As will be shown, child development research has demonstrated the accuracy of Sullivan's theory about this developmental epoch.

Before turning to Sullivan's ideas about the juvenile era, it is important at this juncture to discuss Sullivan's response to the central dynamic of Freud's psychosexual theory, the Oedipus complex (Freud, 1905, 1910b, 1912a, 1918, 1940) and, its female equivalent, the Electra complex (Freud, 1925, 1933), which occurred within Freud's theory during Sullivan's transitional phase between childhood and the juvenile era. In *Conceptions of Modern Psychiatry*, Sullivan specifically noted his familiarity with Freud's (1905) *Three Contributions to a Theory of Sexuality* and the concept of the Oedipus complex, but made little mention of it in *The Interpersonal Theory of Psychiatry*. In both his paper published in 1926 and in a chapter on female psychology in *Personal Psychopathology* written in collaboration with Clara Thompson, Sullivan quite specifically rejected Freud's notion of the Electra complex (see also Thompson's (1943) influential paper on penis envy from the interpersonal perspective). He only alluded to his discontent with the idea of a universal, archetypal Oedipus complex without directly challenging Freud. Instead, Sullivan focused his thoughts about the relationship between sexuality and mental illness on what he termed the deleterious effects of the archaic Western cultural norms on the healthy acceptance of sexuality (1929), which, as will be discussed later in Chapter 6, formed a basis for his thoughts about the dilemma of early adolescence.

Mullahy (1970) stated that Sullivan very much rejected Freud's idea of natural sexual longings of the child toward the parent without directly criticizing Freud. In a position similar to Ferenczi (1933), Sullivan reasoned that love (*philos*) and tenderness was different from lust (*eros*) and that the boy's (and girl's) desire for tender, emotional ties to the mother should not be confused with lustful urgings. Additionally, instead of seeing the mother as the child's first seducer (Freud, 1940), Sullivan believed that the child was someone to be loved, but not lusted, by the parents. Sullivan explained the seeming tension between same-sex parent-child dyads came from a feeling of familiarity with the same-sex child, leading the parent to be more comfortable in making socialization demands on the same-sex child and more indulgent of the less familiar, opposite-sex child. The conflict between the same-sex parent and child dyad arose from these additional authority issues occurring between them. Sullivan believed that this pattern of authority relationship was what happened in general, suggesting that other kinds of patterns could be present as well as other determinants of the pattern such as peer relationships. Sullivan believed that it was a mistake to assume common patterns of social and cultural interaction as universal ones. Additionally, he thought it was a misunderstanding to assume that, when certain men compared the wives (unfavorably) to their mothers, these men lustfully desired their mothers. Instead, Sullivan reasoned that these men were likely caught up in long-standing patterns of dependency and suggestibility with their mothers. As Youniss and Smollar (1985) have suggested, the Freudian notion that reawakened Oedipal wishes in adolescence determined authority relationships was conceptually difficult to square with the child social development research. This research supported Sullivan's more complex, interpersonally based notions of adult and peer authority relationships found in the juvenile era and preadolescence.

Instead of Oedipal issues being of dominant importance during the period of time before latency, Sullivan's concern about the transition from childhood into the juvenile era involved problematic interpersonal patterns that could impede the necessary socialization during the next developmental epoch. Problematic interpersonal patterns established in childhood such as "as if" performances, resentment, and malevolent transformations could contribute to an *arrest of development*, which for Sullivan was a slowing of the acquisition of social skills necessary for the next epoch's much more complex interpersonal demands. In addition, idiosyncratic family patterns, acceptable in childhood, where for example the parents attended to the child's every whim, be it day or night, interfered with the task of learning to share in peer relations and could lead to the new juvenile's exclusion from the group. Sullivan paid special attention to the dilemma of what he called the *lonely child*. The child with few playmates and limited opportunities to experience the world outside the family entered the juvenile era socially underdeveloped. The lonely child by necessity constructed a rich phantasy life in compensation for his or her lack of social interaction. By the end of childhood, there was a growing social necessity for the child to distinguish between the inner phantasy world and socially agreed upon reality. While more socially active children gradually learned the distinction between phantasy and consensual validated "reality" through social interchange, the lonely child's rich phantasy life, which had not been subject to consensual validation, could easily become the object of misunderstanding and ridicule by peers in the juvenile era. For Sullivan, his dilemma led the lonely child to a tentativeness with peers that even further contributed to a partial arrest in development.

Sullivan stated that childhood in Western civilization ended for almost everyone with the abrupt introduction of the child to school. The school became a new major instrument of socialization and offered an unparalleled opportunity to correct problematic patterns of interpersonal cooperation established in childhood. Behavior tolerated or encouraged by the family was now unacceptable in the juvenile world of new authority figures and peers, creating inner tension about, and new motivations to modify, existing interpersonal patterns, personifications, and self-system dynamisms. For Sullivan, the *juvenile era* was the first period of development where the maturing person became really social. Imbedded in Sullivan's notion that inappropriate aspects of the personality likely underwent important modification during the juvenile era was the idea of the relative plasticity of interpersonal behavior and experience. While Sullivan conceptions about the conservative nature of self-system and security operations modified his position, his thoughts about social adaptability and growth was more in keeping with Kagan's (1984) findings that patterns of socialization were very often more predictive of child development than the impact of arrest at supposedly age-specific developmental periods, as Freud believed.

Sullivan postulated two major conditions contributing to change during the juvenile era, the first of which what he called the *correction of parental educational patterns by comparison*. Instead of the childhood world largely organized around parental authority, the juvenile world was populated by a much wider variety of adult authorities. Sullivan believed that this social reality led to one of the most important developmental influences, an expansion of the experience of *social subordination*. In childhood, parental or family authority was absolute, unquestioned, and open to relatively little influence from other authority. New authorities in the juvenile era, especially teachers, exerted considerable influence on the juvenile and offered experiences of social subordination to authority quite different than found with the parents. Teachers introduced juveniles to new, intelligible structures and routines to the organization of their learning and work, with significant limits over the kind of authority they can impose. The authority relationship between teacher and juvenile was markedly less personal than between the parents and the juvenile. Teachers could offer the juvenile new opportunities to increase his or her self-confidence and self-esteem, often mitigating against impoverished or destructive family influences.

Of course, the teacher introduced new influence in the juvenile's life, the broader society beyond the family. As Mullahy (1970: 389) stated, "a teacher who likes to teach and who likes her pupils will help many unhappy youngsters learn that there is something better in life than what they have seen or lived through at home." Of course, Sullivan recognized the ability of an insensitive or cruel teacher to contribute to unfortunate family influences or to introduce a new source of anxiety into the juvenile's life. Sullivan also pointed out that teachers could provide socializing influences such as prejudice and stereotyping on the basis of race, religion, and gender which were deleterious to the juvenile's growing sense of self. This introduction to a range authority figures, including the parents of his peers, allowed juveniles to compare and contrast their parents' behavior with others, leading to increased differentiation in patterns of social subordination. Juveniles figured out that their parents were not god-like figures, that different authorities varied in their estimable and troublesome features, and, in more fortunate cases, that some parents or other authorities could have a special feeling for the juveniles' special attributes and abilities. Sullivan approached this situation of learning about the variations of good and bad in others, including parents, in a way vastly more clear, complex, and understandable than complicated notions of Klein's concept of the depressive position and Kohut's concept of transmuting internalizations.

Sullivan postulated that the other major of social contribution to change during the juvenile era was the advent of *peer relationships*. The experience of social subordination (which also included the observation of how other peers related to authority figures) was essentially asymmetrical regarding the juvenile's and the adults' contributions to interaction, with greater restrictions on the juvenile's participation and far greater weight given to the authority of the adult. While juvenile-adult authority relationships underwent considerable change during the juvenile era, they were still asymmetrical, subordinate-superior in nature. In fact, family relations based on social subordination remained a fact of life throughout a person's development. For Sullivan, the juvenile's need for his parents, so central in earlier phases of development, was complemented during the juvenile era with what he called the need for *compeers*, otherwise known as *peer relations*. This change coincided with a critical shift in role of playmates from the more egocentric patterns of play in childhood to more cooperative pattern of interaction in the juvenile era.

An entirely new and exceedingly important pattern of relationship emerged with peer relationships, which Sullivan termed the experience of *social accommodation*. In addition to the kind of unilateral, top-down authority the juvenile experiences with adults, peer relations offered the juvenile the opportunity and requirement to interact with peers with direct or symmetrical reciprocity (Rubin et al., 2013; Youniss, 1980). Because peer relationships were not limited by unilateral authority, peers could seek out other peers who were willing to interact in similar ways. Peers were much less constrained in the nature of their interactions. Unlike with parents and other adults, the juvenile peer could respond to aggression from another peer with aggression or can revert to the older pattern of social subordination, but later withdraw from the relationship. Juveniles learned that satisfaction of the social need for compeers required the juvenile to modify more egocentric patterns and take into consideration the needs of the other. Social accommodation between peers required each other to learn how many slight differences existed in life regarding what others thought was correct and acceptable and to make adjustments accordingly.

Through the give-and-take of concession, while maintaining their own positions, peers in the juvenile era learned the critical social process of *cooperation*, through which juveniles develop patterns of friendship and *compromise*. Additionally, Sullivan noted that the juvenile quickly learned the social importance of **competition** and the social rewards brought by being the best student, the best athlete, the best practical jokester, or a member of the winning team. The social judgment of the juvenile by his peers was a significant concern during juvenile era, a process which Sullivan called *establishing a reputation*. By comparison and contrast within juvenile society, based on the judgment of peer leaders and members of various in-groups, the juvenile found the various advantages and disadvantages of being superior, average, or poor in a given arena of activity. Sullivan believed, particularly in Western society, that the overemphasis on the value of competition led to unfortunate consequences for those juveniles who were poor in competitive areas that were in fashion, such as sports, or superior in areas that were out of fashion, such as academics. Without the balancing processes of cooperation and compromise, the person could over-rely on competitive strategies and become "chronic juvenile," one who saw everything in life centered around getting ahead of the next fellow. Adding to the interpersonal cooperation patterns of infancy based on empathy and tenderness of the parent toward the child and of childhood based on the social compliance and theorem of reciprocal emotion, Sullivan now included critical peer interpersonal cooperation patterns based on friend-ship, competition, and compromise in the juvenile era. The success of learning these new juvenile era patterns became factors critical to the new elaborations on self-esteem and a feeling or self-worth.

Sullivan noted several other social patterns, which had debilitating effects on development of social competence and healthy self-esteem, occurring throughout much of social existence, but which were especially found in the juvenile peer culture. As part of the processes of competition and compromise in the juvenile era, juveniles continually made social comparisons and con-trasts between the self and one's peers. Because juveniles placed much sig-nificance on the social judgments of peers in forming their sense of self, Sullivan believed that the social processes of *ostracism* and *stereotyping* could have a devastating impact on necessary interpersonal development during the juvenile era. Sullivan stated that, whenever there are large groups of juveniles, some juveniles would suffer from social **ostracism**, the experience of being outside of valued peer groups (in-groups) and being devalued by in-group peers because of it. While out-group peers hopefully found their way to other out-group peer groups, taking some of the potency away from being excluded by desired in-groups, even being a member of such a group carried with it the experience of inferiority with respect to other peers, handicapping the development of positive self-regard. If the out-group peer, whom Sullivan often called the lonely ones, was unable to find any group, he or she suffered intense experiences of inferiority, which led to the need for extreme ela-borations of the self-system in order to maintain a fragile sense of good-me. Frieda Fromm-Reichmann (1959) and Edith Weigert (1960), close colleagues of Sullivan at Chestnut Lodge and the Washington School of Psychiatry, expanded on Sullivan's ideas about the extraordinarily disorganizing power of loneliness in personality development and everyday experience.

In addition, the juvenile era was a particularly critical time for another aspect of ostracism, the experience of *stereotyping*, i.e., attribution of inferred differences based on a variety of factors such as gender, race, religion, social status, occupational group, mental and physical handicaps, and the like. Sullivan, who wrote earlier wrote important articles on racism (Sullivan, 1938a; 1940, 1941) and anti-Semitism (1938a), believed that these crude classifications of people impeded the rational development of personifications and were of significant source of difficulty for both the holder and recipient of the stereotype in later life. Sullivan also mentioned the often-related process of *disparagement*, security operation which lowered anxiety arising from low self-regard by noting how unworthy everyone else was. The juvenile got temporary relief from his feelings of unworthiness by using disparagement, but paid a high cost for this relief by alienating himself from others and by learning less from them. If this pattern survived much beyond the juvenile era, where it was a relatively common aspect of juvenile society, Sullivan believed that disparagement could be socially crippling. While Sullivan focused on the role of parents in the learning of disparagement, the concept could be easily linked to peer influences as well. Sullivan's concept of disparagement was similar to the psychoanalytic concept of devaluation, which played such a critical role in the later theories of Kohut on narcissistic defense and of Kernberg on splitting in borderline and narcissistic personality. While Kohut and Kernberg regarded devaluation as a primitive defense arising from disturbance in early object relations, Sullivan saw disparagement as an all too common and unfortunate pattern of interpersonal relationship arising in the juvenile era as a result of a cultural overemphasis on the value of competition.

In addition to the impact of new interpersonal patterns in the juvenile era, Sullivan commented on important cognitive changes, which reflected changes in the development of the self-system and personifications. Sullivan noted that the juvenile's world underwent a geometric leap in the level of social complexity and the juvenile was bombarded with increased social expectations and requirements. As such, occasioned by the increasing shift from the parataxic to the syntaxic mode of experience, juveniles began to use their increased capacity to *control focal awareness* to exclude patterns of interpersonal cooperation required during and appropriate to childhood. As a result, much of what went on in childhood was "forgotten." A concept mentioned in his discussion of the beginnings of the self-system during infancy, Sullivan called this operation *selective inattention*, the process of shifting awareness away from anxiety-laden interpersonal situations as if they did not exist. As noted by Erdelyi (1990), Sullivan's concept of selective inattention in the juvenile era has a double-edged meaning that it encompasses both positive and negative aspects of the control of focal awareness. On the positive side, selective inattention allowed the juvenile to forget patterns which no longer mattered, freeing his or her awareness to work on the new, complex social world. On the negative side, when selective inattention worked to ignore or exclude important aspects of experience from focal awareness because of anxiety and insecurity, the juvenile was cut off from directing himself to important needs. If too many aspects of unmet needs overloaded processes of sublimation, they manifested into peer relationships and authority relationships in a troublesome manner, especially because they lay outside focal awareness and conscious self-control. For example, a juvenile overloaded with selectively inattended anger towards his parents unwittingly may be defiant towards teachers or aggressive with peers. Failing to attend to the social cues which serve as a warning sign about the unfortunate interpersonal consequences of these angry behaviors could lead the juvenile to be rejected by others. As Singer (1990) has noted Sullivan's concept of selective inattention was conceptually similar to Freud's (1915a, 1923a) defense of repression. Singer regarded Sullivan's concept to be more specific and transactionally focused than Freud's, which had advantages in describing its relationship to character formation.

Another cognitive operation of the self-system which Sullivan saw developing during the juvenile era was what he called *supervisory patterns*. Supervisory patterns were "illusory 2 group patterns," which were the cognitive representations of the juvenile's anticipated or imagined disapproval or rejection from peers and others in reaction to the juvenile's words and actions. *Supervisory patterns* served to focus awareness on the experience of anticipated social disapproval by means of an internal dialogue in which the juvenile as a result could control his or her behavior to avoid the disapproval by "listening" to the criticism of imagined others. As will be discussed further in the next chapter, in more extreme examples of the use of this pattern, Sullivan believed that sub-personalities could emerge in which the juvenile experienced the imaginary others as a real voice who was always with the juvenile. In the pattern Sullivan called the *"hearer,"* the juvenile judged the relevancy, i.e., social acceptability, of what he or she said regarding how the juvenile believed others would hear himself or herself. Sullivan's other supervisory pattern, the *"spectator,"* paid attention to what one shows to others. As mentioned in Chapter 1, Sullivan discussed a third pattern called the *"reader,"* revealing his intensely critical, self-condemning inner voice which made writing all but impossible for him in his later years. Sullivan's concept of supervisory patterns is remarkably similar to the automatic negative thoughts and overly critical self-judging process in the concept of dysfunctional schemas that Aaron Beck and other cognitive therapists (Beck et al., 1979; Beck & Emory, 1985; Beck & Freeman, 1990) have implicated in the causation and treatment of depression, anxiety, and personality disorders.

By the end of the juvenile era, Sullivan postulated that the developing person constructed a concept of an *orientation in living*, defined as a generic, recurrent set of patterns or tendencies of interpersonal relations that were manifest in most spheres of life. Sullivan took the position that the child did not have an orientation to living in the larger world beyond the family. Instead, he believed that the extensive social experiences of the juvenile, with the complex of relationships with parents, peers, and adult authorities beyond the family, were required to establish an orientation to living. Sullivan described someone as *adequately oriented* if they developed a good grasp generally of their own needs and motives; insight into how to adequately meet these needs, while avoiding undue anxiety; the capacity to set medium and long-range goals, foregoing momentary impulsive satisfaction; and the ability to enhance the opportunity for prestige. *Inadequately oriented* individuals failed to have the organizing tendencies such that important needs went unmet, the person engaged in security operations at the cost of increasing competency and learning, found delay of gratification difficult, and had a sense of self marked by low self-esteem and inadequate sources of social acclamation. Singer (1990) stated that Sullivan was a pioneer in the study of character formation, whose emphasis on characteristic patterns of recurrent experiences and situations presaged the psychoanalytic work of Shapiro (1965, 1981) as well as modern concepts of personality disorder (see Millon & Everly, 1985). For Sullivan, the concept of an *orientation to living* represented his thinking on the formation of character, noting clearly and explicitly that much important personality growth occurred after age of ten. Sullivan's emphasis on post-childhood development put him at sharp variance with almost all psychoanalytic thinkers, with the exception of Erikson (1950, 1959) who himself may have borrowed liberally from Sullivan's writings.

# Chapter 6

# Developmental Epochs of Adolescence

## The Long Transition to Adulthood

With characteristic complexity and clarity, Sullivan's writings on adolescence paved the way for modern psychoanalytic and psychological understanding of this critical period of development. Previously, the vast majority of psychoanalytic thinking about adolescence focused on Freud's genital period with its dependence on concepts of the oedipal complex, castration anxiety, and penis envy. Perhaps the best-known psychoanalytic work on adolescence by Blos (1962) viewed the development of character during this period as a result of resolving oedipal conflicts. By moving beyond a Freudian intrapsychic perspective to an interpersonal model, Sullivan's work stands as a transformative contribution to understanding of adolescence. While credit is often given to Erikson's (1950, 1959) psychosocial model displacing Freud's theory, there is evidence to indicate that Erikson richly borrowed from Sullivan's earlier ideas, though perhaps without sufficient credit. Sullivan divides what is usually considered as adolescence into three successive epochs of development – *preadolescence, early adolescence,* and *later adolescence.*

## Preadolescence

Sullivan next turned to the description of an epoch of development, which was a distinctive and unique contribution to psychodynamic/psychoanalytic theory. He called this next epoch of development *preadolescence*, which was distinguished by a significant transformation in peer relationships and interpersonal relatedness. Preadolescence began with the appearance of a different kind of peer relationship than with playmates in the juvenile era. This interest was a new, more specific relationship to a particular member of the same sex who becomes a *chum* or a close friend. For Sullivan, the coming of the *chumship* relationship represented the first step in the maturation of interpersonal relations in which the other person's (in this case, the chum's) needs were keenly felt as relatively as important as one's own. Sullivan believed that there was a critical difference in the nature of peer relationships in the juvenile era from those experienced in preadolescence. For Sullivan, juveniles were often insensitive to the importance of other people.

DOI: 10.4324/9781003305712-8

Relationships in preadolescence did not have the "how do I get what I want from this other person" focus found in juvenile peer relationships, but instead involved a mutual understanding, acceptance, and desire to satisfy each others' needs for connection and security. He stated that the juvenile entered preadolescence no earlier than eight and a half years of age and usually later.

Sullivan proposed that this shift occurred because of the appearance of the *need for interpersonal intimacy*, which he defined as "the type of situation involving two people which permits validation of all components of personal worth" (1953: 246). Sullivan was very specific in distinguishing interpersonal intimacy from what he called lust. He stated that "interpersonal intimacy can really consist of a great many things without genital contact" (1953: 246). Quite unlike other psychoanalytic theories, love was not first felt toward a member of the opposite sex; in fact, the attainment of (later) heterosexual love was severely hampered without the experience of chumship. Sullivan speculated that failure to find a same-sex chum during preadolescence might be a contributor to the development of what he called a homosexual way of life, although he saw this process far too complex to ascribe it a single determinant. While Sullivan did not specifically state why the need for interpersonal intimacy arose at this time in development, he stated rather that interpersonal intimacy was the next step in the inexorable movement toward the highest form of interpersonal connectedness, which he called love. Underlying Sullivan's conception of the need for interpersonal intimacy was the idea that the humans were primarily oriented toward interpersonal connection.

Next, Sullivan described the social processes involved in the preadolescent shift to intimacy. He defined the concept of *collaboration* as a preadolescent pattern of interpersonal cooperation as distinct from the juvenile era patterns of competition, compromise, and cooperation. Unlike the more impersonal or self-centered juvenile social operations, collaboration involved making sure each other's satisfaction and security were met and taking satisfaction in the success of each other as part of the maintenance of prestige, status, and freedom from anxiety. The social structure of preadolescent society consisted primarily of two-groups of chums that interlocked with other two-groups to form the preadolescent gang. From these interlocking two-groups vital to developing interpersonal intimacy and security, some one or two of members of the gang arose as the most highly admired group members, who became the leaders of the group. The essential difference between teams and other groups found in the juvenile era and preadolescent gangs, referring specifically to boys, involved meeting the growing need for intimacy through collaboration. Sullivan strongly disagreed that preadolescent gangs were fundamentally antisocial (see Golding's, 1962 *Lord of the Flies* as an example of this assumption), emphasizing that truly antisocial gangs were focused on group leaders and were organized around the competitive, disparaging, and egocentric assumptions, with a malevolent twist, of juvenile groups. In such antisocial groups, peer leadership enforced group loyalty as protection from social insecurity and from low self-esteem.

Just as new possibilities for significant modifications to the self-system occurred with increased freedom from the influence of the family during the juvenile era, the development of interpersonal intimacy with a chum during preadolescence provided new freedoms from a self-image based on juvenile self-personifications derived from the ability to compete and membership in an in-group. Because of closeness found in chumship, preadolescents were now able to see themselves through the eyes of a valued other. Sullivan (1953: 247) stated, "remarkably fantastic ideas about oneself" based for example on juvenile group ostracism or personification of parents are "subject to influence through new experience ... at each of the developmental thresholds." Sullivan vehemently disagreed with the Freudian "all-too-prevalent idea that things are pretty well fixed in the Jesuitical first seven years" (1953: 248), especially as it pertained to preadolescence.

The need for intimacy became a powerful driving force to establish a relationship with another. Sullivan believed that the fact that one significant person was all who was needed to form this new pattern of interpersonal cooperation was a distinct advantage. In the context of this dyadic relationship, ineffective patterns of self-deception and deception of others in the juvenile period may be remedied through interaction with the chum, resulting profound changes in the self-system. Sullivan gave numerous examples of the kind of unfortunate patterns that could be corrected under the influence of a close relationship with a chum. Egocentricity and malevolence could be given up at least partially to establish and maintain closeness. Two ostracized juveniles could find each other, alleviate the need for socially objectionable patterns of relationship through an intimate bond of friendship, and become better accepted into the larger social group. While Sullivan was clearly not naive about the influence of destructive early patterns of interpersonal relationships and their impact on the individual's self-system, he believed that it was a disservice to the individual to fail to notice fortunate opportunities and influences throughout the course of life. Interestingly, Levinson's (1978) study of adult development revealed alternating periods of change and stabilization in life structure of his subjects similar to what Sullivan suggested in earlier development, indicating a natural, progressive tendency during men's life course to constructively reorganize social circumstance and self-concept, in contrast to reductionistic and pessimistic perspective of psychoanalysis.

Sullivan's last comments on preadolescence pertained to what he described as the *experience of loneliness*. He believed that loneliness, though difficult to describe, was a very important motivation in interpersonal development. While tributaries to the experience of loneliness could be traced to earlier parental difficulties with tenderness and respect for the child's uniqueness, as well as frustrations in the need for compeers, Sullivan believed the actual experience of loneliness was a phenomenon which came only in preadolescence and afterward. Sullivan noted that the experience of loneliness was more powerful than anxiety, in that people would search for companionship even though it caused considerable anxiety. Loneliness as an organizing concern began in the preadolescent period but became a much more intense driving force in the next epoch of development, early adolescence. While his observations on how loneliness contributed to interpersonal development and psychopathology were penetrating, he had difficulty with fully understanding phenomenon similar to his earlier formulations about anxiety, which Bowlby and Ainsworth achieved more successfully in attachment theory and the experience of separation anxiety (Bowlby, 1961).

How accurately did Sullivan observe the value of peer relationships? While his conceptualizations carried a great sense of intuitive accuracy, they were at considerable variance with Freudian psychoanalytic theory's emphasis on the overriding importance of child-parent relationships, especially mother-child or triangular relationships. Freud's idea about the central role of Oedipus complex in personality development and the psychogenesis of treatable psychopathology characterized the period between the phallic and genital stages as latency, the stage where the Oedipal struggle remained dormant. In fact, the whole concept of latency, with its mildly derisive portrayal of the latency age boy as the agreeable Boy Scout, indicated the general disregard Freud had for this period of development. As Youniss (1980) pointed out, peer relations live in the shadow of psychoanalytic theory, if at all, and do not play a significant role in personality development. In contrast, Sullivan accorded vital roles in his interpersonal theory to the *juvenile era*, "the actual time of becoming social," and *preadolescence*, the time for establishing intimacy. Relationships with peers were at the core of his thinking and were seen as essential to interpersonal (personality) development. Unlike Freud whose concept of mature love came from belief in the resolution of Oedipal striving by renouncing attachment to the opposite-sex parent, Sullivan gave considerable weight to the influence of peer relations, particularly in preadolescence, to the development of the capacity to love. While Kohut's (1971, 1977) descriptions of the change from selfobject to whole object relatedness are similar to Sullivan's concept of interpersonal intimacy during preadolescence, Kohut, like Freud, put an almost exclusive emphasis in the quality of parent-child relations as determining factors. Fairbairn's (1952) discussion of Stage 3 of object relations, the mature relational phase, emphasized the mutual giving and receiving between differentiated persons was closely akin to the Sullivan's thoughts about the successful resolution of preadolescence. On the other hand, Fairbairn's writing neither described specific operations required for this shift to occur nor considered the contributions of the two-stage evolution of peer relationships central to Sullivan's theory. Discussions about the role of peer relations in the development of mature object relations were largely absent from the writings of such major object relations theorists as Klein, Mahler, Jacobson, Winnicott, and Kernberg.

While it is beyond the scope of this book to offer a complete review of the considerable experimental literature on peer relations, research in child social development has strongly supported Sullivan's theory. In his groundbreaking, intensive study of the relative roles of parents and peers in six- to fourteen-year-old children's social development, Youniss (1980) found that the quality of parent-child relations alone during the juvenile era and later in preadolescence could not adequately describe the rich fabric of children's social behavior. His research uncovered two distinct kinds of relations, one with parents and another with peers, each with a distinct and different social structure, structures very much in line with Sullivan's observations. Additionally, Youniss discovered that, while children tend to see parental authority as all-knowing at the beginning of the juvenile era, their beliefs underwent a change by the time of adolescence, with peer influences contributing significantly more to the preadolescent's view of reality. Youniss' research revealed that, as Sullivan had hypothesized, peer relations contributed more heavily to the development of the social processes of cooperation and compromise than relations with adults, through the practice of co-construction and symmetrical reciprocity. Rubin et al. (2013) summarize the empirical research supporting Sullivan's concept of peer relations along with Youniss's and others' early research (e.g., Bigelow, 1977; Bigelow & LaGaipa, 1975; Gottman, 1983; Hartup, 1993, 1992, 1989, 1979; Selman, 1980; Shantz & Hartup, 1992; Smollar & Youniss, 1982; Youniss & Volpe, 1978).

Youniss also found that the development of intimacy grew largely from peer relationships during preadolescence in much the same fashion as Sullivan described chumship (see also the supporting research of Berndt, 1982; Buhrmester & Furman, 1987; Furman & Buhrmester, 1985; LaGaipa, 1979; Selman, 1980). Intimate peer relations have been found to be essential for healthy psychological adjustment in adolescence (Townsend et al., 1988) while impaired peer relationships were implicated in later psychopathology (Parker et al., 2006). In summary, child research studies have pointed out that, while parental relations retained an essential role in the child's social development, peer relations had a similarly important influence, while the kinds of influence of each relationship differed in the direction postulated by Sullivan.

## Early Adolescence

Sullivan's next epoch of development, *early adolescence*, arrived with "eruption of true genital interest, felt as lust" (1953: 263) and continued until the integration of the complex interpersonal and physical events of puberty became organized into socially acceptable patterns of sexual relationships. Sullivan saw *lust*, the last of the truly zonal tensions of need, as the experiential component of the genital need culminating in genital activity leading to orgasm. Like all tensions of need, lust requires interpersonal cooperation around which dynamisms of lust must develop. Much as the external social event of entrance into school abruptly shifted the child into the juvenile era, internal physical maturational changes leading to genital interest launched the preadolescent into *early adolescence*, whether ready or not. Sullivan believed that the eruption of the need for lustful satisfaction in early adolescence collided with the developing interpersonal needs for personal security (freedom from anxiety) and for interpersonal intimacy (collaboration with at least one other person leading to freedom from loneliness). Additionally, as part of the change from preadolescence to early adolescence and undoubtedly due in part to the advent of lust, Sullivan noted a shift in the need for intimacy. He described this event as the shifting from the isophilic (same sex intimacy) to the heterophilic (opposite sex intimacy) relationships or from seeking someone like oneself to seeking someone quite unlike oneself. As Buhrmester and Furman's (1987) research confirmed, this change in focus was really an additional interest and attraction, since isophilic relationships continued to play an important role in early adolescence. Awakening curiosity about a member of the opposite sex heralded changes in the early adolescent's covert processes which filled the new adolescent's mind with feelings of longing and desire.

Sullivan formulated that this most biologically natural change in interest collided with powerful cultural influences, which made a smooth developmental transition into early adolescence difficult. Early adolescents discovered that their interest in the opposite sex met with a wide variety of group and cultural prohibitions. The role of sexual repression in society (see Coleman (1988) and Henriques (1959) on moralistic and naturalistic sexual cultures) became a significant concern for Sullivan in many ways. While one of the important problems of adolescence is how to avoid procreation, the societal strictures about birth out of wedlock were clearly communicated through use of the term *derision* to describe the situation and the legal status, i.e., illegitimacy, accorded a person born into this situation. Additionally, the early adolescent was confronted with a confusing double standard for men and women concerning the expression of lust. With these conflicts, a new kind of social awkwardness entered relationships with others. Discussions of whom one likes and does not like became a new part of relationships with chums and the objects of one's interest were open to public scrutiny by, and potential ridicule from, the gang. The early adolescents' self-esteem was closely associated with their choice of love/lust interest. To complicate matters further, there was often a significant difference in timing for boys and girls in coming to puberty, leading to, in the earliest stages of this period, to a mismatch in experience.

In early adolescence, this complex interplay of biological, psychological, and social forces brought upon what Sullivan eloquently described as the ***collision between the needs for lust, security, and intimacy***, the three major and equally powerful dynamisms of integration and disintegration of interpersonal situations. Sullivan quipped, in an indirect criticism of Freudian theory, that, if one overlooked loneliness, one might think lust was the most powerful human dynamism. Beginning in preadolescence and increasing in importance in adolescence, Sullivan accorded the need for intimacy and the avoidance of loneliness the central, though by no means exclusive, motivational role in his interpersonal theory. Also, given his emphasis on the importance of the self-system throughout his writings, Sullivan believed that the arrival of lust clashed with interpersonal security and freedom from anxiety. For Sullivan, adolescence was a particularly turbulent period of development because of the enormous interpersonal complexity involved in the integration of these three highly important human motivations. Before detailing the important dimensions of the lust dynamism, he systematically highlighted some of the complications in integrating lust, security, and intimacy.

Sullivan believed that self-esteem and personal worth came under tremendous stress as the early adolescent tried to find means to satisfy the dynamism of lust, leading to the *collision between lust and security dynamisms.* Societal prohibitions represented in parental attitudes about sexuality, group reputation with one's peers about display of sexuality and choice of love/lust interest, and anxiety about this particular zone of interaction were formidable threats to the maintenance of self-esteem. In highly repressive families, the adolescent's autoerotic discharge was invariably accompanied with various guarding operations to prevent parental discovery or suspicion. Sullivan was clearly ahead of his time in his discussion about masturbation, that highly disapproved of, but very common, act which peaked in adolescence. He saw masturbation as quite valuable in preventing lust from becoming too great, while the more difficult process of establishing heterophilic or other intimacy took place. For Sullivan, the unfortunate severe societal prohibition against masturbation, and adolescent shame and anxiety accompanying it, was the cause of much unfortunate human misery. He also noted that the failure to resolve severe primary genital phobia from early in life, which was organized with the prototaxically organized, not-me personification, was especially psychologically dangerous to the early adolescent. The appearance of lust collided with the overwhelming anxiety of barely understood earlier prohibition and erupted in a severe disturbance during personality, usually frank psychosis or dissociative phenomena.

Additionally, Sullivan recognized that the shift in the early adolescent's intimacy from isophilic to the heterophilic relationships could collide with need for security. The early adolescent's interest in forming companionships with members of the opposite sex could sometimes evoke strong repressive influences from parents, who confused early adolescent's interest in intimacy with interest in genital sexuality. If the parents disapproved of the early adolescent's heterophilic interests, the early adolescent was faced with the dilemma of retreating from his or her new interest in intimacy with a member of the opposite sex, which led to loneliness and resentment, or defying parents, which resulted in severe anxiety and lower self-esteem within the family. Sullivan believed that, if the parental disapproval was charged with jealousy and ridicule triggering significant guarding operations, the early adolescent could enter a profound state marked by anxiety, confusion, and suspicion in relation to his or her parent, which in severe instances led to paranoid states.

Sullivan also gave special attention to the *collision between lust and intimacy* during early adolescence. He noted that establishing intimacy with a member of the opposite sex was often accompanied by the variety of kinds of awkwardness, including embarrassment, diffidence, and excessive precautions. Overt and covert measures to conceal lustful feelings from others, and sometimes unfortunately oneself, accompanied the desire to overcome loneliness. Additionally, some early adolescents used what he called the *not* technique, a reversal of diffidence into a bold (and interpersonally insensitive) approach to meeting the need for lust, thereby underemphasizing motivations toward intimacy. What Sullivan called the segregation of object persons, the creation of distinctions between persons toward whom one did or did not discharge his lust, provided additional evidence for this collision of lust and intimacy. This distinction was particularly applied to women who, in Sullivan's opinion, faced the dilemma of either being a good girl, with whom one could establish Platonic intimacy, or 'the bad girl' or 'whore,' with whom one satisfies lust. Sullivan thought that such a culturally determined division or separation of lust from intimacy fabricated self-esteem difficulties for female early adolescents, who literally were forced to split off lust and intimacy motivations. The lack of natural integration of lust and heterophyllic intimacy could also lead to "homosexual" play between chums (lust and isophyllic intimacy) or a primary autoerotic orientation in the earliest stages of adolescence. Sullivan believed far too much was made of casual "homosexual" play between chums or autoerotic behavior in the earliest stages of adolescence and that the need for lust combined with the need for intimacy and the need for security (finding a societally appropriate mate) usually led to correction of these earlier warps. He became concerned when these alternative operations became longtime patterns, which then made it especially difficult for the adolescent to break down societal barriers to intimacy and reach out to an intimate heterosexual partner.

Sullivan accorded importance to the role of fortune and misfortune when the early adolescent began heterosexual experimentation. Sullivan (1953: 271) stated, "The number of wretched experiences connected with adolescents' first heterosexual attempts were legion and the experiences are sometimes very expensive to further maturation." Because society was sexually repressive, much anxiety attended heterosexual experimentation, leading to numerous and various kinds of initial sexual failure, such as erectile insufficiency or premature ejaculation in young adolescent males or vaginismus and anorgasmia in young adolescent women. Such difficulties with sexual performance could be devastating to the young adolescent's self-esteem, leading to ideas that he lacked virility or she lacked responsiveness. Feelings of guilt, shame, aversion, and revulsion for one or both partners could be attached to heterosexual experimentation and severe preoccupation with one's sexual identity could ensue. Sullivan parenthetically mentioned that alcohol was undoubtedly useful as an anti-anxiety agent and a convenient excuse for difficulties, but could also lead to an overreliance on it as a way to deal with difficulty. In the most severe instances, a marked manifestation of the separation of lust from intimacy, which he called dissociation, could appear.

Sullivan discussed two other ways to cope with the anxiety about sexual performance that emerged in early adolescence. First, the adolescent could withdraw from attempts to meet both lust and intimacy through social isolation. The isolated adolescent used reverie (daydreams, phantasies, and dreams) as a substitution for actual interpersonal experience. While such methods could be initially useful, the isolated adolescent could eventually retreat permanently into the safety of this method of need discharge. Changes could occur in the reverie process which created highly idealized, imaginary companions which posed a severe barrier to meeting others. This process made it difficult to break down obstacles in reaching out to real and imperfect intimate others, leading to what Sullivan called the schizoid problem. Secondly, if the lust dynamism appeared before the adolescent achieved isophyllic intimacy, the chronic juvenile pattern led to a need to be envied and competitive, non-intimate stance regarding lust manifested as being, in the juvenile male adolescent, a Don Juan or "ladies' man" or, in the juvenile female adolescent, a "teaser."

After first describing associated interpersonal dilemmas with it, Sullivan next defined the *lust dynamism* as a psychobiological integrating apparatus which he called "the last and most conspicuous and illuminating of all the dynamisms" (1953: 281). At the biological level, he saw lust as a complex physiological process involving the autocoid or endocrine system (physiochemical), autonomic nervous system (physical arousal), and the central nervous system (interpretation of meaning and signs), involving zones of interaction including tactile erogenous zones and genital-visceral erogenous zones, which would become integrated into the full range of activity leading to the sex act. Sullivan revealed his detailed knowledge of the phases of intercourse (well before Masters & Johnson's, 1966 research on the stages of sexual arousal) which he called the effector apparatus. He also discussed the importance of the eductor apparatus, his term for the cognitive aspect of sexual performance such as knowing the goals of lust motivation, including faciliatory, precautionary, and inhibitory knowing.

At the interpersonal level, Sullivan viewed the *lust dynamism* as a pattern of overt and covert symbolic events in different modes of experience and as a system of integrating tendencies of security, intimacy, and lust. Sullivan's definition of the integrating tendencies of the lust dynamism involved a highly complex and detailed formulation of its operations. The lust dynamism required psychological maturation through earlier stages of development, modified by experiences of satisfaction and anxiety and, in unfortunate circumstances, of disintegrative change or dissociation. Each individual's particular anxiety about, and responses to, lust varied widely (i.e., it did not fall into an archetypical pattern such as the Oedipus complex) and was influenced by both family and peer manifestations of cultural inadequacies. These culturally induced anxieties created a situation where the cognitive operations of misinterpretation, concealment, selective inattention, and dissociation of the experience of lust were ubiquitous, which led to distortions in living and disturbance of self-esteem. Sullivan believed that excessive anxiety and resulting experiential distortions were particularly handicapping, that the integrating tendencies were channeled at best into partial satisfactions, and that these satisfactions were experienced as overwhelmingly important. In such patterns of partial satisfaction, the person would have residual motivation which would be discharged in anxiety-tinged dreams and waking phantasies, which undermined self-esteem and led to elaborate self-system operations or social distancing. The greater the need for self-system operations around lust in early adolescence, the lesser the opportunity for the person to make changes which could correct the warp in his or her personality, which the integrative aspects of the lust dynamism could provide.

Having emphasized the self-system (interpersonal security) aspects of his definition of the lust dynamism, Sullivan next described the types of *integrating tendencies for intimacy and lust,* which made up the rich array of sexual relationships and behaviors found in society. Sullivan believed that loneliness and excessive lust were powerfully unpleasant experiences in adolescence. In terms of intimacy, the need for friendship and acceptance in preadolescence was redefined into the need for a loving relationship with a member of the opposite sex by late adolescence or else other patterns of lust and intimacy would have to be found. Sullivan classified the integrating tendencies patterns of intimacy set down in early adolescence as autophilic (self or narcissistic love), isophilic (love of a person of the same gender), or heterophilic (love of a person of the opposite gender). He next classified lust by the preferred partner as autoerotic (masturbatory), isoerotic (lustful expression with a member of the same gender), heteroerotic (lustful expression with a member of the opposite gender), or katasexual (lustful expression beyond a living member of the human species, e.g., bestiality or necrophilia). He lastly referred to six varieties of genital participation or substitution, including orthogenital (genital participation with the genitals of a person of the opposite gender), paragenital (genital participation as if seeking genitals of the opposite gender, with no possibility of procreation, e.g. passive role in fellatio, cunnilingus, or manual masturbation; active role in pederasty), metagenital (no genital participation oneself, only genital participation of the other), amphigenital (such as *soixante-neuf*), mutual masturbation, and onanism (solitary masturbation). Sullivan classifications gave him an extensive set of possible integrations of the lust dynamism (Sullivan noted 45 possible and six highly unlikely patterns) from which to explore what interpersonal experiences lead to this particular organization of the lust dynamic.

Sullivan ended his discussion of the epoch of early adolescence with a strong admonition to his fellow psychiatrists not to attend simply to a person's sexual behavior, but to see sexual behavior in its interpersonal context. As Sullivan (1953: 295) stated, "lust cannot be eliminated from personality any more than hunger can ... but to think that one can remedy personality warp by tinkering with the sex life is a mistake." He believed that the way to understand the dilemma of early adolescence was to focus on the extraordinary collision of the main motivators of human experience – security, intimacy, and lust. For Sullivan, interpersonal dilemmas were primary and the failure to find an appropriate solution to the dilemma of early adolescence led to grave problems in living. These problems led to failure to attain an integration of these basic needs that led to a positive self-identity, an important step toward accomplishing a mature capacity for love.

### Homosexual Way of Life

Throughout the chapter on early adolescence in the *Interpersonal Theory of Personality*, Sullivan addressed a particular aspect of the integrating tendencies of the lust, which he called *the dilemma of homosexuality*. Sullivan's views on homosexuality were exceptionally lucid and compassionate, even by today's standards. In his unpublished book *Personal Psychopathology* written in the 1930s (eventually published in 1972), he rejected the idea that homosexuality was inborn. Instead, throughout his writings and lectures he took the position that what was called commonly called homosexuality was not a single concept, but a poorly defined and complex set of integrating tendencies, which came from a variety of different needs.

Sullivan's classifications of possible integrations of the lust dynamism gave him a rich diagnostic tool to understand more deeply the tapestry of sexual orientation in general and what is broadly called homosexuality in specific. For Sullivan, the most serious problem about homosexuality was that it met with overwhelming social ostracism. He compassionately elucidated what he called *abhorrent cravings* (often involving images of iso-erotic practices) and the person's high degree of anxiety when his urges were societally defined as repulsive. When he explored with his patients the nature of their cravings, Sullivan helped them find out where the experience came from in their lives as well the real and symbolic meaning of the phantasies. Sullivan believed that the cause of much of what was called homosexuality developed earlier in life, leading to failure to change the preadolescent direction of the need for intimacy.

For Sullivan, the greatest problem associated with homosexuality was not the behavior itself, but the low self-esteem, the need to conceal the experience, the interpersonal isolation, and the intense loneliness resulting from the security operations they needed to use to avoid severe societal disapproval or even violent repression. In a statement startlingly ahead of his time, Sullivan asserted a **homosexual way of life** was not a hopelessly disordered mental condition, (i.e., a sexual perversion), but could be a relatively secure way of living, if same sex emotional intimacy was also involved. His position was markedly different from Freud's (1905) view of homosexuality as a psycho-pathological condition brought about by narcissistic regression from the Oedipal situation. Perhaps even more remarkable, Sullivan published his opinions about homosexuality when it was criminalized by the prevailing homosexual sodomy laws in most places in the U.S. (Eskridge, 2008) and pervasively vilified by religious groups (Hamblin & Gross, 2014). Further, in his role as the psychiatric consultant to the Selective Service System during World War II, Sullivan actively tried to abolish homosexuality as a dis-qualifier from military service. Unfortunately, his proposal was rejected by the Director General Lewis Hershey and he was eventually fired (Bérubé, 1990). Indeed, nearly 100 years ago, Sullivan proposed more open and ac-cepting attitudes toward Lesbian, Gay, Bisexual and Transgendered (LGBT) individuals in a social context far more repressive than today's standards and his thinking remains surprisingly modern. As stated in the first chapter, it is likely that one reason Sullivan's ideas were dismissed, forgotten and disavowed was his clear-eyed and courageous stance about homosexuality.

Since Sullivan's time, much has been learned about homosexuality, espe-cially the groundbreaking and at times controversial work of John Money (1986, 1988, 2012). Money's extensive research on the biopsychosocial complexity of sexuality led to important modern concepts such as gender identity, gender role, gender-identity/role and lovemap. *Gender identity* refers to the extent to which a person experiences oneself to be like others of one gender. Whether people view themselves as being male or female or gender neutral largely determines their self-identity and provides a significant foundation for their interactions with others. Perhaps most importantly, Money introduced the term *sexual orientation* in place of *sexual preference*, arguing that attraction is generally not a matter of free choice or preference. What Money called the *lovemap* was the interpersonal and sexual patterning for the individual that can be relatively enduring throughout the lifespan. He also promoted the diagnostic term *paraphilia* as a more accurate and useful diagnostic label that was eventually adopted in the DSM III (American Psychiatric Association, 1980), replacing the term perversion which reflected the prevailing societal moral ostracism.

It is important to note that Money's (1988) genetic research findings predominately refuted Sullivan's belief that homosexuality was not biologically determined. On the other hand, for example, Hunter's (1990) research found that a high number of men with childhood sexual abuse histories later led homosexual lifestyles. While this may lend some support to Sullivan's assertion of a psychosocial causation of homosexuality, the question of genetic and psychosocial pathways remains complex and raises difficult questions that are unanswered today. However, Sullivan and later Money's pioneering work has helped remove the social stigma and moralistic denunciation of LGBT ways of life. They opened the door to a deeper, more complex, and science-based understanding of human sexuality as well as provided excellent concepts to examine sexuality beyond simplified labels of heterosexual and homosexual.

A relatively recent addition to Sullivan's legacy as a psychiatric pioneer of an open attitude toward human sexuality in general and homosexuality specifically has been the literature on "the gay Harry Stack Sullivan" (Blechner, 2005). Most notably interpersonal psychoanalysts Michael Allen (1995) and Mark Blechner (2005) researched Sullivan's personal sexual background, while historian Naoko Wake (2006, 2008, 2019) explored the impact of his sexual orientation on his clinical work and theory. Allen and Blechner found evidence that Sullivan likely adopted a homosexual way of living, which they believed was given short shrift in Perry's (1982) biography and appeared to be a source of embarrassment among many of early Sullivan's followers. Blechner in particular notes the relationship between Sullivan and his adopted son Jimmie as an example of both a well-integrated loving relationship and a daring example of using adoption as a way for Sullivan to legally protect Jimmie's rights of survivorship. Interestingly, both authors omitted evidence from Perry that Sullivan also had sexual relationships with women. More importantly, Allen and Blechner believed that Sullivan's homosexuality was central in his formulation of interpersonal theory. While Allen and Blechner suggested a likely aversion among Sullivan's followers about Sullivan's homosexuality, Perry (1982) clearly acknowledged his sexual relationships with men, but also with women. In retrospectively re-fashioning the "gay Sullivan," these authors leave out part of the complex story of this remarkably complex man and the possible role of bisexuality in his theory. In his work on bisexuality, Eliason (2000: 139) speaks about 'bi-negativity' ...

> "the reduction of sexual identity to an either/or, "us versus them" framework helped lesbians and gay men to organize politically and socially, based on the belief that they were a cohesive minority group, the assumption of sexual sameness ignored important differences of race, class, age, religion, and other aspects of identity. It also contributed to a number of bi-negative attitudes, including the notion that bisexuality doesn't really exist."

Careful reading of Sullivan's writings about the complexity of sexual identity and behavior beginning in early adolescence demonstrates an interest in the complexity of analysis similar to Eliason's.

In her research and extensive writings, historian Naoko Wake further explored the significance Sullivan's therapeutic treatment of patients as a "gay psychiatrist" and "the intellectual and institutional paradigm in psychiatry that influenced his practice and its limited confrontation with the social stigmatization of homosexuality" (Wake, 2006: 325). Based on her review of old clinical files from Sheppard Pratt made available to her, Wake argued that Sullivan's well-noted successes with who were called schizophrenic patients at that time was largely determined by the selection of young male homosexual patients to be treated by a compassionate homosexual psychiatrist and male homosexual ward aids. Wake (2008: 188) further stated, "he kept his compelling practice hidden, not bringing it into open discussion to confront the definition of homosexuality as 'sickness.'"

Though it is beyond the scope of this introductory book to provide a comprehensive analysis, I will share some of my thoughts about the "gay" Sullivan literature, especially my critique of Wake (Evans, 2011). In particular, Wake's main conclusions are oddly ahistorical on the one hand and factually incorrect on the other. Frankness and openness about homosexuality in the U.S. and United Kingdom is a relatively recent historical and societal advancement, perhaps beginning in 1969 with the Stonewall Riots in New York City. The punitive social stigma attached to admission of homosexuality also can be seen in the forced chemical castration and later suicide of the great Alan Turing, a father of modern computer science (Hodges, 2014). Previously, and for years after Sullivan's life, homosexual behavior between consenting adults was a criminal act in the U.S. (Eskridge, 2008), laws from which the U.S. Supreme Court did not begin to provide relief until the 1960s and 1970s (Weinmeyer, 2014). Even so, same sex sodomy laws continued in numerous states and were not ruled unconstitutional until the 2003 U.S. Supreme Court decision *Lawrence v. Texas*. Wake's view that Sullivan publicly exhibited a "limited confrontation with the social stigmatization of homosexuality" is not carefully or compassionately contextualized in the history of his time. Further, her claim is further weakened by Sullivan's work in the Selective Service System referred to earlier, where he did publicly confront this stigma against homosexuals in the military. Further, his writings on homosexuality quite specifically addressed the trauma of stigmatization for homosexual individuals.

Additionally, it is abundantly clear that Sullivan's published writings were not a limited confrontation of the stigmatization of homosexuality, especially for the time when he wrote and presented. Sullivan was quite openly affirmed that homosexuality should not be considered a mental disorder and stated, "to talk about homosexuality's being a problem really means about as much as to talk about humanity's being a problem" (Sullivan, 1953: 294).

Sullivan's statements were unique and revolutionary, opening the door for the careful reader to view homosexuality and relationships with the rich complexity they deserve. In fact, Sullivan persuasively attempted to move beyond overly simple labels.

> I would like you to realize, if you realize nothing else, how fatuous it is to toss out the adjectives "heterosexual," "homosexual," or "narcissistic" to classify a person as to his sexual and friendly integrations with others. Such classifications are not anywhere near defined enough for intelligent thought; they are much too gross to do anything except mislead both the observer and the victim.
>
> (Sullivan, 1953: 294)

A good example of this problem in using simplified classification is found in Wake's (2006) analysis of records of patients treated by Sullivan at Sheppard Pratt Hospital. She noted that Sullivan spoke openly and acceptingly with patients who struggled with homosexual thoughts and he encouraged the introduction of physical contact between male patients and Sullivan's specially trained male ward aides such as hugging, touching, and kissing. Wake reasoned that Sullivan's openness about discussing homosexual thoughts arose from his own personal experience as a gay man and that encouraging physical contact between male patients and male ward aides was similarly motivated.

Unfortunately, Wake's analysis either was not informed by Sullivan's own writings about the reasons for his ward structure, or, having read them, she failed to understand and incorporate them in her analysis. As summarized in the first edition of this book (Evans, 1996), Sullivan carefully selected and trained ward aides to work with ward patients on how to model appropriately warm and supportive interpersonal behavior to alter earlier severely problematic problems in living. Sullivan chose not to use hospital nurses because their gender and authoritarian training could be oppressive to young schizophrenic men whose difficulties existed in large part because of severe problems with early mothering and overwhelming anxiety about lust. Sullivan greatly focused on training and supervising his carefully selected male attendants to understand and respect the patients' anxieties and to create a private, warm, and accepting group for the patients. Specifically, by integrating touch into the treatment of lonely, isolated troubled men at Sheppard Pratt, Sullivan defied the cultural and psychoanalytic taboo against touching, especially same-sex touching. Whereas Wake thought Sullivan used touch because of his experience as a gay man, she missed the point. He integrated touch within an attachment-based treatment consistent with his interpersonal theory of psychotherapy by strengthening interpersonal security through reassuring physical gestures and ultimately enhancing a sense of intimacy between persons. Further, it is not far-fetched to imagine that such taboo breaking may have engendered considerable apprehension in some staff at Sheppard Pratt, giving rise to anxiety-driven conjecture about homosexual impropriety on Sullivan's ward. A re-analysis of Sullivan's Sheppard Pratt records might shed light on alternative hypotheses. Unfortunately, Wake (personal communication 2022) confirmed that the valuable clinical records at Sheppard Pratt on which she based her research are gone, reportedly shredded because of space issues.

## Late Adolescence and Adult Maturity

In his last epoch of development, Sullivan attempted to formulate what lay beyond the resolution of the complexities of early adolescence. Sullivan's conception of *late adolescence* began, not with a biological or societally induced change, but the achievement of an interpersonal capacity, which he called "preferred genital activity" (1953: 297). Once the late adolescent completed the difficult task of forming a relatively clear sexual identity, he or she was free to work on "the establishment of a fully human or mature repertory of interpersonal relations, as permitted by available opportunity, personal or cultural" (1953: 297). He believed that many of us failed to achieve our potential inherent in being fully human, which resulted in an arrest of development marked by a late adolescent and in an adult life of inner conflict, boredom, and ongoing turmoil and conflict in work, family, and intimate relationships. Sullivan commented that the opportunity to move beyond late adolescence could be dictated by events beyond the control of the individual, such one's socioeconomic status and other real-life restrictions, or may have to do with longstanding personal problems which came from warps in development. He noted an explosion of growth of experience in the syntaxic mode during late adolescence, which created situations to better able to understand oneself and others, which in turn could provide very useful corrections in problems in living. Sullivan described how new autonomy available during late adolescence, found in high school, new work circumstances, and especially college education, could offer expanded opportunities to broaden the late adolescent's awareness of other people's attitudes toward living, of the degree of interdependence in living, and of different ways of handling interpersonal problems.

From Sullivan's perspective, the major interpersonal barrier to benefiting from such new opportunities naturally came from inadequate and inappropriate elaborations of the self-system created by unfortunate early developmental experience. All too often people arrived in late adolescence with a derogatory view of themselves in some or many areas of their life. Such individuals viewed themselves as inferior, inadequate, or not capable or deserving of intimacy and love. In contrast, for Sullivan, mature individuals were self-confident, assertive without being aggressive, good judges of others, and able to establish intimacy and easy communication. The interpersonal consequence of inadequate self personifications was that others found it difficult to establish satisfying relationships with the inadequate late adolescent, thus confirming the inadequate individual's worst fears. Sullivan also believed that "self-respect is necessary for the adequate respect of others" (1953: 308). Conversely individuals with an inadequate sense of self were likely to distort and misrepresent the thoughts, feelings, and motivations of others. Inappropriate representations of others found in the use of stereotyping and disparagement were at the core expressions of low self-esteem. Overcoming these patterns was critical for the late adolescent to develop into a mature adult, literally coming to grips with anxiety and its impact on one's self-regard rather than being in the grip of anxiety. If fortunate circumstances did not intervene, Sullivan believed that, short of extraordinary intervention, only psychotherapy could restore the individual to the path of mature development.

By his own admission, Sullivan was vague about what it meant to be fully human or mature. He reasoned that mature people are unlikely to come under the scrutiny or study of the psychiatrist. Sullivan hypothesized that the mature individual was compassionate, understood the limits of himself or herself and society, and was adroit at handling minor experiences of anxiety in the self and others. He emphasized the capacity to observe and handle anxiety as a corrective to previously ignored or misinterpreted experience in such a way as to make use of it. Sullivan held that life's goal was to secure collaboration with a least one other person and hopefully more. In such collaboration, mature individuals held the valued other as important as themself, enjoyed the other's successes and good fortune, and encouraged the other to widen his or her world with new interests, curiosity, and competence. For Sullivan, this mutual sharing and deepening of interests promoted feelings of vitality and vibrancy, the essential experience of being fully human. Sullivan perhaps did not live long enough, or was not developed enough himself as an adult, to develop a bigger picture on what lay beyond late adolescence. It might be said that the extension of Sullivan's thinking on adult maturity and the attainment of full human capacities can be seen later in Erikson's (1950) theory on the eight stages of man, Maslow's (1962) self-actualization theory, and Levinson's (1978, 1996) theory of adult development.

As one can sadly see from his vagueness about adult maturity, Sullivan's own limitations as a person operating in the real interpersonal world must have been most painfully clear to him. It is a testament to Harry Stack Sullivan that his honesty, humility, and extraordinary powers of observation of the human condition carried him so sublimely far with what he had. Sullivan's interpersonal theory of psychiatry, and in particular his incisive and compassionate perspective on human development, was a unique reworking of the field of psychodynamic theory. It is a great paradox that

Sullivan, a profoundly lonely and isolated man, would liberate psycho-dynamic theory from a more egocentric perspective to one which viewed persons as inextricably interrelated with the interpersonal world around them. In the next three chapters, we shall turn to the way in which Sullivan put his troubles to best use, his uncanny ability to understand deeply troubled individuals and the creative therapeutic ways in which he established understanding and intimacy with them.

# Section III

# Applications

# Chapter 7

# The Interpersonal Theory of Mental Disorder

In approaching the subject of mental disorder, I must emphasize that, in my view, persons showing mental disorder do not manifest anything specifically different in kind from what is manifested by practically all human beings.

(Sullivan, 1940/47: 3)

Historically, major advances in psychodynamic theory have been catalyzed by breakthroughs in the treatment of mental disorders thought to be untreatable by the preceding generation. While, as Stern (1985) and Brazelton and Cramer (1990) pointed out, there are problems with basing theories of normal development entirely on data from retrospective reports obtained in clinical work, clinical experience treating complex disorders has been the richest source of information for theory building within psychodynamic theory. Examples of psychodynamic treatment advances birthing new theoretical concepts are numerous: Freud's discovery of psychoanalytic theory and technique arising from his study of hysteria, Fairbairn's recasting of psychoanalytic theory from his work with schizoid phenomena, Klein and Mahler's contributions to psychoanalysis based on their work on childhood psychosis, Bowlby's discovery of attachment theory coming from his work with war orphans and adolescent delinquents, and Kohut's and Kernberg's advancements in theory deriving from their clinical work respectively with narcissistic disorders and borderline disorders. The roots of Sullivan's interpersonal theory, perhaps the most novel and significant advancement in psychodynamic theory since Freud's original work, came from a similar clinical breakthrough – his success in treating schizophrenia and paranoid states.

When Sullivan began his work as an in-patient psychiatrist, initially at St. Elizabeth's Hospital and especially at Sheppard-Pratt, there were two prevalent theories of schizophrenia and severe mental disorder, Kraepelin's (1918) descriptive psychiatry and Freud's (1911b) psychoanalytic theory. Both theorists held that psychosis was essentially untreatable, but their reasons for this belief were quite different. Kraepelin believed that schizophrenia resulted from an intractable biological and genetic abnormality, while Freud

DOI: 10.4324/9781003305712-10

believed that schizophrenics were unable to form a transference with the analyst, thereby rendering psychoanalysis impossible. At St. Elizabeth's, Sullivan was influenced by William Alanson White's compassionate perspective of the problem of mental disorder and embraced White's experimental attitude in intelligently adapting aspects of psychoanalytic theory to the treatment of psychosis. At Sheppard Pratt, Sullivan developed a highly successful approach to the in-patient treatment of schizophrenia, which dramatically challenged the prevailing thinking about the treatment of psychotic states and about the nature of mental disorder in general.

This chapter turns to Sullivan's perspectives on the problem of mental disorder, which he defined variously as *difficulties in interpersonal living* or *patterns of inadequate or inappropriate interpersonal relations*. The passage from Sullivan's developmental theory to his concept of problems in living was intentionally quite seamless, because of his belief that the psychosocial processes underlying the "normality" and "pathology" of interpersonal relationships were much more similar than otherwise. Expanding on William Alanson White's (1935) ideas about the commonalties between normal individuals, the mentally disordered, and criminals and advancing Freud's (1901) thinking behind *The Psychopathology of Everyday Life*, Sullivan elevated his concept of the *one genus hypothesis* into a unique perspective on the problem of mental disorder. Sullivan believed that those who come to the attention of the psychiatrist have problems of interpersonal living which vary from so-called 'normals,' not in the kind, but in the degree or pervasiveness, of difficulty. This extraordinarily compassionate orientation toward people struggling with painful and problematic patterns of living was an emblematic achievement for Sullivan and is a perspective that still today raises serious questions about the way mental health professionals are commonly taught to think about their work.

Sullivan established a model of mental disorder that systematically challenged barriers between what is normal or pathological, including the behavior of doctor and patient, and offered the outline of a more sophisticated model for understanding problems of interpersonal living. While aspects of Sullivan's interpersonal approach to mental disorder are found throughout all his writings, especially his edited and posthumously published lectures *Clinical Studies in Psychiatry*, *The Interpersonal Theory of Psychiatry* (Chapters 19–21), and *The Psychiatric Interview* offer the most advanced and focused statement of his ideas and serve as the primary references for this chapter. For those interested in exploring Sullivan's perspective in greater breadth and depth than can be encompassed in this chapter, the author strongly recommends reading these primary source materials. This chapter contains two major sections: first, Sullivan's critique of the models of the psychopathology found in descriptive (Kraepelinian) psychiatry and Freudian psychoanalysis; second, Sullivan's description of the primary psychological processes important to problems in living and his explanation regarding how these processes coalesced into patterns commonly referred to as clinical entities or psychiatric diagnostic categories. This latter section will begin with the role of anxiety in problems of living and will then emphasize Sullivan's thought on three major dynamisms of difficulty-the schizophrenic dynamism, the obsessional dynamism, and the paranoid dynamism.

### Sullivan's Critique of Kraepelin and Freud

One of the unique contributions of interpersonal theory was Sullivan's critique of the two dominant models of psychopathology (Kraepelin's and Freud's) and his distinctive reframing of the concept of psychopathology into problems of living. Perhaps in no other area did Sullivan more markedly differ from Kraepelin's tradition than in the area traditionally called psychopathology or mental disorder. As mentioned earlier in this book, Kraepelin's model of mental disorder is widely regarded as the oldest trend in modern psychiatry. Kraepelin saw mental disorders as fixed medical entities of biological and genetic etiology and as such the mentally ill could be clearly differentiated from normals. As Havens (1968) pointed out, Kraepelinian psychiatry focused on the careful description of symptoms grouped within a clinical syndrome and followed their course over time, while noting which factors accompanied the syndrome, such as frequency, distribution and heredity was well as its phenomenal and cognitive manifestations. The end point of this research was a clear, definable taxonomy of mental disorders like disorders of the body. As Mullahy (1970) noted, Sullivan strongly objected to the traditional categories of mental illness and saw them as a hindrance to the true understanding and treatment of "difficulties in living."

Sullivan's voiced numerous objections to the Kraepelinian model of mental disorder. First and foremost, Sullivan saw mental disorder as an expression of inadequate or inappropriate patterns of interpersonal relationships, not primarily of disordered biology and heredity. For Sullivan, these problematic patterns originated from psychosocial etiology, principally from difficulties in development due to societal and parental restrictions the child's attainment of important needs. Next, classical descriptive psychiatry tended to focus on various signs of disorder as objective indication of a disease, instead of examining the experience of the patient to ascertain what meaning it had to the patient and what particular interpersonal experiences caused and maintained the symptoms. For Sullivan, a danger with traditional psychiatric diagnosis was that the psychiatrist could fix on a particular label, assume the diagnosis to be the person, and not see variations in the patient's dynamisms of difficulty in different situations and changes over time. For example, Sullivan often noted that his experience with patients who were strikingly obsessive indicated that they were prone to schizophrenic operations under certain circumstances. A static diagnosis could lead to a failure to note the change in the particular dynamism, leading to the formulation of an inappropriate treatment approach. As an application of his one genus hypothesis, Sullivan believed that everyone from time to time could show evidence of all dynamisms of difficulty. For example, Sullivan insisted that even psychotic phenomena were present in nearly everyone, just as non-psychotic phenomena were abundantly present in schizophrenics. Similar to Sidman's (1960) critique of the problems of normative research, Sullivan concluded that Kraepelin's over-reliance on traditional medical diagnosis could readily obscure the underlying complexity of how specific psychological processes arising from an idiosyncratic developmental history led to the individual's difficulties. Wilfred Bion's (1976, personal communication) perspective on psychiatric diagnosis rather succinctly summarized Sullivan's point of view. In response to my question to him about the absence of a formal diagnosis in his case formulations, Bion replied that diagnosis told you what was obvious, which was not of much use in really understanding a person.

Additionally, Sullivan believed that traditional descriptive psychiatry's emphasis on classification of mental disorders said little or nothing about the specific way to intervene in the individual's particular difficulties or about how the psychiatrist's own processes influenced the course of treatment. When the psychiatrist (by which he meant psychotherapist) focused on observing symptoms and syndromes and determining diagnostic labels, his interpersonally "neutral" stance could readily lead the patient to feel objectified. This fundamentally unempathic position distorted the psychotherapist's relationship with the patient and was antithetical to Sullivan's notion of the participant-observer nature of all psychotherapist-patient interaction. On a more ominous note, Sullivan observed that some psychotherapists stressed the importance of certain symptoms and labels which carried greater professional prestige. As Sullivan (1956: 194) stated, "So they are inclined to fight for it, and sometimes to influence the patient insidiously in the direction that the label requires the patient to move." As confirmation of Sullivan's point, anyone closely observing a modern case conference will sadly notice the application of *au courant* diagnostic formulations about patients which may be relatively unencumbered by fact and may be part of a covert competitive process among psychotherapists. Lastly, Sullivan believed that traditional Kraepelinian diagnosis could be iatrogenic in that it came dangerously close to causing problems in living which it purported to ameliorate through the harmful social process of stereotyping (see Sarbin & Mancuso, 1980).

Drawing on Leary's (1957) and Carson's (1969) elaborations of the patterns of interpersonal reciprocity suggested by Sullivan's theory, Carson (1982) discussed the unfortunate tendency for psychotherapists to use stereotypic psychiatric labels such as borderline to personify problematic patients who stirred up feelings of inadequacy in the therapist. This stereotyping could set up a self-fulfilling prophesy in which the therapist behaves towards the patient within the stereotypic confines of the diagnostic label, evoking a reciprocal disturbed response from the patient, which in turn "confirms" the therapist's personification of the patient. While Sullivan did not reject wholesale the idea of clinical syndromes, he viewed them as frames of reference which could be a useful tool (along with knowledge of the dynamisms of difficulty, assets in interpersonal relationships, and developmental context) in formulating therapeutic intervention and possibility for change for a given intervention. For Sullivan, the objectifying stance of traditional descriptive psychiatry in the diagnosis of mental disorder failed to sufficiently include the psychotherapist in the interpersonal field of the psychotherapist-patient relationship, which could lead to unfortunate, countertherapeutic mismatches.

Much has happened in the world of psychiatry since 1996, especially the emergence of the neo-Kraepelinian (NK) direction in contemporary psychiatry focus on the medical model especially as seen in the DSM IV (APA 1994) and DSM 5 (APA 2013). Beginning with the DSM III (American Psychiatric Association 1980), the diagnostic manual aimed to free diagnosis from psychoanalytic assumptions and was designed to offer supposed atheoretical descriptive categories instead. Thus, the primary approach became untethered from a comprehensive view of what it was to be human and the troubles humans experience, a fundamentally impersonal take on the most personal part of medicine and health care. Instead, DSM IV and DSM 5 emerged to become the hallmark of modern biological psychiatry's search for the ...

> need to address the various expressions of an illness across developmental stages of an entire lifespan, and the need to address differences in mental disorder expression as conditioned by gender and cultural characteristics. The opportunity to evaluate the readiness of neuroscientific advances in pathophysiology, genetics, pharmacogenomics, structural and functional imaging, and neuropsychology was also a priority.
>
> (Regier et al., 2009: 645)

The goal of NK psychiatry has been to increase reliability in diagnosis in research and clinical practice globally, using unambiguous criteria "in the absence of etiological understanding" (Regier et al., 2009: 645). The NK ideal therefore is to categorically isolate largely biologically driven mental illnesses determined by physical dysfunction and heritability of genetic abnormality. Of course, the assumption of biological syndromes is an etiological one, so this desire to develop a non-etiological classification creates an unacknowledged bias in the assumptions of a diagnostic system like the DSM 5. As a result, nearly the entirety of the interpersonal approach to "problems of living," including the psychosocial impact of genuinely biological disorders, is absent from the thrust of modern neo-Kraepelinian psychiatry, replacing compassionate psychotherapy and sociotherapeutic institutional care with medication and other biological treatments. While certain advantages may accrue from a deeper understanding of the biological person, what is lost is dropping interpersonal focus on individuals' problems of living, including family dynamics, developmental experiences, and social and cultural influences on what is called mental disorder. Understandably, however some may wish, there is no medication to ameliorate these powerful influences. Even more problematic for NK psychiatry is the assumption that psychological disorders, even with a biological component, need not be understood from a comprehensive view of what it is like to be human.

This radical expansion of the Kraepelinian model of mental disorder in the DSM IV and especially the DSM 5 has brought forth substantial criticism even among mainstream psychiatrists. For example, renowned schizophrenia psychiatrist Nancy Andreasen (2007) expressed serious concern that the DSM does not provide a truly comprehensive description of a given disorder, and undercuts serious psychiatric research by valuing reliability of diagnosis over validity. Further, this approach overvalues short-cut checklists over comprehensive interviews and history taking and as such is reductionistic and "has had a dehumanizing impact on the practice of psychiatry" (Andreasen, 2007: 111). Allen Frances (2014), who led the American Psychiatric Association task force that produced the DSM IV, roundly criticized the DSM 5 for expanding the psychiatric categories to include many millions of people currently considered normal. He notes the vastly increased influence of the DSM in determining treatment decisions and in driving the direction of psychiatric research with a strong bias toward psychiatric medication. Further, Lekka et al's (2022) comprehensive literature review revealed that the DSM 5 increases the stigma of mental illness and contributes heavily to patients with mental disorders experiencing dehumanization.

In a more far-reaching challenge to the medicalization of psychiatry, alternative diagnostic models have arisen. Perhaps the most comprehensive approach is the *Psychodynamic diagnostic manual, 2nd Edition* (PDM-2; Lingiardi & McWilliams, 2017). Originally published in 2006 (PDM Task Force, 2006) as a collaborative effort between five psychoanalytic organizations with strong conceptual underpinnings, the PDM-2 integrates the clinical complexity of well-thought-out psychodynamic conceptualization with strong empirical and methodological validity to support it. Unlike the DSM approach, the PDM-2 diagnosis is a multiaxial model that begins with a rich, empirically supported description of its Personality Patterns and Disorders (P) axis, including the level of psychological organization ranging from normal to neurotic to borderline to psychotic. This is followed by the Profile of Mental Functioning (M) axis, an assessment of overall metal functioning including nine mental capacities – for example, capacities for relationships, self-regulation, affective experience, and self-confidence. Only after a comprehensive assessment of patients' personality and mental functions do psychological symptoms and syndromes (and their subjective experience of them) enter the assessment on the S axis. In effect the PDS-2 flips the DSM 5 on its head, emphasizing the person and their symptoms over the DSM 5's focus on symptoms alone. As Lingiardi et al. (2015: 98) stated

> The *PDM* considers each disorder as a constellation of signs, symptoms, or personality traits that constitute a unity of meaning. It attempts to capture the gestalt of human complexity while combining the precision of dimensional systems and the ease of categorical applications.

It should be noted that this approach of putting the psychological problems in context of the person's overall functioning is similar to Sullivan's approach to problems in living with the advantage of many years of quality empirical research to back it up.

Reflecting a reaction to the biological assumptions and oversimplicity of the NK DSM model, a number of other alternative diagnostic systems have emerged to capture a greater complexity of the human condition and struggles. Four such systems with strong empirical support and phenomenological appeal will be reviewed. Perhaps the closest of the DSM, the Hierarchical Taxonomy of Psychopathology (HiTOP: Kotov et al., 2017; Kotov et al., 2020) is a dimensional diagnostic approach that is based on personality trait psychology is an effort improve the organization, description, and measurement of psychopathology. It is designed to capture the whole person in terms of self-reported set of observable characteristics or traits of an organism called phenotypes. HiTOP aims to address limitations of the DSM-5 and ICD-10, such as arbitrary boundaries between psychopathology and normality, blurred boundaries between mental disorders, frequent disorder overlap and comorbidly, and diagnostic instability. Beginning with research about psychopathology rather than under-supported conceptualization, individual mental health symptoms are merged into similar components or traits and arranged into clinical syndromes. These clinical syndromes are then grouped together into overarching psychopathology continuums, such as internalizing and externalizing difficulties. This approach describes mental disorders dimensionally rather than categorically, thus reducing boundary problems and diagnostic variability. HiTOP has already developed dimensional measures capable of research and clinical applications for eleven classes of DSM disorders with the hope of eventually supplanting the DSM with a more evidence-based and clinically useful system. HiTOP is a highly collaborative research effort involving many scholars with a strong emphasis on making the system applicable to clinical problems (Ruggero et al., 2019).

Another promising alternative approach to the DSM with a strong interpersonal focus similar to Sullivan's interpersonal theory is the Power Threat Meaning Framework (PTMF: Johnstone & Boyle, 2018b), a project of the Division of Clinical Psychology of the British Psychological Society.

Their approach integrates the interplay of Power (including biological, interpersonal, social, cultural coercive; legal; economic, and ideological forces); Threat (the negative action of power may pose to the person, the group and the community leading to emotional and physical distress); Meaning (the person's particular experience of these forces): and Threat Responses the person has learned and resources they can use for emotional, physical, relational and social survival. This model does not emphasize the concept of psychopathology as in the DSM, but rather looks at coping strategies as more or less functionally adaptive based on past experience. It further focuses on the totality of the person's particular situation without favoring biological, psychological, social, or cultural factors, with an emphasis on understanding and assisting individuals rather than labeling and treating. Johnston and Boyle (2018) note many adaptations of their model with a special emphasis on treating the effects of psychological trauma. Interestingly, PTMF has many striking parallels to Sullivan's Interpersonal Theory, including the importance of the interpersonal context, the influence of development, the centrality of meaning, and the emphasis on common patterns of adaptation with a de-emphasis of psychopathology terminology, though appears to have no knowledge of him.

A third important alternative model has been directly influenced by Harry Stack Sullivan. Pincus, Hopwood and Wright (Hopwood et al., 2011; Pincus, 2005; Pincus & Hopwood, 2012) have further elaborated empirically the interpersonal core of psychopathology and the interconnectedness of patient, therapist, and expression of problems in living. In very recent writing, Wright, Pincus & Hopwood (2020) and especially Wright, Ringwald, Hopwood & Pincus (2022: 2) "the field of psychopathology is transitioning away from discrete categories of mental disorders and shifting towards understanding psychopathology using dimensions that cut across traditional dimensions." They proposed Contemporary Integrative Interpersonal Theory (CIIT) as a model that has both theoretical elegance along with substantial research to support its many advantages over other models of psychopathology and their diagnostic systems. In essence, they adopt the Sullivanian conception of psychiatry as the science of interpersonal living …

> virtually all domains of personality and psychopathology implicate interpersonal functioning and vice versa. CIIT elevates the interpersonal not only because humans are a social species but because functioning cannot be defined in a vacuum; it must serve some purpose, it must have an object.
>
> (Wright, Ringwald, Hopwood & Pincus in press: 4)

Following Sullivan's recommendation for Bridgman's (1945) principle of operationalism P.W. principle of operationalism, Pincus, Hopwood, Wright and others in CIIT have applied complex empirical and statistical methods to the study of interpersonal living and its impact on psychopathology. As a result, their research yields a higher level of evidence-based theory and practice than found in other diagnostic schemes. While it is beyond the scope of this introductory book to explore the depth and complexity of CIIT, the interested reader is encouraged to explore their work.

Sullivan also challenged Freudian psychoanalytic theory and model of psychopathology and was indeed the major proponent, along with Eric Fromm, Karen Horney, and Clara Thompson, of the shift to relational psychoanalysis which largely dominates contemporary psychoanalysis (see Mitchell & Black, 2016). While Sullivan and Freud (1901) had similar positions regarding the ubiquity of psychopathological processes, Sullivan believed that Freud placed far too much emphasis on early development, the supposedly archetypal conflict of the Oedipus complex, and sexual behavior in accounting for the genesis of mental disorder. As Stern (1985) noted, Freud started with specific mental disorders and worked backward to elaborate a model of fixations and arrests in development to account for the disorders. Sullivan challenged Freud's emphasis on what Sullivan called the "Jesuitical first seven years" of development, believing instead that the preadolescent period (which Freud called latency) and adolescence was frequently more important in determining the nature of mental disorder than earlier periods. Sullivan did not place the same credence on the Oedipus complex and, in fact, questioned Freud's assumption about its universality and the classification of all mental disorder as either oedipal or pre-oedipal.

Clearly, Sullivan did not believe that mental disorder was due to distortion in sexual development per se, but the collision of the needs for lust, security, and intimacy. Sullivan downplayed the relative contribution of innate or inherited constitutional factors to mental disorder, which also put him at variance with Freud (see Sulloway, 1979), instead emphasizing social and cultural contributions to the inadequate or inappropriate patterns of interpersonal living in what was called mental disorder or psychopathology. Finally, while Sullivan and Freud both acknowledged the contribution of the psychiatrist's perceptions and actions in diagnosis and treatment, Freud (1912b) believed that the fully analyzed psychoanalyst could be free from countertransference. To say that one could be free from the interpersonal influences of anxiety, loneliness, and fear was unbelievably arrogant from Sullivan's perspective. He saw such self-deception as a security operation and an example of selective inattention within the analyst for which the patient would likely suffer. In addition to Sullivan's frequent cautions about the power of self-system as a conservative aspect of personality which led people to not profit from experience, he also posited a "powerful drive toward mental health" (1956: 57). He saw this potential even in people with serious mental disorders, which differed significantly from Freud's (1920, 1930) pessimistic concept of the death instinct. In fact, probably based on his own personal experience, Sullivan strongly believed that personality could change for the better, and mental disorder could be overcome, throughout the course of life.

## Basic Processes in Problems in Living

Sullivan's theory of mental disorder primarily focused on how interpersonal processes, common to all persons, operated to form problems in interpersonal living. As with his interpersonal theory, Sullivan's analysis of the processes of mental disorder began with the experience of the patient, using interpersonal concepts (especially the concepts from his epochs of development) as a frame of reference for what the signs (i.e., symptoms) of interpersonal difficulty meant to patient. His goal in elaborating these processes was to collaborate with the patient to describe signs and patterns of problems in living, and to uncover their meaning to the patient in a way that was comprehensible to both the psychotherapist and the patient. His thinking about mental disorder was inextricably woven into his ideas about normal development and treatment. The role of the psychotherapist was not to list symptoms and establish the correct diagnosis in a detached and objectified way, but to expertly and empathically engage the troubled individual in the syntaxic mode of experience, with the patient's benefit being the goal. As such, in describing mental disorder, Sullivan emphasized interpersonal processes, not clinical symptoms or syndromes. Salzman (1980) saw Sullivan as the founder of the study of personality disorder, because of his concern about elucidating recurrent patterns of interpersonal living in terms of their effects of relationships and the self. In their research and conceptualization, Pincus et al. (2020) further elaborated on personality disorder as essentially an interpersonal phenomenon that could not be understood outside this context.

Because of his theoretical orientation and emphasis on functional language, Sullivan tended not to use the term psychopathology and used the term mental disorder at most sparingly. Parenthetically, Sullivan's use of the word psychopathology in the title of his first book, *Personal Psychopathology* may have been one of many examples of the way he used irony to get across his point of view. Instead, he redefined the concept of mental disorder as the *dynamisms of difficulty* or *inadequate or inappropriate patterns of interpersonal relations ...*

> Mental disorder as a term refers to interpersonal processes either inadequate to the situation in which their personals are integrated, or excessively complex because of illusionary persons also integrated into the situations. It implies sometimes a greater ineffectiveness of the behavior by which the person is conceived to be pursuing the satisfactions that he requires.
>
> (1938: 128)

*Dynamisms of difficulty* were problematic patterns of interpersonal relations arising from experience with intense anxiety and the serious and
relatively unresolvable conflict between the satisfaction of physical and
interpersonal needs and the expectations and requirements of significant
others which restricted the expression or satisfaction of these needs. This
collision between need satisfaction and interpersonal security led to actions
that did not achieve a motivational goal or achieved a partial and
unsatisfactory goal. The over-dependence on a particular inadequate or
inappropriate pattern led to increased frustration and an ever-increasing need
to utilize various security operations to alter unsatisfactory experiences.
Sullivan used the concept of *dynamisms of difficulty* for a whole range of
situations, from habitual patterns he called *warps in personality* to special
types of patterns which were not carried out consistently or over a large area
of living. The primary difference between a general warp in personality and
more prescribed and infrequent dynamisms of difficulty was the former's
pervasiveness; the actual processes underlying the dynamism of difficulty
were similar. As Sullivan stated ...

> I am now beginning a discussion of the patterns of inadequate or
> inappropriate interpersonal relations, which are ordinarily called mental
> disorders, mild or severe. By adding "mild or severe," I wish to indicate
> that the topic of mental disorders covers all sorts of things, from minor
> accidents, such as unhappily being unable to remember an important
> person's name when you are about to request a favor from him, to the
> most chronic psychosis in the mental hospital. And so ... if the term
> mental disorder is to be meaningful, it must cover like a tent the whole
> field of inadequate or inappropriate performances in interpersonal
> relations.
>
> (1953: 313)

Reflecting his growing belief in the problems of psychiatric jargon, Sullivan
later became disenchanted with his term dynamism of difficulty and switched
to the term *inadequate or inappropriate patterns of interpersonal relations*.

### Anxiety, Security Operations, and Mental Disorder

Sullivan believed that anxiety, the experience of interpersonal insecurity, was
the primary cause of inadequate or inappropriate patterns of interpersonal
relations. Because of his belief that much of human motivation was directed
toward attaining interpersonal experiences of tenderness, understanding, and
later intimacy, Sullivan asserted that anxiety exerted a powerfully distorting
effect on development and personality. Like all interpersonal processes,
anxiety was experienced in different ways at different periods of development.
In Infancy, because the texture of the interpersonal relationship between the

infant and the mothering one was primarily the felt distinction between nonanxious-attached and anxious-separated states, anxiety in the mothering one induced an experience of anxiety in the infant which was inescapable and incomprehensible. The infant could only respond with very primitive processes such as somnambulant detachment, dissociation, and selective inattention to modify unbearable affects by "ignoring" the awareness of needs with which anxiety collided. In Childhood, anxiety arose from overly prohibitive, restrictive, and punitive parental responses to the child's expression of important interpersonal and physical needs. The child's unwitting behavioral substitutive processes such as sublimation and early language-based substitutive processes such as verbalisms and "as if" performances served to escape parental punitive attitudes and behaviors. While these substitutions shifted the expression of the child's need to parentally approved behavior, they only partially satisfied the need and concealed it from others and the self. When punitive parental behavior was especially intense and cruel, Sullivan posited another dynamism, malevolent transformation, in which the child learned to treat his, her, or others' need for tenderness as a sign of weakness to be manipulated.

With the Juvenile Era came the need for compeers and the frustration of this need, i.e., the experience of ostracism arising from peer social disapproval and exclusion from then juvenile gang. As sources of anxiety expanded beyond child-parent relations, increasingly complex security operations (such as regressive overdependence of parents, supervisory patterns, disparagement of others, and social isolation) were employed to fend off the anxiety of peer social disapproval. The brief, but critical period of Preadolescence was marked by the need for a chum, a person with whom to establish isophilic (same sex) intimacy. The anxiety associated with the frustration of this highly important interpersonal need was the experience of loneliness, which for Sullivan was one of the most powerful and underestimated of human motivations. The experience of loneliness was responsible for a multitude of intricate security operations, based on the individual's particular social situation.

Sullivan believed that Early Adolescence became the focal epoch for testing the integrity of all prior interpersonal adaptations. The powerful interpersonal integrative tendency of lust collided with the moralistic and prohibitive cultural values about the expression of lust, potentially leading to severe anxiety. As lust was the engine for establishing heterophilic (opposite sex) intimacy, prohibitive attitudes towards its expression also created intense loneliness. The anxiety and loneliness created by unsatisfactory integrations of lust, interpersonal security, and intimacy caused regressions to earlier, less complex patterns or revealed and intensified more or less chronic arrests and warps in personality. Sullivan described many patterns of inadequate interpersonal relations separating lust, intimacy, and security (such as the chronic juvenile, the homosexual adjustment, the sexual double standard, and the isolated adolescent) as ways to control anxiety during the early adolescent period. With the formation of a relatively clear sexual identity, Late Adolescence was the period for establishing a full repertoire of mature interpersonal relations, as permitted by available opportunity, personal and cultural The anxiety attending this period has been called existential anxiety by others and involved reduced self-esteem resulting from the failure to attain deep level of intimacy, to find a deeper sense of meaning in life, to fully utilize one's potential, or to meet important inner dreams (see Levinson, 1978).

While the person was particularly vulnerable in infancy and childhood, frequent or prolonged experiences of anxiety at any stage of development profoundly disrupted the person's sense of interpersonal security (and later need for intimacy) and, limited by self-system dynamisms employed to minimize anxiety, interfered with his or her ability to establish satisfying interpersonal relations. For Sullivan, the study of mental disorder was the investigation of the impact of anxiety at different developmental epochs, the ensuing security operations of the self-system, and the recurrent inappropriate or inadequate interpersonal relations resulting from these processes. Given Sullivan's emphasis on the importance of experience in the syntactic mode, the earlier the person's experience of significant anxiety, the more problematic it became to understand the person and collaborate with him or her about what was troubling.

Because of the role of anxiety in forming inner representations of self and other, Sullivan believed that excessive experience of anxiety damaged the person's ability to develop a positive self-concept and to anticipate positive cooperation with others. As a result, personifications of the self appeared as customarily low self-esteem (bad-me) and minimized anxiety by concealment and social isolation, exploitative attitudes and substitutive processes, or dissociation of important motivations (which in the extreme formed the not-me). Additionally, personifications of others were marked decreased expectations for positive interpersonal cooperation (bad mother experiences) or by fear or terror of others (primitive bad or malevolent mother experiences). The cognitive development of foresight, a necessary capacity for problem solving, was impaired by anxiety as well. Sullivan repeatedly stated that anxiety operated in opposition to meeting both zonal needs (such as hunger, eliminative processes, and lust) and general needs (such as needs for tenderness, empathy, and intimacy).

While mild forms of anxiety, such as disapproval, were useful for socialization beginning in childhood, Sullivan believed that anxiety unleashed processes called *security operations*, such as sublimation, selective inattention, dissociation, and substitutive processes, which were the foundation of inadequate or inappropriate patterns of interpersonal relations when used pervasively. A highly related experience, loneliness, the experience of frustration of the need for intimacy due to excessive security operations, which emerged in preadolescence and early adolescence, was similarly involved in the establishment of dynamisms of difficulty. Sullivan believed that the experiences of anxiety and loneliness lay at the heart of all mental disorder.

Sullivan's conceptualizations of self-system and security operations, the operations of the personality that avoid anxiety, were central to his understanding the dynamisms of difficulty. As Sullivan stated,

> The self-system is struck off in the personality because of the necessity for picking one's way through irrational and un-understandable prescriptions of behavior laid down by parents; in other words, the child has to be educated into a very complex social order, long before the reason and the good sense of the whole thing can be digested, long before it becomes understandable, if it ever does. The self-system comes to be the organization that controls awareness; all operations that are not primarily of the self go outside awareness.
>
> (1940/1953: 4)

Sullivan saw self-system as one of the three basic aspects of the personality along with the waking, aware, and active self, which consciously sought interpersonal situations to mutually engage in meeting needs, and the period spent in sleep, which provided relief from the vigilance of security operations and satisfied unmet needs from the day through symbolic operations in dreaming. Because the function of the self-system was to avoid and minimize anxiety, most of its operations were not readily accessible to awareness, which severely hampered learning from later life experience. Sullivan's *dynamisms of difficulty*, mild or severe, were essentially operations of the self-system which led to inadequate and inappropriate patterns of interpersonal relations.

While Sullivan described a great variety of operations of the self-system throughout his writings on personality and mental disorder, it is beyond the scope of this book to outline all of them. Instead, the rest of this section will highlight six security operations important to severe dynamisms of difficulty – *selective inattention and dissociation* (important to his conceptualizations about schizophrenia); *sublimation*, *verbalisms*, and *as if performances* (substitutive processes central to his thinking of obsessionalism); and *malevolent transformation* (his major contribution to the problem of human cruelty and criminality). Part of the management of focal awareness, *selective inattention* was the process of shifting awareness away from anxiety-laden interpersonal situations and served a dual function. Usefully, this process would allow earlier interpersonal patterns which no longer mattered to be "forgotten," i.e., placed out of awareness, freeing awareness to focus on the newer, more complex social world. On the other hand, when selective inattention operated to ignore or exclude aspects of experience from focal awareness that really did matter, the process excluded material from the person's awareness that could be valuable to learning more effective patterns of interpersonal cooperation. Selective inattention (and security operations in general) operated "backwards," that is, when interpersonal situations in the present triggered recall of a past anxiety-laden situation, selective attention operated to exclude the experience, even if attending to it was important. As Sullivan (1956: 42–43) stated, "The thing that determines whether this is done well or ill, from the standpoint of long-range results for the person, is how smoothly the control of awareness excludes the irrelevant and includes the relevant."

A common example of selective inattention seen in clinical practice involved the patient, who, having experienced especially aggressive or hostile parenting during childhood, repeatedly fails to see such behavior in adult intimate relations. While selective inattention of the parent's behavior was necessary in childhood to control anxiety and preserve necessary attachment, the patient cannot communicate or behaviorally set appropriate expectations for the adult relationship, even though to do so would be exceedingly important in the present adult circumstance. The patient may experience intermittently severe distress about serious episodes of hostile behavior in the present relationship, but quickly shifts focus away from the experience as if it never occurred. The intermittent experience of distress is not available to the active and aware part of the personality to assess the overall value of the relationship. Rather than describing the situation with diagnostic terms, such as a self-defeating or masochistic personality, Sullivan would focus on how, and under what circumstances, the process of selective inattention of mistreatment by another operated.

While a ubiquitous process, Sullivan's believed that *dissociation* was the underlying, previously adaptive, process overutilized in severe mental disorders. As Mullahy (1970) stated, Sullivan used dissociation in two major ways – first, as the complete inhibition of motivation toward satisfying certain needs with the total exclusion of any recognition of their existence and, second, as an aspect of the personality functionally separate from and completely unacceptable to the self. For Sullivan, like sublimation, dissociation involved a motivational component and, like selective inattention, it contained the element of exclusion from focal awareness. Sullivan believed that dissociation was the mind's response to overwhelming experience (beginning with overwhelming anxiety in infancy) and operated as an interpersonal process in which later motivations associated with these experiences prevented uncanny emotion. The person was blithely unaware of dissociated behavior and its impact on others. Sullivan included such phenomena as fugue, automatic writing, and certain hysterical paralyses and tics as indications of an underlying massive dissociation. He saw the appearance of abhorrent cravings (entrance into awareness of increasingly intense and unsatisfied longings for something perceived by others as abhorrent), automatic writing, and tics as the first step of breakdown of dissociated motivation. This failure of dissociation was attended by overwhelming, unbearable anxiety, the kind found primarily in psychotic decompensations. While it was perhaps his most important concept for understanding severe mental disorder, Sullivan was uncertain about what dissociation was and where it fit in the overall personality. Until late in his writing, he thought the dissociation was not part of the self-system, but a system of operations 'outside of the self.' Sullivan later conceptualized it as the part of the self-system, the primary operation of the 'not-me' personification, in which experiences and motivations were so anxiety-ridden that they needed to be excluded from all awareness. Like his concept of anxiety, Sullivan's thinking about the process of dissociation, though unclear, anticipated critical advances (see Kluft, 1985, 1990; Putnam, 1985, 1989; 2016) in the study of trauma and dissociation which have confirmed Sullivan's notions of traumatic causation of dissociation and its function to contain massive anxiety and decompensation. Though largely unacknowledged for his contribution, Sullivan eloquently elaborated a number of theoretical ideas about the effects of overwhelming life experiences that can be found throughout modern conceptualizations of the human response to trauma (e.g., Herman, 1992; van der Kolk, 1987).

As the infant matured and had a greater ability to affect the social environment, substitutive processes became the primary mode of operation of the self-system, especially sublimation, verbalisms, and 'as if' performances. While selective inattention and dissociation were processes of the control of focal awareness, Sullivan emphasized the behavioral component of the process of sublimation. As a consequence of coping with an irrational culture, Sullivan saw sublimation as an automatic pattern of behavior, outside of awareness, in which the direct and complete satisfaction of a need was given up for a partially satisfying, socially approved pattern. Interestingly, Sullivan stressed that, for sublimation to work well, this substitutive pattern of behavior could not restrict too much need and unsatisfied need must discharged during sleep through the process of dreaming. Inadequate patterns of sublimation led to disrupted patterns of interpersonal relations. For example, in what might today be called passive-aggressive personality, anger is insufficiently sublimated to prevent interpersonal relations which are highly frustrating to important others, or, in what is sometimes called inadequate personality, need satisfaction was overly restricted which leads to chronically impoverished interpersonal relations. When sublimation patterns were recurrently threatened by the breakthrough of severe anxiety, the profoundly disturbed sleep, dissociative processes, or schizophrenic dynamisms of severe mental disorder could erupt.

As the of the child matured and language in the syntaxic mode replaced private reverie and the earlier verbal behaviors of autistic verbalizations and gestures, the substitutive processes of verbalisms and 'as if' performances developed as a part of the necessity to conceal and deceive. Sullivan used the term *verbalism* to describe how words were used to fend off anxiety, by what is commonly called lying and insincerity or in more severe instances obsessive verbalizations. A discovery so important that it was deeply embroidered into the fabric of social convention, the child learned early about the magical properties of language to ward off punishment and disapproval. Instead of the unwitting character of sublimation, verbalisms were verbal behaviors occasioned by increased awareness and cognitive ability. This awareness did not extend to the long-term consequences on interpersonal cooperation, as evidenced by the chronic use of verbalisms by individuals whom Sullivan called psychopaths. He noted that psychopaths seemed shocked when they were not believed or entrusted based on their verbal behaviors, rather than for their deeds. Under the duress of severe anxiety, for some individuals the utterance of words retained the more primitive and magical ability to ward off anxiety without the direct manipulation of others, a pattern Sullivan related to obsessionalism. Sullivan thought that both psychopathy and obsessional states were closely related to schizophrenia, all representing very early disturbance in interpersonal relations.

"As if" performance was another of major substitutive processes seen be Sullivan as important to the understanding of mental disorder. Similar to verbalisms, the person employed "as if" performances to mentally and behaviorally ward off perceived punishment and anxiety. The individual acted like or sounded like what others expected of them as a way of concealing other behavior (dramatizations) or by pretending to do something to evoke sympathy or feign intimacy (personae). Sullivan's concepts of verbalisms and especially "as if" performances described the behavioral operations which revealed an underlying psychological state similar to Winnicott's (1960) concept of the false self. While an ineffective interpersonal pattern found all too commonly in daily life, Sullivan saw the need to deceive and conceal as the root of preoccupations and compulsive behaviors that later developed into obsessional states. In the extreme, the process of "as if" performances combined with dissociation to develop a variety of sub-personalities found in dissociative identity disorders.

The last of Sullivan's conceptualization of operation of the self-system implicated in severe mental disorder is *malevolent transformation*. It concerned the processes by which the individual organized early experiences of cruelty in parenting figures and involved the development of the personification of experience with malevolent others. Based on the person's unfortunate association of the need for tenderness with anxiety and pain, he or she came to perceive the interpersonal world as an essentially dangerous place where he or she was constantly in the presence of enemies who would prey upon any expression of the need for sympathy and understanding. As a result, the experience of the need for tenderness in the self or others came to be experienced as a sign of weakness and helplessness to be disdained, used, and exploited. For Sullivan, if this childhood pattern went relatively unaltered by later good fortune, then malevolent transformation became the core operation of the self-system, a warp in personality that expressed itself in cruelty towards others that would be the parents' sad legacy to the next generation and generations to come. Research demonstrating the high prevalence of the perpetrators of family violence and child abusers who themselves were abused as children (see Finkelhor, 1984; Groth, 1979; Starr et al., 1991; Toch, 1992) and prevalence of family violence and child abuse history in the etiology of later psychopathy (Farrington & Bergstrøm, 2018) has amply confirmed Sullivan's ideas about intergenerational transmission of malevolence.

## Dynamisms of Difficulty

As discussed earlier, Sullivan had significant problems theoretically with the idea of clinical entities in psychiatry. While Mullahy (1970) suggested that perhaps Sullivan overstated his concerns about psychiatric diagnosis, Perry (1964: xi) stated that Sullivan was reluctant "to set schizophrenia apart from living itself; in part, also, he came to feel, increasingly over the last ten years of his life, that the main implication of his work was in the area of social psychology – in the wide spectrum of preventive measures within society itself." With this orientation in mind, this section will explicate the three dynamisms of difficulty for which Sullivan was best known – the schizophrenic, the obsessive, and the paranoid – from Sullivan's perspective about how the processes underlying these dynamisms coalesced into experiences with patients that psychiatrists labeled psychiatric diagnoses. It is important to keep in mind Sullivan's view that these dynamisms of difficulty could arise anywhere from transient regressions to earlier interpersonal patterns or from more enduring warps in personality that comprised an overall orientation toward living. Additionally, the section will include two new dynamisms of difficulty that are embedded in his work but never fully elucidated by him – the dynamism of psychological trauma and the dynamism of personality disorders.

### The Schizophrenic Dynamism

Sullivan was, and continues to be, best known for his early work with schizophrenia at Sheppard Pratt Hospital. He formulated perhaps the first psychodynamic theory about schizophrenia that led to successful psychosocial treatment. Sullivan's ideas about schizophrenia are interwoven throughout his writings on personality, mental disorder, and psychotherapy and his papers on schizophrenia fill an entire book, *Schizophrenia as a Human Process*. While space does not permit a full discussion of his many thoughts on schizophrenia, reading Sullivan's original writings offers a fertile source of surprisingly contemporary insights about this baffling human dilemma.

In present times the predominate fashion in psychiatry is to consider schizophrenia as a genetic and biological disorder (e.g., Horváth & Mirnics, 2015; Van de Leemput et al., 2016), while others have recently found considerable research data to understand schizophrenia in a broader social context (e.g., Van Os et al., 2010). Interestingly, Sullivan distinguished between two broad types of schizophrenia – *dementia praecox*, as proposed by Kraepelin, which was an organic degenerative disorder that had an insidious onset often called simple schizophrenia, and *schizophrenia proper*, which was an outcome of severe problems of living that erupted more or less abruptly, though patterns leading to it may have been evident for years. He did not consider the treatment of the first disorder to be within the province of psychiatry as he conceptualized it, except to the degree to which the social stigma of any biological disorder may be helped by psychiatric intervention. Frederickson (2021) also differentiates what he calls fragile patients from those with biologically based psychiatric disorders where the patient's capacity to form relationships is fundamentally compromised. It is also interesting to note that, while he has been criticized for ignoring the importance of biology in severe mental disorder, Sullivan speculated, back in the 1940s, that manic-depressive disorder, unlike schizophrenia, had a primarily biological origin. Additionally, Sullivan suggested that manic-depressive disorder would eventually be better treated by psychopharmacological intervention than psychotherapy many decades before the discovery of lithium therapy.

Sullivan (1962: 261) focused on schizophrenia proper as an especially difficult problem in living. "Some ten years' rather close contact with sufferers of schizophrenic disorders culminated in the firm conviction that not sick individuals but complex, peculiarly characterized situations were the subject-matter of research and therapy." Sullivan used the word schizophrenia differently from psychodynamic theorists and Kraepelinian psychiatrists, focusing on schizophrenia, not as a "so-called clinical entity," but on a set of underlying processes which he called the dynamism of schizophrenia. While Sullivan noted that the processes underlying the **dynamism of schizophrenia** were found in everyone, he used the term schizophrenia primarily to describe an overall orientation toward living that represented a serious warp of personality. He saw the unusually inadequate or inappropriate patterns of interpersonal relations as indications of the person's need to rely on psychological processes manifested at the earliest developmental level. Frederickson (2021) greatly advanced Sullivan's concept of schizophrenia proper to what he calls the fragile patient, a significant innovation in interpersonal thinking, which detaches the worn label of schizophrenia from the treatment of very troubled patients.

Etiologically, Sullivan conceptualized the *dynamism of schizophrenia* as an extreme warp in personality which resulted from very inadequate socialization (parenting). Because of idiosyncratic familial expectations, the individual was effectively cut off from both his or her own interpersonal needs and never learned to integrate these important needs with others outside the family. Because the existence of the child's needs did not fit into the family belief system, the individual perceived both important others as fundamentally unempathic and many aspects of the self as debased and unworthy. Fearful in his or her approach to others and woefully under-socialized, the individual experienced extraordinary difficulty interacting with adults and peers outside the family. This interpersonal incompetence reinforced the low self-esteem acquired from family interactions and led to profound further isolation. During juvenile and preadolescence eras, the person's opportunity to correct an unrealistic and idiosyncratic view of the world was hampered. The person withdrew increasingly into an inner world of compensatory fantasy, fraught with tension and longing beyond what could be understood by others. Because of an extremely brittle self-concept and self-system operations favoring avoidance and interpersonal isolation over learning and interpersonal connection, the person's need for peers and later the need for intimacy with other was ineffectively either poorly sublimated into fantasy or massively dissociated. Sullivan noted the schizophrenic individual, in contrast to the person with a healthy development of personality, exhibited disproportionate dissociated aspects of the personality.

As these important interpersonal needs were increasingly dissociated and integrating tendencies with others went undeveloped, the person's capacity to meet the developmental tasks of adolescence was seriously compromised. Because the individual grew up in a family environment where he or she developed fantastic ideas about relationships with others and about sexuality, it was not especially surprising that the appearance of the lust dynamism occasioned enormous complexity in the person's inner experience and relationships. Because lust dynamism was extremely difficult to sublimate or dissociate and required integration with previously dissociated needs for intimacy, the individual's characteristic security operations of sublimation (social isolation and fantasy) became inadequate. Hence, the failure of sublimation caused an increased use of selective inattention and dissociation, security operations which were highly vulnerable to disorganization. For Sullivan, this inadequate pattern of interpersonal living culminated in a situation which marked the first of two stages of the schizophrenic dynamism – the loss of faith in self, fear of the interpersonal world, and the excessive reliance on dissociation of needs as part of the not-me personification.

Because lust and intimacy were too powerful to effectively sublimate or dissociate, these major impulse or motivational systems could not be totally divorced from the aware self and literally came out in the night.

> The individual, with serious impairment of the dependability of his self and the universe, progresses into a situation in which the dissociated parts of the personality are the effective integrating agencies ... The result is a condition which I cannot distinguish by any important characteristic from

that undergone by an individual in attempting to orient himself on awakening in the midst of a vivid nightmare.

(1962: 243)

Characteristically, sleep became disrupted as the breakthrough of dissociated impulses entered dreaming in undisguised manner, leading to what Sullivan called profound and ominous dreams. While the massive anxiety of experiencing aspects of the not-me during sleep is conspicuously encountered by most of us during an occasional vivid nightmare, it was very emphatically encountered by people at the beginning of a severe schizophrenic episode. The eruption of dissociated impulses into the person's sleep life led to severely disrupted sleep or to severe nightmares from which the person could not "wake up," i.e., could not contain in sleep.

Sullivan described a great variety of ways in which dissociated motivations spilled over into waking life and integrated interpersonal situations. Sullivan theorized that abhorrent cravings, hallucinations, and delusions were mental representations of dissociated urges which broke through into consciousness, which at the same time needed to be disowned. Sullivan saw abhorrent cravings in schizophrenia as the entrance into awareness of increasingly intense and unsatisfied longings for something which was repulsive to the person, for example, homosexual impulses (representing desire for both lust and isophilic intimacy) or death wishes toward someone. Hallucinations came from highly dissociated, self-deprecatory ideas, which were expressed usually as hallucinated perceptions of accusatory "voices" from illusory others or occasionally as visualizations of the unacceptable impulse. Schizophrenic delusions were disowned representations of the primitive bad-mother personification, which were unsystematized and autistic beliefs that people were dangerous or had malignant intent, which often was experienced as coming from other powers. Sullivan saw these *autochthonous thoughts*, contents of mind which seemingly came from outside of oneself with no feeling of ownership, as the first step of the breakdown of dissociated motivation. *Automatisms*, active behavioral attempts on the part of individual to meet dissociated needs such as fugue states, automatic writing, and tics, were more severe failures of dissociation. As dissociated parts of the self came into awareness (i.e., as not-me personifications and severe bad-me personifications became inescapable), the failure of dissociation was accompanied with overwhelming, unbearable anxiety and was a disaster to self-esteem. A state which Sullivan called *panic*, the experience of the disorganization of the personality, ensued, which was terrifying and could not be allowed to last for long. Because all aspects of awareness were interrupted by overwhelming experiences of uncanny emotion, the person's need to escape this experience (often called psychotic decompensation) became inexorable, leading to the second stage of the schizophrenic dynamism.

For Sullivan, the second stage of the dynamism of schizophrenia was distinguished by the processes of escape from unbearable anxiety (see Garfield, 2018 on the role of unbearable emotion in psychosis), with behavior almost entirely directed to avoid anxiety rather than engage in social interaction. Because of the failure of the self-system and especially the failure of dissociation, Sullivan believed that the most primitive operations of regression into parataxic and prototaxic modes of experience and somnolent detachment became necessary to separate from awareness needs that met with uncanny emotions. Regression in the second phase of the schizophrenic dynamism was marked by the person's significant withdrawal from interpersonal functioning below the level of normal socialization and by the appearance of primitive referential processes. As Sullivan stated, "the self-system has lost control of awareness, so that it cannot exclude these earlier processes and restrict awareness to late, highly refined types of thought" (1956: 24) and "the schizophrenic process is of a piece with the referential operations of very early life" (1956: 13). Early referential processes such as autistic reverie and autistic speech rendered interpersonal consensually validated experience irrelevant, allowing the person to escape the social world for the world of autistic fantasy.

Sullivan did not believe that the various presentations of the schizophrenic dynamism (catatonic, hebephrenic, and paranoid) were separate clinical entities, but were typical courses of events to be observed in the schizophrenic condition. Sullivan saw the almost total withdrawal from the social world marking the catatonic variation, while the hebephrenic existence appeared to be a regression to early magical language and pre-social behavior. The paranoid variation seemed to Sullivan to be more organized than the other two, indicating a greater systematization of the paranoid coloring found in all severe mental disorders and a strong reliance on the security operation of projection of blame to relieve anxiety. Sullivan noted that close observation of the course of the schizophrenic dynamism revealed that what were called separate sub-categories of schizophrenic could be seen at different times in the same person and were simply different patterns of security operations to deal with the same underlying problem – the containment of unbearable anxiety. Additionally, Sullivan vehemently disagreed with Kraepelin and others who stated that schizophrenia was an ecstatic escape from the pressures of reality and that the difficulty with treatment revolved around bringing the schizophrenic back to the less pleasant world of responsibility. Sullivan believed that, while the person did escape the pressures of social interaction with the protective shell of schizophrenic regression, he or she lived in a nightmarish, irrational, and incomprehensible world in which the menacing, primitive interpersonal experience of bad-mother personification was omnipresent. Sullivan stated that the schizophrenic person's inordinate need for sleep was due to the use operation of somnolent detachment (the need for sleep as a regressive devise to escape unbearable experience), which attested to the terror of schizophrenic existence.

Sullivan spoke compassionately about the severe dilemmas faced by the schizophrenic person who attempted to move from the second stage of schizophrenia into greater social integration. Because the dynamism of schizophrenia developed in response to immensely low self-esteem and highly painful interpersonal experience, the relationship with others, including the psychotherapist, was colored by paranoid processes and the contagion of anxiety. Additionally, the primitive referential processes and regression of social behaviors were exceedingly difficult to understand by others, who lived largely the syntaxic mode of experience. Sullivan also noted that the use of regression as a security operation was itself demoralizing for the schizophrenic and added to the person's already chronically low self-esteem. Sullivan believed that the schizophrenic dynamism was difficult for the person to change and could usually only do so with fortunate experience with a compassionate other who worked to empathically understand the schizophrenic person's experience. While recovery from the second stage of schizophrenia was often perilous, Sullivan also reminded his colleagues that the schizophrenic dynamism as an episode or series of episodes in one's life among people, but not the sum total of who the person was.

### The Obsessional Dynamism

Surpassed only by his contributions to understanding the schizophrenic dynamism, Sullivan's conceptualization of the *obsessional dynamism* was a signature clinical contribution, leading Salzman (1980: 283) to state that "Sullivan was the undisputed model" for the conceptualization and treatment of obsessive individuals. As with all mental disorders, Sullivan focused on the processes underlying this complex dynamism of difficulty, relying on his understanding of the security operations which he called substitutive processes as the basis for his conceptualization of the obsessional dynamism. As recalled from the earlier discussion, substitutive processes, such as sublimation, verbalisms, and as if performances, were ways that the self-system kept anxiety outside of awareness. Sullivan saw verbalisms and "as if" performances as the underlying root of preoccupations used to mentally and behaviorally ward off perceived disapproval, punishment and anxiety. For Sullivan, substitutive processes of the obsessional dynamism relied on the use of words and acts to conceal the expression of unacceptable needs from the self and others. In these processes, language and behavior were utilized to obscure, distance, and misdirect, rather than communicate direct intent. Sullivan noted the similarity between the primitive operations in the use of language in the obsessional dynamism and the autistic character of speech and the magical power of words from early childhood. The obsessional's preoccupation with trivial and irrelevant details, which rendered communication uncommunicative, led Sullivan to theorize that rumination itself absorbed the person's inner experience during times of stress as a way to escape anxiety. One of Sullivan's main contributions to treatment of the obsessional dynamism was his insistence on the necessity for psychotherapists to shift their preoccupation with the content of the verbalisms, focusing instead on the style and function of language to avoid or distract direct interpersonal communication. While Sullivan believed that the obsessional dynamism was frequently found in a variety of states from normal to pre-schizophrenic, the dependence on these operations as the predominant mode of interpersonal relationship was what characterized the so-called clinical entity of obsessive-compulsive neurosis or disorder.

In terms of etiology, Sullivan believed that the person employing the obsessional dynamism grew up in a family whose relationship with children was marked with hostility and hypocrisy. Sullivan (1972: 123) saw "loveless marriages complicated with hypocrisy and impotence as the prime source of this distortion." While lip service was given by parents about caring for members of the family, these parents actually behaved in a belittling, controlling, and demeaning manner toward their children and each other, which belied their spoken word. Because of the acute dependence on the parents for attachment and tender connection, children needed to selectively inattend from hostile behaviors and give greater credence in their awareness to their parents' magical use of words to obscure reality. Because of the atmosphere of little tenderness, excessive demands, and an unattainable contingency for acceptability, communication in the family functioned to ward off disapproval and punishment rather than communicate human needs. As Salzman (1980: 279) stated, obsessional tactics were used "to overcome great uncertainty in a world of malevolence and unfriendliness ... managing in a hostile world which is rejecting and threatening."

As a result, the obsessional person experienced significant difficulty in interpersonal relations, because of the need to use power operations to maintain control of others. The self-system of the obsessional person was marked by extraordinarily low self-esteem and a sense of "jittery security among one's fellows" (1956: 30). While intimacy was an experience to be avoided, the obsessional sublimated this need into interpersonal connection through intellectuality, control, and perfectionism. Specifically, Sullivan spoke of what he called the flypaper technique or obsessional stickiness in which the obsessional used long speeches, "befogging arguments," and other circumlocution functions to avoid being held to an idea that could lead to criticism or embarrassment, but which at the same time maintained a sticky connectedness with others.

The obsessional's attitude of seeming invulnerability and requirement of certainty about acceptance revealed to Sullivan an underlying experience of pervasive powerlessness. The main interpersonal experience of the obsessional was the feeling of intense vulnerability in relationships with others. Their obsessional substitutions which were the most conspicuous and troublesome aspects of their lives were simply directed towards keeping others at bay to protect themselves from their extraordinary vulnerability to anxiety. While Sullivan agreed with Freud's observations about the need for control in the obsessional dynamism, he strongly criticized Freud's (1905) formulation about this need for control as a way to deal with hostile and aggressive drives related to underlying feelings of hatred and anger. As Sullivan (1953: 267) stated, "But to interpret the obsessional neurosis as a mask of hatred is, I think, just dreadful hokum – the cart has been on top of the horse." Sullivan believed that this need for control arose from the fear of humiliation and the need to maintain acceptability and status. While he saw how the obsessional could be seen by others as hostile, Sullivan characteristically separated the function of the interpersonal operations from their appearance, i.e., as adaptive, not retaliatory. As Salzman (1980: 280) stated, the obsessional's need for control came "not (from) hostility but the danger of exposing one's weaknesses, helplessness, humanness, and ineffectiveness that is a component of every ritual and obsessive tactic."

Unlike the dynamism of schizophrenia, Sullivan believed that the ...

(obsessional) dynamism is quite adequate to meet the ordinary run of life events, and therefore the person does not suffer any great accumulation of tensions and unsatisfied needs, nor any great onslaughts of anxiety from acute insecurity.

(1956: 30)

It was only when the security operations of the obsessional dynamism were seriously challenged that its shaky developmental foundation was exposed. Based on his considerable experience with both disorders, Sullivan saw a clear relationship between the dynamisms of schizophrenia and obsessionalism. Because of the primitive, though stable, organization of the obsessional dynamism, it was extremely vulnerable to schizophrenic processes when substitutive operations no longer worked effectively. When self-esteem and interpersonal security were seriously challenged or the needs of lust and intimacy could not be circumvented, the obsessional dynamisms could undergo regression. The failure of sublimation could instigate the increased use of dissociation and, with it, vulnerability to schizophrenic dynamisms. Sullivan believed in the idea of the "logical progression of dynamisms," which operated in characteristic ways to changing circumstances, fortunate and unfortunate, in the interpersonal environment. Sullivan's concept of the relative fluidity of dynamisms of difficulty (as opposed to the more fixed nature of the concept of "mental disease") has been especially born out in the study of the interpersonal processes of the so-called borderline personality (see Evans, 1992, 1993) and empirically validated by the research of Wright, Ringwald, Hopwood & Pincus

(2022) indicating the fixed personality disorder categories are simply inaccurate. Sullivan believed that this progression could work in both directions, that fortunate circumstances (such as a good psychotherapist or therapeutic community) could be harnessed by "the drive toward mental health" existing in practically everyone, allowing the person who heavily relied on obsessive dynamisms to develop more adequate patterns of interpersonal relations.

### The Paranoid Dynamism

Though often seen as a type of schizophrenia, Sullivan saw the *paranoid dynamism* – his last dynamism of difficulty explored in this chapter – as having distinct, though related, processes which he believed were valuable for elucidating this inadequate or inappropriate patterns of interpersonal living. As Sullivan (1956: 145) stated, "The paranoid dynamism is rooted in (1) an awareness of inferiority of some kind, which then necessitates (2) a transference of blame onto others." The paranoid dynamism was essentially a progression of painful experiences and security operations to modify these experiences. The person utilizing this dynamism must first have had the experience of chronic insecurity, which, he hypothesized, originated from significant developmental misfortune.

Sullivan believed that the likely parenting style in the development of the paranoid dynamism was one in which the parents took out their own disgruntlement with themselves on the child and consistently blamed the child for their own failings. Naturally, the child accurately sensed the unfairness of the parents, but, if the child challenged this unfairness, the parents "compounded the felony by defending themselves, by claiming they were so fair" (1956: 147). Instead of providing the child with experiences which anticipated tenderness, reasonable expectations, and clear communication from significant caretakers, the parents surrounded the child with hostility, capricious standards, and incomprehensible verbalisms, which required the child to sacrifice his or her own experience of reality for a tenuous interpersonal security. The necessary empathic linkage with parents during late infancy and early childhood was broken, leaving the child with experiences of interpersonal disconnection and fearfulness, helplessness, and a debased self-concept, a state later described by Erikson (1950) as one of fundamental mistrust.

Sullivan outlined cognitive changes required to adapt to this hostile and mystifying parental environment. A fundamental dilemma for the child arose from the distortion in learning to differentiate the source of the child's feeling of resentment. The development of a reliable sense of how the child felt about himself or herself or others, especially whether the source of one's discomfort was "inside (being a person worthy of scorn) or outside (resenting the parents' unfairness)," was severely hampered by the parents' requirement that the child conceal and distort his or her inner feelings about the parents. As a result, in order to provide a sense of interpersonal security, the child initially accepted the parents' debased view of himself or herself. Sullivan speculated that this pattern of interpersonal relationship made it extremely difficult to distinguish what was inside the self and what was outside, resulting in a profound confusion about the self and frequent cognitive misinterpretation of the interpersonal environment, which was an experiential hallmark of paranoid dynamism. Because awareness of chronically and severely low self-esteem and cognitive confusion were not tolerable and could not continue to be experienced, security operations were required to decrease feelings of inferiority. Having experienced the shifting of blame from parent to child, the child learned to shift blame to others for his or her own feelings of inferiority. The security operation of *shifting of blame* was both an immediate relief from distress and a seriously flawed pattern of interpersonal relationship that reinforced the feelings of inferiority it served to alleviate.

In describing the paranoid dynamism, Sullivan distinguished between a "paranoid slant on life" and the paranoid state. A *paranoid slant on life* developed in response to profound insecurity, anxiety, or jealousy of feeling constantly disrespected for aspects of the self, which the person cannot "fix," all the while seeing that others engage in respectful, easy intimacy with others. The loss of self-esteem and jealousy of others became intolerable and the shift was effected from a malignant or punitive self to a self who is blameless, noble, and expanded in worth. This paranoid distortion often provided a welcome relief. If taking a "paranoid slant on life" was not adequate to relieve the feelings of inferiority and jealousy, a more pervasive and systematic misinterpretation (including delusions of grandeur and persecution) of interpersonal events became necessary, marking the progression to the paranoid state and possibly paranoid schizophrenia.

Sullivan described the *paranoid state* as the wholesale transference of blame which became systematized in a rational seeming manner, "a misinterpretation of events to constitute an explanation, usually rather transcendental in nature, of what is troublesome" (1956: 145). The very severe paranoid elaboration protected against massive inferiority, marking the transition from "unhappy sanity" to "the relatively more comfortable psychosis of the paranoid state" (1956: 146). The paranoid person's malevolent attitude towards the world served to hide extraordinary suffering and vulnerability. As Sullivan (1953: 361) stated, "the only impression one has is of a person in the grip of horror, of uncanny devastation which makes everyone threatening beyond belief." Such a state was so intolerable that the person needed to ...

personify the specific evil (and) begins to put blame on these others ... he begins to wash his hands of all those real and fancied aspects of his own personality which he has suffered up to this point (and) arrived at a state that is pretty hard to remedy – by categorical name the paranoid state.

(1953: 361–362)

Sullivan observed that the security operations of paranoid dynamism were inherently unstable in that they prevented the possibility of developing any satisfactory interpersonal relations. The highly systematized nature of the paranoid state constituted a set of operations to lessen this instability. The paranoid transformation of the personality used substitutive processes similar to the obsessional state, which allowed the individual to become preoccupied with an elaborate system of persecution that becomes a completely absorbing occupation of the self. Nearly every interpersonal event was scrutinized through the lens of paranoid system.

In his later writing, Sullivan elucidated another developmental tributary to the paranoid dynamism. He observed that a particular form of parental disapproval with the pre- and early adolescent's establishment of intimate relations outside the family could be malignant to the developing pre- and early adolescent's sense of self. Particularly, if this parental disapprobation was charged with jealousy and ridicule toward their son's or daughter's increased freedom to establish intimacy outside of the family, the early adolescent could experience a profound state of anxiety and shame about his or her need for intimacy and sexuality and could experience confusion and suspicion toward his or her parents. In severe instances of parental ridicule, the young adolescent's distress over the collision of needs for intimacy and lust, on one hand, and the need for security, on the other, led to a retreat from usual adolescent integrations and to the elaboration of the distinct paranoid process of jealousy.

Sullivan reasoned that jealousy, representing the envy of another's capacity for intimacy, was often found in paranoid individuals. As a result of parental debasement and severe difficulty in establishing intimate peer relations, the isolated adolescent's sense of self-esteem was riddled with intolerable experiences of inferiority and inadequacy. To compensate for feelings of inferiority, the individual fantasized about, and became obsessively attached to, a desired mate or mates, who had high social status and developed easy intimacy with others. Whether the isolated individual attempted to establish a relationship with this desired mate and was rebuffed or the individual relied only on fantasy operations, his or her experience of inferiority underwent a paranoid shifting of blame. In severe instances, the paranoid individual shifted the difficulty in establishing an intimate relationship to a paranoid distortion that jealous others plotted and schemed to deny him or her the object of his or her longing. The operation of jealousy both established a connection with others and also kept them at bay. Grandiose beliefs about one's worth to others alternated with persecutory ideas about others' jealousy or jealous attachment to an unattainable other. An unattainable love object could become tied into the individual's angry, paranoid systematization, sometimes with tragic consequences.

While Sullivan recognized that individuals in the paranoid state were vulnerable to regression into schizophrenic dynamism, he thought that the paranoid dynamism was used as a massive adaptation security against schizophrenic decompensation and could be remarkably stable over time. He believed that the so-called clinical entity of paranoid schizophrenia constituted a failure of the paranoid dynamism to relieve or remove chronic anxiety. He remarked on important differences in the delusional systems in paranoid schizophrenia and the paranoid state, noting the relatively unsystematized beliefs in paranoid schizophrenia when compared to the more systematized, better rationalized, and more consensually plausible cognitions found in individuals in a paranoid state. Sullivan reasoned that the paranoid state came in response to later problems in the developmental process which distinguished the predominant use of the paranoid over the schizophrenic dynamism. The more organized and seemingly syntactic mode of the paranoid state revealed to Sullivan a relatively stronger self-system than found in schizophrenia. Sullivan also believed that *paranoid coloring*, i.e., a general wariness and suspiciousness of others, was a phenomenon common to most mental disorders, but did not necessarily indicate the use of the paranoid dynamism. Paranoid coloring indicated the person's chronic low self-regard and a general anticipation of interpersonal disapproval which he believed was a ubiquitous experience in mental disorder.

Sullivan fiercely disagreed with what he called Freud's "doctrine of homosexuality." In the famous Schreber case, Freud (1911b) hypothesized that repressed homosexual desires were the primary causal factor in paranoia. Sullivan believed that, while extreme anxiety and panic over isoerotic reveries, acts, and abhorrent cravings were frequently found in individuals with paranoid states, so-called homosexual panic was only one possible manifestation of experiences about which the person felt debased and deeply inferior. In fact, Sullivan found that "homosexual panic" indicated far more serious, prior developmental difficulties than anything having to do with lust and represented anxiety and confusion caused by an unacceptable expression of unmet needs for isophyllic intimacy which collided with lust. Sullivan stated that the psychoanalytic technique, which suggested an attack on paranoid beliefs to get at underlying homosexual motivation led to a psychiatric treatment stance which could be stated, "Abandon all hope of a feeling of interpersonal security, and then we might be able to do something" (1956: 164). Sullivan's approach to the understanding of individuals suffering from the difficulties of the paranoid dynamism was but one more example of his extraordinary capacity to discriminate clinical presentation (signs and symptoms) from its underlying function in the personality. Sullivan's empathy and compassion for the interpersonal dilemmas and intense suffering of individuals with severe problems in living, as well as his understanding of the part that the psychotherapist played in maintaining or alleviating this trouble, were the foundation of his unique approach to psychodynamic psychotherapy.

## Personality Disorder: An Interpersonal Perspective

As previously noted, Salzman (1980) and Singer (1990) saw to Sullivan's central approach to explicating recurrent patterns of interpersonal living as the foundation of the modern study of personality disorder. His dynamisms of difficulty described chronic patterns of difficulty in interpersonal trans-actional, rather than symptomatic, terms. Even the term dynamism, and its implication of a dynamic and unfolding processes, has great advantages over the term diagnosis, which provide static and reified symptom clusters without an etiological basis. Among the most controversial elements of the changes in psychiatric diagnosis was the introduction of a second diagnostic category in DSM III (American Psychiatric Association, 1980) called Axis II Personality Disorders. These disorders were set apart from the symptomatic Axis I Mental Disorders, such a depression and anxiety disorders. Heavily influenced by Theodore Millon's biopsychosocial theory (1969, 1981), the DSM III adopted personality disorders as a class of chronic and pervasive mental disorders characterized by engrained maladaptive patterns of behavior, cognition, re-lationships, and inner experience exhibited across many contexts that diverged from acceptable cultural norms. Such patterns began in early development, were rigid across situations, and caused significant distress or functional dis-ability. The goal was developing a systematic diagnostic scheme that differ-entiated distinct personality disorders much the same as other mental disorders in the neo-Kraepelinian tradition.

While Millon's approach was a commendable attempt to marry person-ality theory with modern psychiatric diagnosis of psychopathology, in practice research beyond a few personality disorders has been sparse, clear treatment direction has not emerged for most personality disorders, and what research exists shows limited scientific validity and clinical utility (Clark, Livesley & Morey, 1997). Wright, Ringwald, Hopwood and Pincus outline CIIT's bold alternative, which is to acknowledge that what are called per-sonality disorders are at their core interpersonal disorders. Inspired by Sullivan's interpersonal theory and drawing on many research clinicians such as Leary (1957), Carson (1969), Kiesler (1996), and Benjamin (1995), Pincus, Hopwood, Wright and CIIT colleagues have argued for, and demonstrated empirically, that personality disorders, and indeed psychopathology in gen-eral, are only systematically comprehensible in light of understanding inter-personal processes involving adapations of self, interpersonal relationships, and affect.

Wright, Ringwald, Hopwood & Pincus (accepted for publication) has proposed reconceptualizing personality disorders with a direction called *interpersonal disorders.* This CIIT conceptualization has received strong and growing empirical support and is consistent with the modern shift to using transdiagnostic systems of domains, dimensions, or spectra. They define interpersonal disorder as ...

> Adaptive functioning is defined as a sustained ability to engage inter-personally in ways that coordinate and satisfy the agentic and communal needs of self and other, relatively consistent with one's developmental stage and socio-cultural context, through the flexible, stable, and effective regulation of self, affect, and interpersonal behavior, and dysfunction [is] defined as the sustained breakdown in any of the processes that support and maintain the flexible, stable, and effective regulation of self, affect, and/or interpersonal behavior.
>
> (Wright, Pincus & Hopwood 2020: 266).

In contrast to the DSM definition of personality disorder, the advantage to this fundamentally more sophisticated reframing of psychopathology is that it integrates a structural model, the functional purpose of interpersonal behavior, the importance of context, and dynamic processes over static symptoms. Their model incorporates already established methods of psychological assessment and suggests a clear path toward intervention in psychological treatment. Without a doubt, CIIT is a development of interpersonal theory and practice that carries forward the essence of Sullivan's visionary ideas and takes them to previously unimaginable heights. To get a more detailed view of this exciting advance in the science and practice of psychopathology, the reader is encouraged to read the work of CIIT.

## PTSD as a Human Experience: An Interpersonal Approach

No discussion of Sullivan's interpersonal approach to psychopathology would be complete without the inclusion of the one major modern DSM diagnostic category with specific etiology – post-traumatic stress disorder (PTSD). Of all the early psychoanalytic/psychodynamic thinkers, Sullivan and Erich Fromm were the greatest proponents of understanding the impact of real-life events on interpersonal functioning. Unlike Freud, Sullivan in particular saw how unfortunate life events well beyond early childhood affected the person and was particularly sensitive to what he called 'parental insanity' throughout child and adolescent development. Unlike Kraepelin, interpersonal etiology was central to Sullivan's understanding of psychopathology.

While the early history of the PTSD diagnosis was largely tied to the trauma of war (Kardiner & Spiegel, 1947), van der Kolk's (1987) and Herman's (1992/2015) groundbreaking books opened the broader study of

PTSD as the response to interpersonal violence. Freyd's work (1996) on betrayal trauma and the damage to trust in sexual abuse furthered the discourse about PTSD being an interpersonal problem. On the other hand, from the initial inclusion of PTSD in the 1980 DSM III through the current DSM 5, the neo-Kraepelinian thrust for increased diagnostic reliability was to increasingly emphasize the objectivity of the PTSD symptoms in diagnosis in favor of de-emphasizing the subjectivity of the symptoms (DiMauro et al., 2014), often at the sacrifice of phenomenological validity.

On the other end of the spectrum from the DSM and consistent with current thinking and research, Evans et al. (2023) proposed the term of trauma spectrum disorder to cover psychological disorders ranging from PTSD to complex posttraumatic stress disorder (CPTSD) to dissociative disorder (DD). Unlike the current DSM 5 classification, the research literature strongly suggests that these three disorders lie on a continuum of severity of trauma exposure, duration of multiple exposures, and response to this exposure. For example, as originally proposed by Herman (1992/2015) and validated by extensive research (see Brewin et al., 2017), CPTSD results from multiple traumatic events occurring over a period of time. In addition to the symptoms of PTSD, CPTSD includes symptoms of negative self-concept, affective dysregulation, and perhaps most importantly for this chapter, interprsonal disturbance. Further, it is well established in the research literature that DD is a disorder almost exclusively resulting from severe trauma in childhood (Dalenberg et al., 2012; Putnam, 1985, 1997).

Arising from my clinical work with torture survivors, interpersonal trauma survivors and U.S. military war veterans, I developed an interpersonal understanding of psychological trauma called PTSD as a Human Experience (Evans, 2014, 2015). Much the same as Sullivan did with schizophrenia, the intent of this approach was to focus on trauma survivors' *experience* and the *meaning* of their trauma instead of focusing on correcting symptoms. This approach differs from the common evidence-based (EBT) cognitive behavioral therapies such prolonged-exposure therapy (PET) and cognitive processing therapy (CPT), which are frequently seen as preferred best-practices treatments for PTSD. Indeed, Steenkamp and Litz's (2013: 51) review of outcome studies for PET and CPT PTSD treatment approaches in the U.S. Veterans Administration indicates that "current treatment best practices aimed at ensuring that trauma survivors' access, complete, and benefit from PTSD care remain far from ideal." Cloitre et al. (2006) suggested that focusing on the interpersonal aspects of PTSD may offer another valuable avenue for treatment of trauma survivors. While current manualized EBT approaches share in common the replicable reduction of positive symptoms of PTSD, the addition of an interpersonal, "experience near" understanding of the adaptive value of PTSD symptoms can deepen interpersonal connection with and for trauma survivors. It should be remembered that Carl Rogers (1961), an early proponent of EBT, demonstrated that respect, acceptance, genuineness and empathy are critical components of psycho-therapy outcome. Indeed, Roger's work and subsequent research (see Lambert & Barley, 2001) show that the quality of interpersonal relationship between psychologist and client is crucial to therapeutic growth. The main goal of the interpersonal approach to treatment is to empathically help clients understand themselves better and improve their lives as opposed to "cure" or reduce symptoms with the collaborators in this search for understanding. As such a model for understanding a trauma spectrum disorder must be fundamentally empathic, elucidate the trauma survivors' confusing experiences, and help restore interpersonal and community connections.

Like everyone else labeled as having a mental disorder, trauma survivors are sensitive about being labeled as "crazy" and frequently do not find other people able to relate to their traumatic experiences. Further, by definition, traumatized clients experienced powerlessness and helplessness and are emotionally vulnerable when sharing their traumatic experiences and the impact on their lives. Individuals with trauma spectrum disorders approach treatment in a state of confusion and distress about their experience and are likely to be mistrustful and cautious. Psychotherapy by its nature provokes anxiety in both the client and the therapist, which must be addressed if therapeutic change is to move forward (Cohen, 1952; Fromm-Reichmann, 1949). An "experience-near," empathic understanding of PTSD can help diffuse the stigma of mental illness and diagnostic depersonalization so commonly experienced by trauma survivors.

The interpersonal model begins by reframing the meaning of psychological trauma and PTSD from a medical diagnosis to a comprehensible reaction to overwhelming life experiences. Jeffrey Jay (1991) characterized the horrific experiences and memories of psychological trauma as *"Terrible Knowledge,"* a term which focuses attention on the meaning of the survivor's experience. Almost always these traumatic experiences change the person, disrupting what they believed about life (Janoff-Bulman, 1992). To illustrate, I ask the question, "In your worst experience or nightmare before your traumatic experience, could you possibly imagine what you saw and felt then?" Usually, the trauma survivor says that she or he could not begin to imagine the horrors of war, rape, torture, etc. she or he experienced. I share with the survivor my belief that most of us live in a bubble in which we keep out the horror and evil in the world, if we are lucky. In traumatic exposure, a hole is blown in the bubble, forcing us to see unvarnished the evil that is, and always has been, around us. We as humans are changed by this experience, in a powerful way, alienated from the lives we had before, and often live alone with our memories of these traumas, the Terrible Knowledge of what we experienced. I then ask if he or she knew that his or her experiences are universal, experienced by nearly everyone who encounters Terrible Knowledge. Very often the trauma survivor is surprised by this new way of thinking and is open to hearing more.

Once this grounding is established, the interpersonal approach to psychological trauma assists trauma survivors in understanding the various manifestations of PTSD. Starting with the most biologically driven and ubiquitous aspects of the trauma response, hyperarousal, (see Holowka et al., 2012), the function these "symptoms' are reframed as essential responses for staying alive during traumatic encounters, i.e., "Staying Alive." The survival value of hypervigilance, being alert to potential danger and on guard all the time now that one has been exposed to Terrible Knowledge, is easily seen now that basic trust can no longer be taken for granted. Startle reactions, amplified sensitivity to noise and movement, are also comprehensible as remaining on heightened alert during situations of danger. Nearly ubiquitous sleep difficulties post trauma become understandable as difficulty relaxing vigilance and staying partially alert even when asleep. Concentration problems are reframed as the danger of maintaining narrow focus when maintaining a broad focus is more adaptive when in danger. Heightened irritability and quickness to anger becomes functional when considering the fundamental importance of defending oneself in a life-threatening situation.

This inquiry helps trauma survivors become aware that what they thought, or were told, were symptoms of a mental disorder are highly adaptive responses in the context of their traumatic experiences, which undercuts stigma and dehumanization. These mental disorder "symptoms" are comprehensible human survival reactions, which made it possible for the person to survive the dangerous situation. I also share what we know about extended exposure to highly dangerous situations. As van der Kolk (2015) so eloquently shows, the brain undergoes changes that continue its heightened sensitivity to danger long after leaving the dangerous situation, made worse by repeated traumatic exposures. In a very real way, "Staying Alive" patterns are very much battle scars in the same way as a bullet or mortar fragment wound is.

Van der Kolk's (1987) concept of the biphasic response of psychological trauma is also useful in understanding the function of re-experiencing symptoms and numbing/avoidant symptoms of PTSD. He observed that trauma survivors are predominantly in one or the other of these symptom clusters, but rarely both at the same time. From an interpersonal perspective, these symptom clusters are expressions of two powerful human motivations – our human need to understand our experience and our need to avoid pain which we share with all other animals. With this in mind, the model reframes reexperiencing symptoms such as intrusive memories, nightmares, flashbacks, and traumatic triggers and related panic as "Trying to Comprehend the Incomprehensible" and avoidance and numbing symptoms as "Escaping the Pain of Memory."

As an introduction to discussing intrusive, re-experiencing symptoms, one notes that trauma survivors have involuntarily spent much time trying to understand horrific, overwhelming experiences, which they underwent or witnessed. When asked if any of what they saw makes any sense to them, no matter how hard they have tried, not infrequently they related obsessively reliving terrible memories of their experience without any ability to stop. When asked if it is possible that the traumatic experience makes no sense and that is what is traumatic about it, the trauma survivor will quickly and painfully acknowledge that it makes no sense. Since part of being human is to make sense out of, or derive meaning from, what we do and see, re-experiencing traumatic events reveals fundamental damage to the integrity of our meaning of what it is like to be a human with other humans and this Terrible Knowledge never truly leaves us. Because there is no real answer to this question, the interpersonal model reframes traumatic re-experiencing as trying to "Comprehend the Incomprehensible." As suggested by Jay (1991), it is then possible to introduce one clear idea about the meaning of these ex-periences: It is always better to survive. This discussion often brings up powerful experiences of survivors' guilt, questions about why they survived when someone else did. Deeper meaning can emerge out of these terrible experiences when we embrace the question of what it means to have survived. Now that we have our lives, what is it that we have chosen, or will chose in the future, to do with it. Frequently this question leads to an exploration of how the trauma survivor has lived her or his life after the trauma, along with things undone, done poorly and most importantly done well. Some trauma survivors may come to have a deeper understanding of how precious life is and how trauma helped him or her be a better parent, worker, or marital partner as a result of understanding the fragility of life. Also, keeping trau-matic experiences in mind can provide a special understanding of the danger of the world. Indeed, Janoff-Bulman (1992) has shown that trauma victims who "blame themselves" for what happens to them are often engaging in preparatory recognition of dangerous situations so that they, and those they love, are safer from the vulnerability to the evil of the world around them.

Another aspect of "Comprehending the Incomprehensible" involves traumatic experiences that disrupt the victim's deeply held sense of personal morality and spirituality, a concept often referred to as moral injury (see Griffin et al., 2019). In such instances, some trauma survivors are racked with overwhelming guilt for engaging wittingly or unwittingly in an act so horrible that they are unable to forgive themselves, for example in killing a child during combat. Frequently, loved ones, friends and therapists have counseled Veterans to forgive themselves and let go of the past. Often, to the Veterans' great surprise, such well-meaning sympathy only makes him feel them more wretched, confused, and isolated. To provide context, one can share with the trauma survivor that there is only one thing worse than feeling the unbearable guilt for his actions, which is if he felt nothing at all. The interpersonal model encourages discussion of the difference between feeling unrelenting guilt and maintaining moral integrity through remembrance and bearing witness to the terrible acts of war and speaking of the Veteran's unwillingness to "forgive and forget" as an act of moral courage.

Finally, to understand avoidance and numbing symptoms of PTSD, the interpersonal model helps trauma survivors to re-conceptualize this process as "Escaping the Pain of Memory." Avoiding activities that trigger painful embodied feelings and associated memories is part of our natural human motivation to avoid and escape painful experience, something shared with all animals. Because humans are social animals, "Escaping the Pain of Memory" usually involves avoiding social interaction. Social avoidance is frequently exacerbated by the trauma survivors' feelings of guilt and unworthiness to be part of the human group or even to be alive. The increasing avoidance of life situations, especially social interaction, frequently leads to a diminished interest in pleasurable, life-affirming activities. "Escaping the Pain of Memory" can lead to a depressive disengagement from life and can block the trauma survivors' connection to future hopes, aspirations and connections to others. In its most extreme form, past traumatic memories can be so dissociated that the trauma survivor lives in a world where past, present and future remain disconnected and a confused, befuddled and bewildered state of mind predominates. It has long been known that PTSD has the most chronic and intractable course, when the "Escaping the Pain of Memory" or avoidant symptom cluster of PTSD is a principal mode of dealing with Terrible Knowledge (see Feeny et al., 2000; Litz, 1992).

Within the interpersonal model, a second element of "Escaping the Pain of Memory" involves how emotional numbing can be a protective process for trauma survivors in dealing with overwhelming, sudden, horrific, and tragic loss. The normal human grief reaction is similar to depression with deep sadness, lowered energy, and a turning inward (Peña-Vargas et al., 2021) rather than an aggressive, adrenalized focus on externalized danger to essential survival. As a result, as exposure to traumas mount, the trauma survivors learn, "Don't get close so you don't feel loss." Much like avoidant aspects of "Escaping the Pain of Memory," emotional numbing powerfully generalizes to post-traumatic situations, further robbing survivors of their empathic connection to others and to their internal sense of self. Frequently, trauma survivors share how inhuman and "dead inside" they feel when they cannot cry, or feel much of anything, at the funerals of loved ones or during emotional struggles of their children. Helping trauma survivors see that their reactions are an adaptive response to the nearly incomprehensible suffering of trauma can be a first step to engaging in the courageous and painful process of learning to remember their experiences in a different way and regain lost humanity.

A third and different aspect of posttraumatic avoidance is trauma survivors' reluctance, or even unwillingness, to speak about their traumatic experiences. While this behavior can be a way to manage painful memories, not infrequently trauma survivors really never talk about what happened to them with anyone except possibly other than fellow trauma survivors. Many of trauma survivors are able to share excruciatingly painful memories of their experiences with other trauma survivors, but they will not speak about them with their partners, parents or friends. In this way, this dilemma of avoiding conversations reframed as the need to protect others from seeing the "terrible pictures" in the trauma survivors' minds. Many trauma survivors are powerfully motivated to defend and protect others, often at considerable cost to themselves. Acknowledging their motivation for not sharing this information even with spouses can be a powerful way to empathically connect with trauma survivors, reaffirming their good judgment in doing so.

In closing, the interpersonal model of psychological trauma has considerable value in reframing psychiatric symptoms of PTSD into "experience near" statements regarding the adaptive value of trauma survivors' often bewildering experiences. There is no doubt that the diagnostic accuracy and acumen of the DSM 5 and IV Expert Panels based on strong research has advanced our understanding of the sequelae of psychological trauma. It is then up to clinicians to find ways to translate this knowledge to trauma survivors in order to get "in our clients' shoes" (see Finn, 2007a) and re-engage in a narrative about their experience that allows them to see PTSD as a human experience.

Chapter 8

# The Psychiatric Interview and Modern Interpersonal Personality Assessment

In the first edition of this book, the treatment of the psychological assessment and interpersonal psychotherapy was interwoven. For Sullivan, assessment and treatment were virtually indistinguishable as the dynamic unfolding of the interpersonal treatment relationship required the interplay between assessment, intervention, assessing response to intervention, and forming new interventions, and so forth. As Sullivan (1940/1953, p. 180) stated. "Diagnosis and prognosis cannot be dissociated from therapeutic implications." His participant-observation approach to both assessment and treatment is a defining characteristic of interpersonal theory and practice and one of Sullivan's singular accomplishments, one that has been adopted by modern psychoanalysis, though largely unacknowledged. On the other hand, the worlds of psychotherapists and personality assessors are often (I believe artificially) bifurcated and each group may look for something different from each chapter. So, while the division of this chapter from the next chapter is fundamentally artificial, my hope is that the new chapter will draw personality assessors to think about integration with psychotherapy and psychotherapists will be introduced to how modern forms of personality assessment can be relevant to, and enhance, their practices.

## The Psychiatric Interview

*The Psychiatric Interview* (1954) was the assessment method Sullivan used to achieve the elements of the basic stance in interpersonal psychotherapy discussed in Chapter 9 and a model for personality assessment using the clinical interview. This was most accessible of his writings, loaded with practical advice and wise counsel still valuable today regarding the conduct of interviews in which the objective was to be of "use in the service of" the client. He did not believe in a lock step methodology or inflexible approach to the interview, but a deliberate structured procedure. His interview approach both demonstrated the professional's expertise and provided a relatively orderly and systematic interpersonal event against which he could note variations from individual to individual, without stretching or chopping off the client on

DOI: 10.4324/9781003305712-11

a Procrustean bed of rigid technique. No conceptual treatment of Sullivan's psychiatric interview can do justice to the subtlety and richness of his formulations. Instead, the author must be content to discuss Sullivan's definition of a psychiatric interview, the two central processes of participant observation and parataxic distortion, and the four stages of the psychiatric interview with the hope of encouraging the reader to read Sullivan in the original.

### Definition of the Psychiatric Interview

Sullivan characteristically began his discussion of the psychiatric interview by specifying his basic concepts and, in particular, rendering a precise definition of the psychiatric interview ...

> (A)n interview is a situation of primarily vocal communication in a two-group, more or less voluntarily integrated, on a progressively unfolding expert-client basis for the purpose of elucidating characteristic patterns of living of the subject person, which patterns he experiences as particularly troublesome or especially valuable, and in the revealing of which he expects to derive benefit.
>
> (1954: 4)

Sullivan provided an elaborate, dense, six-part definition, the untangling of which reveals a great deal about his view of the nature of personality assessment and psychotherapy.

Sullivan first described that the interview was an event *utilizing vocal communication*, including not only the verbal and linguistic elements, but also incorporating non-verbal elements as well. Sullivan was among the first major thinkers in psychoanalysis and psychotherapy to write about intonation, rate of speech, and difficulty in enunciation, anticipating major psychotherapy research findings on the critical importance of non-verbal elements of therapeutic communication. Sullivan explored the role of non-verbal behavior, taking it out of the realm of "intuition" into the field of scientific study, using wire and tape recordings to validate his clinical impressions (Will, 1954: x). The research of Mahl (1968) and Mehrabian (1972) found strong empirical support Sullivan's ideas, discovering that the non-verbal and vocal components of communication are often more informative than the denotative meaning of words. Beginning with his work with schizophrenics, Sullivan learned to be extraordinarily sensitive to non-verbal signs of discomfort as part of his management of interpersonal security within the interview. Sullivan's emphasis on understanding non-verbal behavior presaged modern body-focused approaches to psychotherapy such as Rothschild (2002), Westland (2015) and Ron Kurtz (Kurtz & Prestera, 1977).

The second aspect of the definition, *the idea of the two group*, contained two distinct components. Ever mindful of the importance of the sociological characteristics of the interpersonal situation of the psychiatrist and client, Sullivan pointed out that the psychiatric interview took place in a dyad. Properties of the dyad were different than other social situations and inferences about processes found in the interview must not be automatically assumed to occur in other social configurations. Implied in this part of the definition was that other social configurations could be useful in psychotherapy, opening the door for milieu, group, and family psychotherapy. Additionally, Sullivan emphasized that the interview took place in a two group to remind the psychotherapist that there were only two real people in the room and that "the number of the more or less imaginary people who get themselves involved in this two-group is sometimes really hair-raising" (1954: 9). Based on his concept of illusory two-groups, Sullivan cautioned the interviewer to remain aware that the processes of personification and parataxic distortion were ever present.

Third, by considering the degree to which the psychiatric interview was *voluntarily integrated*, Sullivan continued to remind the psychotherapist to consider the social context of the person coming to treatment. The psychiatric interview will be greatly affected by whether the client comes in order to better understand him or herself, to suit a parent, spouse, or employer, or to meet a legal requirement. Sullivan understood that, even in the best of circumstances, people entered treatment with mixed motivations about whether they were ready to engage in frank discussion or whether they came to meet outside social requirements. Naturally Sullivan explored the more or less voluntary nature of the psychotherapist's position as well, noting that attitudes of willingness and unwillingness on the part of the psychotherapist were important factors that dramatically affected treatment. What has often been called resistance in the psychoanalytic literature could be seen from an interpersonal perspective as an artifact of the client's assumption of the social setting with the psychotherapist. For example, if a reluctant, troubled adolescent patient perceived that the therapist, who is paid by the family, would share information with a disparaging parent, the patient's uncommunicativeness would continue until his or her concern was aired and the social context was clarified. The patient's "resistance" to speak openly would not be an example of simply clinging to neurotic symptoms, but a real consequence of the social context. Sullivan knew that being clear on the client's social context in coming to the interviewed determined how he or she cognitively formulated the interaction (see Levinson et al., 1967 excellent analysis of becoming a patient). Two studies conducted by Lazare and his associates (Lazare et al., 1972; Lazare et al., 1975) are illustrative. Their research explored why people came for a psychiatric consultation in a walk-in clinic and discovered twenty different reasons for seeking assistance. Of these only two fell under the rubric of what could be seen as traditional psychotherapy, leading Lazare and his associates to recommend that mental health professionals should not assume that the reasons people came had to do with entering treatment and taking an initial interview stance of reaching a negotiative consensus about the services desired and offered. Sullivan was again ahead of his time, taking an approach to the psychiatric interview which grew out of his acute sensitivity to the realities of the social context.

The fourth aspect of Sullivan's concept of the psychiatric interview was the expert-client relationship. In marked variance with Freud's conceptualization of the psychoanalyst, Sullivan's definition established the role of the psychotherapist as an expert in interpersonal relations, a concept that is embodied throughout the later discussion of Sullivan's basic stance. The therapist's expertise was critical in formulating a stance which established and maintained interpersonal security, ascertained the interpersonal learning necessary to correct inadequate interpersonal patterns, and tailored the therapeutic intervention to fit the problem. Sullivan repeatedly emphasized that this expertise was communicated by carefully listening to the client's experience of his or her difficulty and not by hearing therapist's preconceptions about the client. As such, the client was not a "patient" (as in one who waits patiently), but a person who collaborated actively with the therapist-expert. Sullivan believed that such a stance undercut the client's godlike expectations of the therapist, focused the therapist more on the client's experiences and interests, and modeled a more fundamentally sound example of authority. Like Freud (1912b), Sullivan stressed that the psychotherapist should not use relations with the client for gratification, either in a personal or business sense, should not traffic in prestige or standing in the eyes of the client, and should never become the client's companion. A Sullivan stated (1954: 12), "Only if he is keenly aware of this can the expert-client relationship in this field be consolidated rapidly and with reasonable ease." As mentioned above Sullivan's concept of demonstrating expertise was strongly supported by Frank's (1982) research on the common factors of effective psychotherapy.

The fifth component of the psychiatric interview was the *elucidation of characteristic patterns of living patterns which the client experienced as particularly troublesome or especially valuable.* While elucidation of characteristic patterns of living patterns will be discussed extensively in the next chapter's section on facilitating interpersonal learning as the goal of treatment, Sullivan noted that the psychiatric interview emphasized exploration of ...

> obscure difficulties in living which the patient does not clearly understand, that which for cultural reasons-reasons of his particular education for life – he is foggy about, chronically misleads himself about, or misleads others about.
>
> (1954: 14–15).

As part of this process, Sullivan's definition of the psychiatric interview required the psychotherapist to examine "patterns of living, some of which make trouble for the patient"(1954: 13). He warned not to focus exclusively or too heavily on the problems of living without getting a picture of rest of the person in context of the total personality. The expert-client inquiry into the better functioning parts of the personality promoted elucidating inter-personal resources so that the client could "build on sources of existing vitality," to use the words of educator Sampson G. Smith (1972), who like Sullivan was influenced by the philosopher John Dewey. Additionally, Sullivan's insistence on the elucidation of the especially valuable patterns of living served as an invaluable counterbalance to psychotherapists' tendency to look primarily at mental disorder. For Sullivan, by accurately and sys-tematically including and building the client's good-me personifications, the client could more readily tackle the difficult business of confronting bad-me and not-me personifications. Exploring valuable patterns of living oper-ationalized Sullivan's one genus hypothesis (we are simply more human than otherwise) which broke down the division of the well and the sick between the doctor and patient.

The sixth and last piece of Sullivan's definition was *the client's ex-pectation of benefit*. While Sullivan believed that this idea did not sound very impressive, it served as a direct critique and corrective to the growing notion of psychoanalysis as scientific education, which purported that what the patient desired was simple explanatory truth via a scientific exploration of the personality (see Szasz's, 1957 analysis of Freud's position). Sullivan, and later Fairbairn (1958), strenuously objected to this definition of the goals of treatment, stating instead that the client came for relief from conflict and suffering. Sullivan also believed that keeping the expected benefit in front of both the therapist and client sharpened the particular goals of treatment, kept them focused on meeting these goals, and served as a quid pro quo for the considerable trouble of being honest about diffi-culties and personal failure required for effective treatment. Additionally, having a definite idea about what the client expects to gain from treatment made it clear that the therapist worked in service of the client. In Sullivan's approach to treatment, client was not a seeker to be converted to the better reality of the stronger therapist, but an individual employing an expert to assist in understanding and correcting problematic interpersonal patterns. Sullivan believed that this latter attitude led to the best interview, which reduced one-sided expectation that the answer to life's troubles resided in the psychotherapist, if the clients need only to apply themselves to the doctor's prescription. This aspect of Sullivan's model of treatment antici-pated the most important current trend in modern psychotherapy research and social policy, the determination of the effectiveness of psycho-therapeutic approaches (see Leichsenring & Rabung, 2008; Parloff, 1980; Smith et al., 1980; Seligman, 1995b).

Sullivan's definition of the psychiatric interview established a structure for treatment that sensitively outlined the social context of the interview, discussed the roles of the participants, described the work to be done, and established the necessity of a measure of success. It incorporated ideas about important dimensions of the process and outcome of psychotherapy which are taken for granted today, ideas for which Sullivan has received limited acknowledgment. Before turning to the stages of the psychiatric interview, we shall turn briefly to the two important processes found in all interviews and in all human interaction – participant observation and parataxic distortion.

## Participant Observation and Parataxic Distortion

Perhaps Sullivan's most original and valuable contribution to the field of psychotherapy was his explication of the psychotherapist as a *participant observer* ...

> the psychiatrist cannot stand off to the side and apply his sense organs ... without becoming personally implicated in the process ... His primary instrument of observation is his self – his personality, him as a person ... There are no purely objective data in psychiatry, and there are no valid subjective data ... because the material becomes scientifically useful only in the shape of a complex resultant-inference.
>
> (1954: 3)

The determining effect of the therapist upon all interactions and processes in psychotherapy became critical to an in-depth understanding of the therapist's role. Because of this inevitable interpersonal influence, the psychotherapist needed to be ever-alert to his participation in the psychiatric interview, on how his behaviors and idiosyncrasies impact on the client. Throughout the interview, the psychotherapist was charged with understanding through careful observation the client's specific reactions to the therapist, that all the patient does and says is more or less addressed to the therapist. Underlying Sullivan's concept of participant observation was the idea, long since confirmed by social-cognitive psychologists (see Bandura, 1977), that humans actively monitor their social behavior and interactions according to the expectations of social acceptance and rejection.

For Sullivan, even silence was a form of interpersonal participation, and a powerful method of social influence at that. Sullivan believed that the Freudian concepts of therapist neutrality, the blank screen, and free association fundamentally misconstrued the interpersonal nature of all psychotherapeutic interaction. Neutrality, silence, and the blank screen could be easily experienced as indifference by many clients which would affect a distorting influence on the relationship. Sullivan believed if the client could simply sit back and speak freely without being concerned about to trying impress the psychotherapist, maintain esteem in the therapist's eyes, or avoid imagined disapproval, then he or she was unlikely to need the psychotherapy in the first place. The participant observer role of the therapist led Sullivan in a far different direction than Freud regarding therapeutic technique or conduct in the interview. Since participation with the patient was an inevitable part of the role of therapist, Sullivan conceived of treatment as engagement, that is, being engaged to assist client in speaking openly on all matters, including the difficult business of his or her experience of the therapist, without undue effects of insecurity. Sullivan favored the give and take of human dialogue and used consensual validation to clarify meanings of each participant to the other. In essence, for Sullivan, "the concept of participant observation defines psychotherapy" Chapman (1976: 116).

The other significant process within the psychiatric interview was that of *parataxic distortion*, "the really astonishing misunderstandings and misconceptions that characterize all human relations ... (which is) also one way that the personality displays before another some of its gravest problems" (1954: 25). From this definition, it is easy to ascertain the two ways in which Sullivan defined this concept. In the narrower sense of the term, Sullivan used parataxic distortion to describe when the client unwittingly perceived and treated another person as if the other person was similar to a significant relationship from the past. In this narrow sense, parataxic distortion bears a similarity with Freud's (1910a, 1912c; 1915c) concept of transference. Like Freud, Sullivan saw parataxic distortions involving a misapplication of problematic early interpersonal experiences of the past to present relationships, but there the similarities ended. Freud's concept of transference referred to the very specific transfer of repressed, erotic Oedipal feelings toward the parent to the person of the psychoanalyst. Only later did Freud use the term in a slightly broader way, including a vaguely elaboration of negative experiences within the therapeutic relationship. Sullivan had little regard for Freud's notion of the Oedipal complex and focused his concept of parataxic distortion on what he called "illusory me-you patterns" arising from all manner of anxiety-ridden early experience and not simply the so-called "sexual preoccupations of the young." In this narrower sense, Sullivan's concept of parataxic distortion implied a regressive experience in the early parataxic mode of experience. For example, severe, repeated humiliating early experiences with a mother could lead the individual to anticipate pain and humiliation in all relationships with women, a problem that could stunt healthy development of intimacy with women. In the broader definition of parataxic distortion, Sullivan saw this process of as a variant of the human tendency toward misconception or incorrect interpersonal attribution, an aspect of the concept not addressed by Freud. In treatment, Sullivan observed the operation of parataxic distortion in the client's discussions about others as well as in the interactions within the consulting room and believed that failure to observe and clarify these processes would inevitably lead to treatment failure.

## Stages of the Psychiatric Interview

With characteristic humility about the incompleteness of the state of scientific knowledge about psychiatry, Sullivan believed that a structure for developing a relationship with a client was a necessary starting place, which he called a *methodic procedure*. He made no claims that his four stage procedure was necessarily correct; it constituted his best thoughts on the matter, which would be open to modification when a better method was found. He did strongly believe that orderly conduct of psychotherapy was necessary as a way in which the therapist imparted expertise to the client.

### The Formal Inception

The first stage, *the formal inception*, involved the psychotherapist's first encounter with the client. Sullivan believed strongly this initial interaction set the tone for the psychotherapist's and client's work together. The formal inception involved the way the client was initially received by the therapist as well as the inquiry into circumstances that brought the client for consultation. Sullivan began with a respectfully serious greeting of the patient, remembering that the person seeking consultation was a stranger. Sullivan eschewed any gestures of undo familiarity and encouraged the psychotherapist to remember the feelings of discomfort associated with being a stranger. The psychotherapist must be very alert to the impressions that he or she gives to the client, especially given that he or she does not know the client's background or the client's characteristic parataxic distortions of relationships. Naturally, the psychotherapist should be careful to note his or her feelings about and reactions to the client, as these are invaluable information about the client and can assist the therapist in avoiding pitfalls created by the denial of his or her own experience. Sullivan cautioned that, if the psychotherapist could not relatively quickly understand and get beyond initial powerful feelings of dislike for the patient, that it was incumbent on the psychotherapist to either refer the client or end the interview appropriately. As part of this reception, the psychotherapist should give a "brief, but considered" synopsis of any information he or she had received about the client, to promote the client's confidence in the psychotherapist's straightforwardness about interpersonal matters and to give the client the chance to correct any information gathered from other sources. Additionally, this synopsis demonstrated respect for the client's experience and established a model of consensual validation and negotiated consensus (see Levinson et al.'s 1967 study of initial encounters with mental health professionals). Sullivan (1954: 56) stated that the way the psychotherapist conducted the reception of the client "can either greatly accelerate the achievement of the result desired or it can make the result practically unattainable."

The second task of the formal inception was the identification of the client's reason for seeking assistance. Sullivan believed that this task was best accomplished by attending primarily to the client's experience of his or her difficulties or confusions for which he or she sought consultation. For Sullivan, it was critical to get clear very early about what the person saw as the difficulty, how the difficult seemed to develop, how it was affecting the person's life at present, and why the client came for help at this time. While Sullivan was deeply curious about the client's background, he delayed taking a significant interpersonal history until he had a good idea of what troubled the client, stated in terms of the client's experience, and what expectations the client had about the treatment. Sullivan emphasized from the start the collaborative nature of treatment and believed that it was necessary to be able to state, in terms that the client clearly understood, what benefit the client hoped to gain from the collaboration. Sullivan recommended exploring how the client thought that psychotherapy might be of help, including prior experiences with treatment. He thought little could be gained by challenging the client on his or her perception of the prior treatment, suggesting instead that the client's past negative therapeutic experiences be taken at face value. While keeping an open mind that the client's parataxic experience may (but not necessarily) have played a significant role in the difficulty, Sullivan was certainly opposed to the idea of the therapist taking the position of "my profession, right or wrong." Sullivan believed that the formal inception should end with a summary statement by the therapist about the general work that the client and therapist had agreed to undertake, encouraging any disagreements or modifications from the client. Margaret Rioch (1970), a student of Sullivan, more accurately called this aspect of the formal inception establishing of the therapeutic contract. As Sullivan (1954: 69) stated, "By the end of the first stage the patient should come to feel, 'Well, now the doctor knows why I am here.'"

*Case Study – The Hidden Ms. T¹*

To further illustrate the principles of both the psychiatric interview in this chapter and interpersonal psychotherapy in the next chapter, I provide a case study of a 55-year-old woman whom I treated for over four years in intensive interpersonal psychotherapy. I present the case as it unfolded, starting with the informal reception below and continuing through the four stages of the psychiatric interview after a description of each stage. Further, I have also provided case comments after each of the three major elements of interpersonal psychotherapy in Chapter 9. Following the guidance of Gabbard (2000), I have disguised the identity of the "client" to formulate this illustrative case study by amalgamating aspects of several different clients with similar difficulties.

*Ms. T and the Formal Inception*

I was approached by an experienced psychiatrist, Dr. P. at a university psychiatry department clinic for a consultation and possible psychotherapy referral of a middle-aged female, Ms. T, who was in treatment for psychiatric medication and supportive therapy for several years. Dr. P recently heard a Grand Rounds presentation I gave about my interpersonal approach to psychological trauma and she wondered if her client might have a trauma history. Dr. P shared that psychiatric medication had provided some relief for Ms. T, but not to the degree that Dr. P had hoped. Parenthetically, I noted an unusual discomfort in Dr. P as she described her client. Additionally, but she did not appear to have detailed knowledge of Ms. T's personal history. She and I agreed that I would meet with Ms. T for an initial assessment to determine whether I believed I might provide some help for her. After speaking with her client, Dr. P said that Ms. T was somewhat willing to try an initial assessment and I arranged for an appointment time.

On the date of the appointment, I greeted Ms. T in the waiting area, noticing that she sat where she could see all different entrances into the room. From a distance, Ms. T appeared timid and flat emotionally and I was concerned that beginning with too much intimacy might well be experienced by her as intrusive. I decided not to offer her a greeting handshake or make much eye contact and chose instead an initial brief verbal greeting ("I am Dr. Barton Evans. Might you be here to see me?") Once seated in the office chairs at my usual ninety-degree angle, I observed that Ms. T continued to avoid eye contact and waited for me to begin. I began the session by introducing myself as a psychologist and professor and stated that I believed we had two tasks in our first meeting – for me to find out what Ms. T might like my help with and for her to ask me any questions she might have about my approach to psychotherapy and experience that would help her to decide whether she would like to work together. Before turning to these tasks, I said that I first wanted to share what I knew about the background of her treatment with Dr. P and ask her for any corrections or additions to this information. Ms. T indicated that she had nothing to correct (and did not add anything). During my introduction, I noted a brief moment of surprise and interest in Ms. T before she retreated back to her flat emotional front, which I speculated to myself as her fearful and protective defense against interpersonal closeness. I quickly tested my hypothesis by asking her if she had been in individual psychotherapy before and how it had gone. Ms. T impassively shared that she had been in both individual and group therapy and had not gotten much from it, providing me important information that her potential parataxic distortion toward me was to see me as likely to be unhelpful and unattuned. As a counterprojective intervention, I replied that her past unhelpful encounters with psychotherapy were not at all uncommon in my experience. I suggested that we needed to pay close attention together to assess whether our time together was helpful or a waste of her time so that she could decide whether to continue or not. Again, I noticed a fleeting sense of surprise and interest quickly followed by relational retreat.

I next made a mildly abrupt shift, briefly restating our two tasks for the session, and asked where Ms. T would like to start. She became uncomfortable, which I again hypothesized as her fear of intrusion by a more powerful other. I tested my assumption by reducing the relational pressure on her, offering to share something about myself first, if she preferred. Ms. T nodded assent and I shared details designed to hopefully provide some reassurance for her. Laying groundwork for establishing a collaborative expert-client relationship is an important goal of the formal inception. Instilling hope for the client (see Frank, 1973) and confidence in the psychotherapist as an expert in interpersonal living is a central element of successful interpersonal therapy and discerningly sharing expertise can be of significant value with especially reluctant clients. I disclosed that I was a clinical psychologist with over 45 years of psychotherapy experience, who had regularly taught in universities and medical schools. I noted that I had published several books and many professional articles and presented over 200 workshops in the U.S. and around the world. I noticed that Ms. T appeared less physically tense and more interested, with increased eye contact, so I decided next to share that the bulk of my psychotherapy practice was with individuals who did not get much benefit from multiple prior therapies. To my surprise and secret delight, Ms. T asked if I had much success with these clients and I responded quite simply, yes, that most of the time I had. Again, not wanting to provide pressure at this time, I then asked if she would like to know anything further, to which she said no. I followed by saying that I always welcomed questions and disagreements and hoped that Ms. T would feel free to voice them when these arose for her. I shared my conviction that a client sharing her disagreement was always valuable, and even essential, for a psychotherapist to correct misimpressions. I also told Ms. T that I had three different responses to questions, one was to simply answer the question, the other was to first ask the client to elaborate on the question before addressing, and the third was not to answer. This last response meant one thing and one thing only, that the question was a great one, but probably best answered by the client herself.

The remainder of the initial session and formal inception was spent assisting Ms. T to elaborate on what she wished to gain from psychotherapy. As the focus shifted to her, Ms. T's anxiety rose dramatically, making it difficult for her to think and speak. Her reaction again suggested that she experienced a powerful sense of danger in expressing agency. Her distress indicated to me that providing her with interpersonal security in this session and beyond was an essential first step, while slowly enhancing her capacity to speak her suppressed longing for help. As Fairbairn (1958) so cogently stated, psychotherapy is a cure by the hair of the dog that bit you.

Therefore, titrating approaching the interpersonal closeness of Ms. T revealing herself, while maintaining sufficient security against anxiety about intrusion, became paramount. With her permission, I gently questioned her about her current treatment and what she found helpful and less so. I experienced her as becoming less anxious as I shared her considerable burden of revealing what she might want from psychotherapy. What emerged was that Ms. T was taking numerous (six) strong psychiatric medications, including anxiolytic, anti-psychotic and mood stabilizing drugs, which, while somewhat moderating her depression and anxiety, left her mentally foggy and physically logy with little energy to do much. She shared that she had not worked since her last psychiatric hospitalization four years previously and lived in a basement apartment in her parents' home. I invited Ms. T to consider that interpersonal psychotherapy might provide some relief from anxiety and depression in addition to the medications she was taking and that we could take some steps to see if psychotherapy could be of use to her. As the initial session drew to an end, I provided a verbal summary of what we covered and she decided to come back for at least one more session. I experienced Ms. T as leaving a bit more curious and less frozen than upon our initial meeting.

### The Reconnaissance

The *reconnaissance* was the second stage of Sullivan's psychiatric interview. Whereas the formal inception involved greeting the client and finding out the reason he or she came for consultation, the reconnaissance involved obtaining a rough outline of the client's interpersonal and developmental history. As Sullivan (1954: 69) stated, following the formal inception, "The psychiatrist can then say, in effect. 'Well, who are you?'" The goal of the reconnaissance is to discover what kind of person the client is and how he/she came to be this way. Sullivan believed that, while the tasks of the formal inception and the reconnaissance were different, there should be a smooth transition between them, as naturally as possible. Sullivan emphasized that the reconnaissance was not a psychiatric history, but rather a history of the person. Sullivan's outline for obtaining interpersonal data involved asking conventional questions about age, family of origin, birth order of the siblings, and the work history and economic status of family of origin. Next, he shifted the interview from questions of fact to a more interpersonal focus. Sullivan introduced this shift by inquiring what kind of person the client's father was, alerting the client to begin to think more deeply about the nature of his or her interpersonal connections. Interestingly Sullivan recommended that the client describe his or her mother as he found most people had only a vague conception of their mother as a person. He then asked the client about his or her own educational and work history, although with more interpersonal focus than the initial inquiries. Sullivan inquired about marriage with the question,

"Why did you marry?" again orienting the client to examine his or her interpersonal world. This stage of the interview began the identification of characteristic patterns in the client's interpersonal world, especially the client's areas of anxiety and characteristic assumptions about people. The reconnaissance for most interviews was not highly detailed but had the purpose for the therapist to "orient himself as to certain basic probabilities" (1954: 38) about the client. Yet even here Sullivan stressed the importance of accuracy and detail through close, alert listening and inquiry, not simply asking of questions and obtaining answers. As he stated (1954: 38), "The skill of the interviewer in obtaining and interpreting this history may often largely determine the ease or difficulty of the succeeding detailed inquiry."

The reconnaissance could last anywhere from 20 minutes for one- or two-session brief encounters, to over three months in intensive psychotherapy. In intensive psychotherapy, there was not a sharp differentiation between the reconnaissance and the next stage, *the detailed inquiry*. Sullivan believed that, regardless of the length of the encounter, it was sometimes more useful for the client to go into detail when things came up than to artificially move in lock-step fashion through the various stages. An interesting aspect of Sullivan's reconnaissance was his frequent suggestion to clients to write a chronology of important life events, encouraging clients to reflect on their interpersonal experiences outside of the interview. As with the formal inception, Sullivan ended the reconnaissance with a summary. As before, the summary informed the client what the therapist had heard and placed the presenting problem in the context of the person's history and the rest of the personality. Additionally, the summary provided for the client a concise outline of his or her major difficulties in living, which constituted the major direction of treatment. As Sullivan (1954: 88) commented, "Without this statement of a problem of living, treatment situations are apt to be quite defeating." While the establishment of a clear focus was necessary for all good treatment, Sullivan cautioned that some problems were too difficult and too anxiety provoking for the client. In such instances, the psychotherapist used his or her expertise to provide appropriate approximations to the primary problem in living. Sullivan stressed that the psychiatric interview should be problem-focused and economical of the client's time, therefore differing significantly from classical psychoanalytic techniques, the lack of structure of which Sullivan believed often triggered problematic security operations. Sullivan believed that therapeutic summary demonstrated expertise, was very illuminating for both client and therapist, and established the first step in the education about how psychotherapy works.

### The Hidden Ms. T and the Reconnaissance

When I came to the waiting room for her second session, Ms. T was seated in her familiar spot, again where she could see all entrances in and out of the room. She again looked weary and emotionally remote, but I noticed that she made eye contact with me when I entered the room. Once in the office, I asked Ms. T if she had any questions about our first session, or anything in particular she wanted to discuss today (parenthetically, every session hence-forth would begin this way), to which she replied, "No." I then said that I wanted to get to know her better and would she mind if I asked her some questions about her as a person. I quickly added that I wanted to know in depth about her mental health treatment history and what currently troubled her or made her feel better, but I found it more helpful first to get a sense of who she was. Interpersonal diagnosis and psychotherapy emphasize under-standing the person, both her problems in living and advantageous char-acteristics, rather than simply focusing on symptoms of mental disorder so common in psychiatric and other mental settings. Ms. T seemed surprised by this approach, reacting with a mix of anxiety and interest, capturing the dilemma a psychotherapist faced working with her – how to provide sufficient interpersonal security whilst engaging her curiosity and motivation toward personal growth.

I began by asking what I thought were fairly safe questions about her background, remaining alert to surprises by paying particular attention to any rise in anxiety. Ms. T revealed that she had lived with her parents since returning from a psychiatric hospitalization several years before at which time she was no longer able to work in her job. When I asked how things were going with her parents, I noticed a rise in anxiety and Ms. T quickly stated that she was grateful to her parents for providing her a place to stay as she no longer felt safe living in the apartment she owned. To provide safety, I gently switched topics and asked if she had sisters or brothers, to which she replied that she was the oldest of three siblings with a brother and a sister. Her sister, the youngest, lived close by her parents and regularly visited, while her brother lived some distance away and rarely visited because he was busy with work and family. Her brief statement about her brother was accompanied by a rise in anxiety, so I asked about her sister, whom she said was married with two children and a homemaker. I detected a note of sadness in her response and asked her about her marital status. Ms. T rather lifelessly stated that she had never been married or engaged, adding that she was very wedded to her career during her late twenties well into her 40s. I asked what work she did, she matter-of-factly replied she worked as an administrator in a medium-sized company, quickly adding that had not worked in a number of years. I enquired about Ms. T's experience of work to which she replied that she had found it increasingly difficult until her depression and anxiety became too much to continue. She volunteered that she had become increasingly driven during her last year of work, unable to get regular sleep or to maintain concentration on her work, until she reached a point of psy-chological confusion and collapse from which she had been unable to bounce back. I shared that I wanted to know more about this time in her life and what led up to it, but I could see how depressing and frightening this collapse and resulting malaise must be for her. Ms. T appeared more engaged at this point than at any time in our two prior sessions.

As time was ending for this second session, I summarized what I had learned about her, underscoring how her psychological upheaval had so powerfully interrupted her life. In doing so, I was attempting to help Ms. T to separate her severe psychological difficulties from her prior successful functioning as a step towards helping her regain her personal identity beyond her troubles and disturbing psychiatric diagnoses. I stated that I believed that psychotherapy could be of benefit to her, but we would need to proceed carefully for me to understand more about her experience. I suggested that we meet weekly for ten sessions to explore her situation further with the understanding that she could stop any time if the treatment was not helpful. Ms. T agreed and then asked if we might meet less frequently. When I asked her why, she said that her mother drove her to sessions and she did not wish to inconvenience her. I asked Ms. T how far she needed to come to the office (20 minutes) and asked if her mother had expressed being inconvenienced (she had not so long as she was home in time to fix dinner for her husband). I queried Ms. T about whether she had a car and had driven recently. Ms. T said that, while she lacked confidence, she drove herself to psychiatrist meetings numerous times when her mother was unavailable. I expressed my strong preference for regular weekly sessions in order to develop a sense of continuity and wondered if Ms. T might be willing to see how coming weekly went for her. I also offered work together with her to see if we could help her feel freer to drive, releasing her mother altogether from inconvenience, except perhaps on days Ms. T felt especially uncomfortable driving herself. Ms. T agreed to try this arrangement and we set a mutually convenient time for the next week.

In the subsequent ten reconnaissance sessions, Ms. T and I carefully elaborated an outline of her personal and mental health history. I opened each session with an invitation to discuss how the previous session went for her and whether there was something she would like my help with. Each time, and for many months after, Ms. T declined, suggesting that her capacity to tolerate agency without undue anxiety was insufficient at this time. To bind her anxiety, I mimicked a dominant agentic role by leading an increasingly in-depth exploration of her family history, work history and relationship history, while gently focusing on how she experienced these events to allow her inner emotional life to slowly emerge.

Ms. T elaborated on her history, emphasizing her history of psychological difficulties, which I hypothesized was her most prominent self-identity and possibly a way of warding off others' expectations of her. She shared that she had been hospitalized psychiatrically twice as an adult, first in her early 40s for "anorexia" and several years later for "depression and anxiety." Ms. T related that she became obsessed with her appearance in her late 30s and restricted her eating, never able to quell her belief that she was obese, which she maintained to the present. I observed that she was hardly morbidly obese. After her first hospitalization, she lost her job as an administrator for a company and found herself unable to apply for new work. After her second hospitalization, Ms. T was assisted in applying successfully for disability due to mental disorder.

Attempting to balance her self-narrative as a mentally disabled individual, I queried Ms. T about her work life before her hospitalizations. She indicated that she worked as an administrator for a local mid-level size corporation. During detailed questioning, she revealed she was the head of one the corporation's most important division in the role of vice president. Ms. T said that she rose from a staff position right out of university to vice president over the course of six years. She stated that she did "pretty well" at university, disclosing that she graduated with all top marks, again only after careful questioning. Ms. T indicated that she was also a straight A student in school who never caused trouble for her parents. At the age of 17, Ms. T disclosed that she suffered a "mental breakdown" the details about which she was vague and was hospitalized for several weeks. She subsequently remained at home with her parents until her early twenties and was terrified to leave home and be in the company of others. She eventually summoned the courage to complete a high school equivalency diploma and excelled at a local community college. Growing confident because of her successes, Ms. T transferred to a full university several hundred miles from her home and lived on campus, spending almost all of her time studying with very limited social interaction. She appeared noticeably sad as she recounted her past successes, though not with an accompanying rise in anxiety or emotional shutdown. I had a strong suspicion that Ms. T had experienced a horrifying event when she was 17, but I did not think her capacity sufficient to tolerate disclosing this experience.

As our initial ten-week contract, marking the end of the reconnaissance phase of interpersonal psychotherapy, was coming to an end, Ms. T and I agreed that continue on an open-ended basis with the understanding that, if she did not experience psychotherapy as beneficial, she would let me know. At this point in our work, I affirmed that she had had several serious interruptions in an otherwise productive life course, which over time had depleted her and left her riddled with anxiety, loss, and self-doubt. We agreed to work together to understand what was behind her life disruptions with an eye toward helping her reduce her anxiety and depression and perhaps even regain a life purpose, which was now sorely lacking. Throughout the course of the reconnaissance, Ms. T gradually became more present and participated more actively in her psychotherapy.

### The Detailed Inquiry

Sullivan's discussion of the third stage of the psychiatric interview, *the detailed inquiry*, took up about half of *The Psychiatric Interview*, describing the processes of what might be called the psychotherapy proper. As Sullivan stated, what happened in the detailed inquiry depended on the purpose of the interview. Throughout his writing on the psychiatric interview and psychotherapy, Sullivan (1954: 38) insisted on the fact that all therapeutic work must be done in context to the task, "he never carries out a good interview if he forgets what it is really for – namely, to permit an expert in human relations to contribute something to the other person's success in living." This third stage of the interview involved literally a detailed inquiry into the nature of the client's inadequate and inappropriate interpersonal relations, the task mutually agreed upon by the therapist and client. Sullivan described the importance of a broad elaboration of developmental history, which followed closely the developmental model in his interpersonal theory. He explored many of the elements of the client's early life, including toilet training, language development, early school adjustment, and juvenile social development (peer interactions, activities and sports, attitudes toward competition and compromise, ambitions). Additionally, he examined the client's preadolescent and adolescent interpersonal world including presence of a chum, puberty, early adolescent issues, and relationships (body image, sexual preference, use of drugs and alcohol, attitudes about solitude), adolescent school adjustment, sleep functions, and sexuality. Finally, Sullivan inquired about adult adaptation, including adjustment to college, courtship and marriage, parenthood, vocational history, and adult avocational interests. In the formal inception, Sullivan had obtained the client's description of his or her current interpersonal difficulties, which was further examined during the detailed inquiry. Throughout this detailed inquiry into the client's past history and current relationships and social interactions, Sullivan listened for the operation of anxiety, the self-system, and problematic personifications in interpersonal life.

Beginning with Jacobson (1955), a major misconception about Sullivan's approach to psychotherapy has been that he was only interested in the external social events of the client's life and formulated his conception of the patient primarily on social history. While Sullivan did strongly believe in the importance of deeply understanding the client's history and current relationships, he noted his ongoing skepticism on the absolute veracity of this information. He placed far more confidence in the information gained through the observation and examination of the interpersonal process within the interview, that is, the client's relationship to the psychotherapist, as the most reliable source of information about interpersonal disturbance. It was Sullivan's perspective that, because of the effects of anxiety on cognition and memory, much of the important information about the client was unavailable to him or her. The influence of anxiety could be accurately seen by either the deterioration or improvement of communication in the here-and-now process within the interview. The operation of selective inattention, which the therapist noticed by observing the restriction of awareness and the avoidance of painful topics, allowed the therapist to draw inferences about the workings of anxiety. In turn, by skillfully exploring areas of avoidance, in particular what these processes did to interpersonal relations, the therapist could safely interrupt the process of selective inattention and bring back dissociated experience into awareness. Perhaps even more significant for Sullivan was the therapist's experience of reciprocal emotion during the interview. For Sullivan, the therapist was a participant observer whose direct experience of the client revealed the client's characteristic personifications and parataxic distortions. Sullivan (1954: 3) believed of the psychotherapist that, "His primary instrument of observation is his self – his personality, him as a person." It was only through this instrument that the troubled interpersonal expectations of the client could be fully revealed. Within the framework of interpersonal psychotherapy, the therapist had to sufficiently open his person to the client to allow for reciprocal emotion. The therapist had to tolerate being whatever troubled interpersonal perception that client placed on him or her and be aware of his or her own real contributions to the client's anxiety as well (see Mabel Blake Cohen's, 1952 excellent analysis of countertransference and anxiety from an interpersonal perspective). Only through careful exploration of the meaning of the parataxic distortions of the therapist could the client truly and deeply become aware of, and overcome the impact of, this destructive process of interpersonal relations.

For Sullivan, all these information sources (history, current interpersonal relationships, and here-and-now relationship with the therapist) led to the formulation and testing of hypotheses in psychotherapy through both directed and open-ended questioning. Sullivan insisted on getting enough information to attempt to explore with the client as many aspects and meanings of an interpersonal event as possible. He believed that the psychotherapist could not assume that he or she knew what the client was talking about until all sources of information were thoroughly understood. This emphasis on clinical impressions as hypotheses to be tested through consensual validation engaged the competence of both client and therapist, while the shared ownership of the work of psychotherapy ran counter to the myth of the all-knowing therapist. Through this process of hypothesis testing, all three elements of Sullivan's basic stance – maintaining sufficient interpersonal security to address these dilemmas, understanding the learning which needed to take place to move beyond the problems, and tailoring interventions to meet these goals of treatment – came into play most distinctly in the detailed inquiry.

### The Hidden Ms. T and the Detailed Inquiry

What follows is a summary of the main themes and discoveries of what became three years of interpersonal psychotherapy with Ms. T. About one year into her treatment, she took up my invitation to increase her sessions to twice a week, allowing for more intensive exploration and helping her better manage her intense anxiety and ferocious self-attack. In describing each of the themes, I will also discuss the underlying parataxic distortions (called transference in psychoanalysis) in the client-therapist relationship. I also note that this summary of our work together captures working themes without doing full justice to the complexity of the psychotherapy or to Ms. T's courage in addressing serious problems in living.

The first major theme of Ms. T's extended inquiry was exploration of her capacity to recover from her episodes of severe psychological collapse, including sharing her experiences of what she and others had labeled as auditory hallucinations. Like many individuals who suffer both from terrifying episodes of overwhelming psychological distress (and the psychiatric diagnostic terms that accompany them), Ms. T expressed feeling irreparably broken and unable to find her way back to a fulfilling life. Her prominent parataxic distortion of me was as a mental professional only interested in her symptoms and labels. My intervention early in treatment of wanting to know about her as a person beyond her problems did much to counter her expectation of being treated in reductionistic and dehumanized way. As we made our way together through her history, I was able to point out not only problematic interpersonal dynamisms, but also balance these with an awareness of what she had done very capably. This crucial and very Sullivanian assessment had the effect of slowly bring forth hope, where little had existed prior. Additionally, the occasion presented itself for me to refer Ms. T to a psychiatrist with both a lighter touch on psychiatric medication and excellent psychodynamic understanding. Together the psychiatrist and Ms. T were able to restructure medications away from ones (i.e., antipsychotics) causing untoward lethargy and confusion with the effect of providing Ms. T greater energy and clarity.

The second major theme of the detailed inquiry was Ms. T's relationship with her parents, especially her conflict with her father because of his domination and of her mother because of her passivity. Ms. T initially expressed only gratitude toward her parents, but over time she described other aspects of her relationship with them. She slowly revealed how her father was domineering, demanded perfection in others without holding himself to similar standards, and trucked no disagreement with any family member, most frequently using shame for psychological control. Ms. T was the sibling most likely to challenge her father, but she grew acutely sensitive to his harsh criticism. After her hospitalizations and retreat to living at home again, she devolved into defeated passivity and penetrating self-ridicule as her father's denigration of her reinforced her own experience of being irreparably broken and useless. As she was better able to move beyond her devalued sense of self as a "mental patient," Ms. T surfaced and expressed her anger about her father's emotional bullying. She also became more aware of her resentment at her mother's unwillingness to challenge her husband's verbal and, occasionally physical, abusiveness. Beginning in her earliest therapeutic relationship with me, Ms. T had significant elements of parataxic distortion of me as someone with whom she needed to be cautious and docile to ward off possible crushing devaluation. The development of interpersonal security without intrusiveness was my essential first task in psychotherapy, initially providing direction and understated non-possessive warmth in the earliest sessions. Over the three years, Ms. T increasingly took charge of the direction of treatment, coming to sessions with specific concerns she wished to explore.

The third major theme of the detailed inquiry was exploring Ms. T's previously unrevealed history of psychological trauma. As Ms. T found increasing security in the therapeutic relationship, hope for life beyond being a mental patient, and capacity to take on anxiety provoking subjects, I decided to enquire about her first "mental breakdown" at the age of 17. Because this event appeared such a sudden divergence from her previous functioning, followed by extreme social avoidance, I had a strong speculation that Ms. T had experienced a traumatic event. When I asked her what was the first time that she was touched in a way that was upsetting for her, I noticed that she became utterly blank. I enquired gently whether she had just "gone away," which she confirmed, and I shared that blanking out could be a way to protect herself, often involuntarily, from extreme discomfort. I observed that this way of protecting herself came up when I asked about unwanted touch, at which point she detached again. I introduced the concept of dissociation and we agreed that we would both be alert to it and work together as an important way Ms. T communicated that we were in emotionally perilous territory. After helping Ms. T develop the capacity to manage severe anxiety and dissociation, what slowly emerged was her revelation that she had been tricked into coming to an apartment by a man seemingly interested in her and there sadistically gang raped by a group of his friends.

Ms. T shared that I was the first person to whom she disclosed this event as she remained horrified by what transpired. She was also terrified of what her parents would think about her rape and devastatingly ashamed that she "allowed" this to happen. Ms. T stated that no one during her many years of treatment had taken a psychological trauma history and we explored how her resulting symptoms over the years were more consistent with posttraumatic stress disorder rather than schizophrenia or bipolar disorder. Interestingly, while discussing her past trauma was excruciatingly painful, understanding her past "breakdowns" as normal reactions to terrifying events allowed Ms. T to believe that she did not suffer from a hopeless mental disorder such as schizophrenia.

We then set about reconsidering Ms. T's feelings of responsibility for what happened to her, which led her to realize that, as an adolescent, she had been manipulated by evil men who preyed on teenage girls' open-hearted trust. Ms. T was able to share that her verbal "hallucinations" (see Frederickson, 2021 on pseudo-hallucinations) were in fact intrusive memories of disgusting things her rapists said to her, which we discovered were triggered when she felt unsafe in a public area. As a result, she was increasingly able to recognize these "voices" as memories and warnings and became better able to manage her anxiety and expand her world beyond living in her parents' basement. Ms. T and I explored that she courageously and without much help overcame the horrific experience by getting her life on track and excelling academically and in her work life, though at the cost of forming close relationships.

Clearly a compelling underlying parataxic distortion was Ms. T's fear that I would misuse her as men had abused her in the past. This awareness provided validation to my early hypothesis that Ms. T's fear of intrusion was a core projection that made interpersonal collaboration and a declaration of her desire for help so difficult for her.

The fourth major theme of the detailed inquiry was exploring Ms. T's longing for an intimate relationship and her problematic use of the Internet. She revealed that an important aspect of her suffering that led to her two most recent hospitalizations was her growing awareness in her late 30s that she would likely miss out on having a spouse and being a parent, in part because of her obsessive dedication to work. Such concerns are common for her life stage (see Levinson, 1996). Ms. T's trauma-driven avoidance of intimate relationships made it nearly impossible to tolerate meeting men. She disclosed that she spent many hours at night on the Internet in chat rooms, the use of which became increasingly compulsive and risky until her hospitalizations. Ms. T revealed that she wanted help with her recent return to using these sites, with increasing agitated compulsion, which worried her. Together we explored how her behavior was an important step in her successful work in treatment, a compromise between her yearning for connection and her completely understandable fear of close relationships with men. By this point in treatment, Ms. T was able to directly ask for help with her problem, suggesting her parataxic distortion of me had eased to the degree that her capacity had significantly grown to experience the therapeutic relationship in a largely collaborative, syntaxic mode.

### Termination/Interruption of the Psychiatric Interview

The final stage of Sullivan's psychotherapy structure was the *termination or interruption* of the psychiatric interview. Sullivan used the word termination when he did not expect to see the person again and interruption when he came to the end of a particular session in ongoing treatment. Sullivan believed that the purpose of the termination or interruption stage of the psychiatric interview was "the consolidation of what has been achieved in terms of some durable benefit for the interviewee" (1954: 39). For Sullivan, the explicit assessment of the progress of either the whole of the therapeutic work at its end or the work to date focused both the client and psychotherapist on whether the client was obtaining the benefit he or she came for. Sullivan outlined four steps in the termination or interruption of the psychiatric interview – the final statement, a prescription for action, a final assessment of the probable effects of the work of the session, and the formal leave-taking. The final statement concisely summarized what the psychotherapist had learned about the patient. Sullivan advised that the psychotherapist should include in the final statement only what he or she feels confident about, avoiding speculation about areas that have not been thoroughly explored. Sullivan cautioned not to undercut the client's confidence by directly focusing on unfavorable events at the end of a session, but to put them instead in the context of other, more profitable learning. Sullivan placed particular significance on the final statement in the termination of treatment. He recommended that considerable attention be paid to the final statement after a long course of treatment, assisting the client in remembering and reinforcing gains in treatment and accenting the future work to be done after therapy ended. This approach helped strengthen the client's sense of self and encouraged the client to continue the life-long task of increasing interpersonal awareness. In addition to consolidating what the client has learned in the session, Sullivan (1954: 200) specifically counseled that the client "should go away with hope and with an improved grasp of what has been the trouble."

Next, whether for termination or interruption of treatment, Sullivan believed that the therapist should suggest a prescription for action at the end of all sessions. The therapist offered the client a suggestion or some homework for the interval between sessions, something that he or she might try to recall or think about, or some action that he or she might consider taking. Again, not to be mistaken for giving advice which he abhorred, Sullivan encouraged the client to actively participate in treatment by providing a structure that oriented the client toward working between sessions. This therapeutic stance was quite different from Freud's idea of therapeutic neutrality and abstinence and reappeared years later as an important element of behavioral and cognitive-behavioral psychotherapies. The third step of Sullivan's termination/interruption process was the final assessment of the probable effects of the work of the session or of treatment. The client gained increased mastery through the cognitive process of foresight, which Sullivan believed to be a critical capacity in effective interpersonal living. By helping the client assess the impact of what he or she learned in treatment, this mastery was increased and the possible negative aspects of increased awareness could be anticipated. Rooted in his experience of working with dysfunctional families, Sullivan revealed his exceptional wisdom in acknowledging to the client that personal growth could have a disconcerting effect in troubled family and social situations. Finally, Sullivan believed that much damage could ensue from inappropriate interactions at the end of sessions. He suggested a process of formal leave-taking in which the therapist quickly disengaged without awkwardness from the client, blocking the natural tendency to try to do just one more thing or explain a confusing aspect of the work in one more way. The goal of the formal leave-taking for Sullivan was to provide "a clean-cut respectful finish that does not confuse that which has been done" (1954: 205).

### The Not-So-Hidden Ms. T and Termination

The beginning of the third year of working with Ms. T was marked by my decision to retire from psychotherapy and assessment practice. Because my practice was exclusively oriented to open-ended (sometimes called long term), intensive (twice weekly) psychotherapy with individuals with complex problems in living, I decided to inform all of my clients about my retirement eight months in advance. Unlike Sullivan's concept of interruption in ongoing treatment, which provided relevant summary of the work and prescription for action at the end of each session, Ms. T and I entered the termination phase of her interpersonal psychotherapy with the understanding that, when we stopped treatment, she could not expect to see the me again. I said we would continue working as we had, perhaps with a sharper focus on what problems Ms. T wanted addressed as well as her experience of ending an important, close relationship from which she had derived benefit and to which she had made many important changes and invested considerable effort. I noted that, for at least the last four weeks of treatment together, we would summarize out work together in terms of what she had learned and develop a plan for what she wanted to do at the end of treatment, including a decision whether or not to continue with another psychotherapist.

Initially, as expected, Ms. T reacted by becoming remote and emotionally numb and was reluctant to discuss my retirement and terminating treatment. Quite uncharacteristically, she cancelled several sessions at the last minute and, for the first time, forgot a session. I focused on who I might be for her now and Ms. T shared her conflicted feelings about my retirement (e.g., clearly, I was an old man and deserved to retire; how could she be angry after all I had done for her?), which gave way to anger toward me for leaving her. Together we then slowly and painfully uncovered her deep feelings of bitterness and desolation about being abandoned, ignored, and dismissed by the many caretakers in her life. As this awareness emerged, Ms. T was able to see her problems with her parents, her discontent with prior mental health professions and her sexual assault through a sharpened lens of failed attachment. It further became clear that her involvement with others via the Internet was an important way of maintaining distance and safety because of her fear of being hurt and abandoned, while keeping the hope of connection with others alive. As our work together came to an end, we reexamined the history of our work together, using themes from extended inquiry to organize our review. Ms. T and I look at the disillusioning and at times terrible mistreatment she endured, as well as emphasizing her many strengths and successes at moving beyond these problems, which would serve her well going forward. Fortunately, her psychiatrist with whom she had developed a very good relationship around drug management was also a skilled psychodynamic psychotherapist and we were able to easily transfer her care.

## Modern Applications of Interpersonal Personality to Personality Assessment

During Sullivan's career, personality assessment was in its infancy with few measures beyond the Rorschach test so common and useful today. Sullivan was a strong proponent of operationalism, the philosophy of science that endeavored to define all scientific concepts in terms of specifically described operations of measurement and observation. As such, the ability to provide empirically derived assessment of personality patterns found in personality assessment would likely have been of great interest to him, especially those operationalizing interpersonal behavior. Even more so, Sullivan would have been especially pleased by how interpersonal theory and therapy is integrated with empirically based psychological tests into an important modern advance in personality assessment, Therapeutic Assessment, as well as creative personality assessment methods in Contemporary Integrative Interpersonal Theory (CIIT), and an interpersonal approach to the Rorschach test.

## Stephen Finn and Therapeutic Assessment

In recent years, psychological testing has become untethered from its information – gathering origins and the objectification that is a root problem in much of personality assessment (Finn & Tonsager, 1997). Starting with collaborative assessment (Fischer, 1994; Handler, 2006) and especially Therapeutic Assessment (TA: Finn & Tonsager, 1992, 2002), TA is seen by many as the most important trend in personality assessment, especially its integration with powerful therapeutic models, opening up a more organic link between assessment and treatment.

This section will focus on Stephen Finn's Therapeutic Assessment (Finn, 2007a; Fantini, Aschieri ... & Finn, 2022; Tharinger, Rudin ... & Finn, 2022) the most accessible and well-developed model and the one with the clearest link to Sullivan's interpersonal theory and treatment. Finn's delightfully personal chapter (2007b) "Therapeutic Assessment: Would Harry approve?" outlines principal contributions by Sullivan to the development and foundation of TA. Specifically, Finn's TA incorporates basic elements of Sullivan's *The psychiatric interview* including acknowledgement of the inseparable relationship between assessment and treatment; primacy of clients' goals in determining the direction of assessment and treatment; and respect for patients' privacy beyond what is necessary to meet clients' goals. Further, Finn incorporated well Sullivan's participant-observer stance into TA, a crucial innovation in personality assessment that explicitly acknowledges its fundamental intersubjective nature and challenges the illusion of the assessor as an objective observer.

Additionally, Finn replaces the all-to-common emphasis on test scores with what he calls the primacy of careful listening and observing, recognizing Sullivan's often overlooked contribution of attending to nuances in non-verbal communication as key to understanding. TA sees test scores as "empathy magnifiers," that is, a way to understand the client through the process of consensual validation, not as labels for fixed or immutable traits taken outside the context of the client's interpersonal world. As a result, Finn shares Sullivan's deep skepticism about the value of using common psychiatric jargon believing it fundamentally obfuscates clients' concerns and problems in living. The goal of TA and interpersonal treatment is indeed to utilize expertise in interpersonal living gathered through personality assessment to elucidate and demystify. Using core interpersonal concepts of the self-system and the one genus hypothesis ("we are all simply more human than not"), Finn's TA places special emphasis on the importance of managing patient anxiety through establishing collaboration and good will in the assessment setting. This process is greatly enhanced by an acknowledgement of the common humanity shared by the assessor and client, allowing the assessor to get into the "client's shoes." TA has continued to grow and incorporate new understandings such as concepts of epistemic trust and mistrust (Fonagy et al., 2015) into TA treatment of severe personality disorders (Kamphuis & Finn, 2019), in many ways tracking Sullivan's work on the paranoid dynamism.

Hoping to interest personality assessment practitioners and psychotherapists in this important innovation, I provide below a brief overview of TA. In TA, the clinician uses psychological assessment to guide empathic and client-focused treatment interventions, based on clients' own questions about themselves. It has been used to work with a wide variety of clients, many of whom have received limited help with complex difficulties (e.g., de Saeger, 2019). Clients frequently report transformative experiences resulting from these assessment-based approaches. Further, TA and collaborative assessment have been recognized increasingly as an evidence-based treatment model (Aschieri et al., in press; Durosini & Aschieri, 2021; Poston & Hanson, 2010).

In TA, assessors and clients collaborate to explore clients' problems in living by using individualized psychological testing methods to assist in answering their questions. TA begins with eliciting and assisting clients' psychological questions about themselves. Next, clients complete a battery of psychological tests specifically designed to address clients' particular questions and problems. For example, if the client's question involves the effect of a traumatic event on her current close relationships, she may be given a trauma symptom measure, a comprehensive self-report measure like the Minnesota Multiphasic Personality Inventory, and the Rorschach Inkblot Method (RIM), including an explanation by the assessor about how these measures have been shown in research to assess the impact of psychological trauma.

The assessor then scores and interprets the relevant measures independent of the client's questions, then reviews the findings again from the perspective of the client's questions. The assessor then develops the assessment intervention session, perhaps the most creative element of TA. Assessment intervention sessions involve using psychological methods or other techniques to elicit experiences and enactments that can assist the client in reaching a richer emotional understanding of her assessment questions. In assisting a traumatized client who overuses dissociation to manage distress and whose main question is how to manage this process, the assessor might show her emotionally relevant TAT cards that are likely to provoke dissociation in a controlled fashion. The assessor can help the client to recognize her dissociation, learn how to manage it, and become better able to relate to others (see Finn & Kamphuis, 2006). The assessor and the client step back and together discuss and examine how the experiences in the assessment intervention are relevant to the client's outside life.

Next, in the summary/discussion session, the client and assessor collaboratively explore how the TA findings shed light on the client's questions. Unlike feedback sessions in the information-gathering model of personality assessment, the summary/discussion session is a highly collaborative venture, where assessment findings are presented as hypotheses to be explored rather than truths to be pronounced. The assessor is always respectful of the client's self-esteem and approaches this aspect of TA with the therapeutic skill that one would use in interpersonal psychotherapy. After the summary/discussion session is completed, the assessor sends the client a letter in plain language summarizing the main points of the session, making sure to invite the client's contributions regarding the assessor's hypotheses derived from the personality assessment as well as to include her alterations to the narrative. Often, a follow-up session is scheduled four to six weeks later to explore the client's subsequent experiences of the TA and to find out if new concerns have arisen. It should be noted that TA can be used as a short-term therapeutic intervention or as a consultation with referring mental health professionals who have may need help in the treatment of their clients.

## Contemporary Integrative Interpersonal Assessment

Hampering the integration of interpersonal theory and personality assessment, most assessment measures were based on the assumption from trait theory that "individuals can be characterized in terms of relatively enduring patterns of thoughts, feelings, and actions; that traits can be quantitatively assessed; that they show some degree of cross-situational consistency; and so on" (McCrae & Costa, 2008, 160). While somewhat consistent with Sullivan's concept of dynamisms, what is missing in trait theory is the reality of interpersonal context that causes and maintains these patterns. Influenced heavily by Sullivan, Timothy Leary (1957) broke from the trait model of personality assessment to develop the initial model of interpersonal diagnosis of personality. Leary believed that the human potential for growth and personality is best understood in context of interpersonal relationships. His work moved beyond simply categorizing traits to envisioning personality traits on continuum that become activated by reciprocal interactions with others, inspiring the concept of the interpersonal circumplex (IPC). From this truly inspirational work arose important contributors to the theory, research, and measurement of the interpersonal circumplex (see Wiggins, 1996) leading to the robust current work of Contemporary Integrative Interpersonal Theory (CIIT; Pincus, 2005; Pincus & Hopwood, 2012; Pincus et al., 2020). CIIT has provided a high degree of integration between interpersonal theory, research, and evidence-based measurement methodology that transports Sullivan's original interpersonal theory and treatment well beyond its strong beginnings. Of particular interest to this chapter are the new evidence-based personality assessment approaches that arise from CIIT.

As Pincus, Hopwood and Wright (2020) note, the core theoretical assumption is that personality and psychopathology arise from experiences that do not simply involve one person but are the result of interpersonal transactions. The dynamic interpersonal situation, rather than the more static assumptions of trait theory emphasizing stability and generality of personality across situations, redefines how personality assessment and treatment intervention is to be conducted. This radically alters personality assessment from the more standard approaches such as the MMPI, PAI, MCMI, and most other omnibus self-report measures. The central personality assessment methodology in CIIT is the *interpersonal circumplex* (IPC), first introduced by Leary (1957) and much developed through current times (see Gurtman, 2009). The IPC provides the conceptual basis and vocabulary for CIIT personality assessment (see Locke, 2010) and is a model, like Sullivan's IPT, that seamlessly integrates theory, personality assessment and therapeutic intervention.

The IPC assesses *interpersonal complementarity*, i.e., necessary interrelationships in which one seeks aspects in others that may be missing in, or complement, the self, which in turn may attract reciprocal patterns of relatedness from others. As such the IPC is conceptualized as a circle with two major orthogonal dimensions which are called *agency* and *communion*, representing human motivations of becoming individuated and becoming connected. Healthy human relationships occur where the agentic and communal needs of both persons are met in the interpersonal situation. Interestingly, these dimensions track nicely on essential functions expressed by Marvin's Circle of Security model of attachment discussed in Chapter 3, where children repeat the circle of exploring the world from a secure parental base (agency) and returning to connection in the parental safe haven (communion). The two IPC dimensions are further differentiated into complementary dimensions of *dominance* and *submission* on the agency axis and *friendly* and *hostile* on the communion axis. Rather than representing fixed traits, the IPC dimensions involve dynamic circularity and flexibility, with interpersonal behavior in any quadrant being useful and even necessary to fully respond to the wide variety of interpersonal situations and to fully express human potential. Because the IPC is circular, the "pie" can be divided even more finely, with Wiggins (1991) proposing an eight sided or octant model as valuable for IPC personality assessment.

The IPC has given rise to numerous empirically sturdy personality assessment measures, many of which have been used primarily, or even exclusively, for research. It is beyond the scope of this introductory section to provide a comprehensive survey of IPC measures and the reader is referred to Gurtman (2009) and Locke (2010) for a detailed review. Instead, the rest of this section briefly reviews three IPC specific measures and one established omnibus personality assessment measure containing interpersonal traits scales, all of which may be of considerable use in clinical personality assessment and psychotherapy practice from an IPT perspective.

Wiggins (IAS: 1995) Interpersonal Adjective Scales was the first well-validated IPC measure. It included eight scales measuring the fundamental vectors of the IPC interpersonal domain. These IAS scales were (1) ambitious-dominant, (2) arrogant-calculating, (3) cold-quarrelsome, (4) aloof-introverted, (5) lazy-submissive, (6) unassuming-ingenuous, (7) warm-agreeable, and (8) gregarious-extraverted. Rather than components that have no natural conceptual relationship to each other, the IAS provides an approach that is theoretically consistent with the IPC and allows for profile analysis emphasizing dynamic normal interpersonal behaviors rather than static personality traits or psychopathological diagnostic categories. The IAS spurred considerable research and served as the cornerstone for the development of subsequent IPC scales.

The Inventory of Interpersonal Problems (IIP: Horowitz et al., 1988) similarly focuses on interpersonal problems instead of symptoms, which is more suitable to planning therapeutic intervention than symptoms alone. The IIP is a self-report inventory that "identifies systematically the most common problems that people bring to treatment," "differentiate(s) between distress due to interpersonal problems and distress due to non-interpersonal problems," and identifies "what has been achieved through treatment" (Horowitz et al., 1988, p. 888). The IIP served as the basis for a circumplex version (IIP-C, Alden et al., 1990) and a well-validated short circumplex version (IIP-SC Soldz et al., 1995) more adaptable to practical clinical use (see Hopwood et al., 2019). The IIP-SC measures the eight octants of the IIP-C using four items rather than the original eight, which also makes it practical when using as measure for informants as well as the client.

With the Interpersonal Sensitivities Circumplex (ISC), Hopwood et al. (2011) used the IPC model to develop a 64-item, eight-quadrant self-report inventory to differentiate individuals' specific sensitivity to various irritating interpersonal behavior. Where one person might find unwanted personal closeness especially irritating, another may be sensitive to teasing. Interpersonal irritation is found quite generally in individuals with personality disorders, while some specific personality disorders may have particular irritants, such as experiencing indifference from others by individuals with a dependent personality. The ISC was developed to assess both general and specific interpersonal sensitivities, adding to the understanding of an individual as they experienced difficulties in daily living. The ISC also broadens the assessment frame allowing for assessment of specific interpersonal contexts such as with romantic partners, friends, and acquaintances. As such, the ISC offers a greater degree of real-life detail unavailable in broadband assessment measures. In addition to being useful in clinical practice, the ISC has spurred interesting research into such important areas interpersonal functioning as rejection sensitivity (Cain et al., 2017).

The Personality Assessment Inventory (PAI: Morey, 2007) is a comprehensive, multiscale 334 item self-report measure that assesses a variety of psychopathology and personality dimensions. It has increasingly become one of the most valued measures among personality assessment clinicians. A novel feature of the PAI is the inclusion of two interpersonal trait scales, Dominance and Warmth on the IPC. Dominance assesses the degree to which the individual is likely to act in an assertive, dominant, and controlling manner in interpersonal situations. Warmth assesses the degree to which the individual is likely to act in a kind, empathic, and engaging manner in interpersonal situations. Ansell et al. (2011) demonstrated that these PAI Interpersonal Scales accurately taps the two primary dimensions of the IPC. As such, the PAI is an invaluable comprehensive personality assessment from an IPT perspective, expanding the more symptom/ diagnosis-based approach of major omnibus measures to incorporate an interpersonal dimension.

While the original IPC was primarily a two-dimensional structure, and therefore, not entirely unlike a trait approach, CIIT approach to assessment has evolved uniquely to embrace both dynamic and thus multimethod factors (Hopwood, 2023). In particular, CIIT assessment focuses on three additional kinds of dynamics beyond the IPC. The first dynamic is within-person structural dynamics, which enriches the assessment with deeply personal issues like problems, values, and sensitivities. The second dynamic is within-person between-situation dynamics, emphasizing that the same person will exhibit different aspects of his or her self across different situations. The assessment of this intra-person variability can now be assessed with ecological momentary assessment methods such as smartphone apps. The third dynamic is within-person within-situation. This dimension taps the reality that the same person differs from his or her own average interpersonal behavior within the same situation. For example, within a set of interactions, a person can be warm and then rejecting and then warm again, often in a complementary way to the person with whom he or she is interacting. These complex two-person exchanges can now be assessed with computer-assisted tools like the Continuous Assessment of Interpersonal Dynamics (Hopwood et al., 2016).

Together, ICP assessment methods in general and the CIIT model in particular have a distinct chance of revolutionizing the field of personality assessment and the understanding of psychopathology. With Sullivan's IPT as the conceptual basis, CIIT offers a well-researched model that integrates theory, assessment, and treatment into a comprehensible whole. In terms of personality assessment, ICP assessment methods, taken together with previously discussed Therapeutic Assessment and the discussion of the interpersonal approach to the Rorschach discussed next, may well be the future of a responsive and effective approach to personality assessment and psychotherapeutic treatment.

## The Rorschach: An Interpersonal Perspective

Nearly all standardized psychological tests common in clinical practice are developed using a trait model that is different from an interpersonal theory (IPT) perspective. On the other hand, Finn and his colleagues have described the utility of the MMPI-2 (e.g., Finn & Martin, 1997; Finn & Kamphuis, 2006), and demonstrated the potency of Rorschach (e.g., de Villemor-Amaral & Finn, 2020; Finn, 2012a), in Therapeutic Assessment, using a fundamentally an interpersonally based approach to assessment and treatment. When viewed through the lens of IPT, it becomes clear that the Rorschach is perhaps the most fundamentally interpersonal of current psychological assessment methods.

Searls' (2017) history of the Rorschach Inkblot Method provides an important insight into Hermann Rorschach's intent in developing his method. Searles pointed out that Rorschach worked with severely troubled institutionalized schizophrenic individuals with whom most people had trouble communicating. Rorschach tried unintrusive and perhaps even lighthearted approaches that allowed him to communicate with his patients and see their world through their own eyes. As a child, Rorschach was highly aware of a Swiss German party game called 'klexographie' (translated as 'Blotto' [Erdberg & Exner, 1990]), which involved making inkblots and passing them around to guests for playful interpretation. By combining the 'empirical realism of a clinician with the speculative acumen of an intuitive thinker' (Klopfer & Kelley, 1942, p. 3), Rorschach's method is collaborative and by its nature interpersonal. The Rorschach is administered personally to the client by the clinician while sitting together side by side. The method essentially forgoes intrusive interpretation and direction by the clinician by asking the patient "what might this be" or "what does this look like to you." After collecting responses to the ten cards, the next step is an inquiry, a practice in empathy, participant observation, and consensual validation, where the goal is to "see what you saw as you see it." Methods such as extended inquiry (see Evans, 2012) allow for delving deeper into the clients' meaning beyond their responses.

As a direct application of Sullivan's theory to personality testing, Evans (2017) offered a reconceptualized interpersonal model for Rorschach Inkblot Method (RIM) interpretation. Exner's Rorschach Comprehensive System (CS: Exner, 2003) conceptually organizes RIM interpretation into eight clusters that are especially strong on perceptual and cognitive variables (Mihura et al., 2013). The CS also includes empirically based variables of interpersonal functioning and self-concept within two clusters, but Exner eschewed a theoretical orientation to CS, limiting its practical utility for integration with interpersonal theory (IPT). As a step to fill this gap between the CS and Sullivan's IPT, Evans reorganized relevant RIM variables into four main core interpersonal factors for Rorschach interpretation.[2]

1  Meaning of the individual's inner interpersonal world
2  Personifications (inner representations) of interpersonal relations and the sense of self as seen in the reflected appraisals of others
3  Capacity for interpersonal cooperation and consensual validation
4  Interpersonal anxiety

Rather than fit the individual to a predetermined set of constructs, as in ego psychology, the elegance of IPT is its emphasis on "centrality of individual experience," i.e., an individual's experience as something to be discovered and not assumed. Equally, or perhaps even more, important to these empirically determined RIM variables are the phenomenological aspects of the inter-personal process of the Rorschach. As suggested by Finn (2007a), through careful listening and observing, nuances in non-verbal communication during the RIM process add greatly to the understanding of the meaning of the client's responses and scores. Further, conducting an extended inquiry of especially meaningful responses (Finn, 2007a; Evans, 2012) and reading the content of responses (see Schafer, 1953) can be key to discovering together the underlying meaning of the client's RIM communication beyond what is available in objective scoring.

The RIM is a rich source for understanding personifications (inner representations) of interpersonal relations and the sense of self as seen in the reflected appraisals of others. Important CS variables can provide important clues and such personifications can be assessed by the Human Representations and Hypervigilance Index, along with the renamed Affective Difficulty Index and Coping Vulnerability Index in the Revised Comprehensive System (CS-R: Exner et al., 2022). For example, HVI can bring to life the client's inner world regarding fearfulness and wariness (hypervigilance) about interpersonal relationships. The closer the relationship, the more the individual becomes inwardly alarmed, setting in motion interpersonal dynamisms that keeps distance from others by guarding personal space and having difficulty revealing her inner life to others. In IPT language, such an individual has a highly vulnerable self-system, and security operations are quite easily activated by the personification of relationships as likely to be hurtful, if not damaging. Another example would be when the individual has a positive Coping Vulnerability Index and Affective Difficulty Index. A positive CVI strongly suggests a person who is interpersonally inept, puzzled and confused internally about how people think, feel, and behave, leading to difficulty negotiating interpersonal relationships in a satisfying way. In combination with a positive ADI, the individual is likely to be aware of interpersonal ineffectiveness, giving rise to self-doubt and deeply painful feelings. From IPT, the person is likely mystified about how interpersonal relationships work due to ineffective early parent-child experiences (which Sullivan drolly termed "parental insanity").

In terms of inner representations (personifications) of interpersonal relations and the sense of self seen in the reflected appraisals of others – good me, bad me and not me, the CS is rich with relevant variables. Such variables include the Egocentricity Index; Human Contents; Morbid Content; Trauma Content Index; the anger and aggressivity triad of Space, Aggressive Movement and Aggressive Content: and Active versus Passive Human Movement can provide invaluable information about one's sense of self (self-esteem) and how one interprets others (personifications of others). For example, an individual with a low number of whole human responses relative to partial or imaginary representations is likely to have personifications are largely made up of unrealistic understanding and idealized expectations of others. Further, such an individual with high Morbid Content and a positive Trauma Content Index is likely to see herself as internally damaged and fearfully anticipate emotional harm by others. With elevated Space responses and Aggressive Content, the individual likely anticipates aggression as a frequent and normal part of relationships and unsurprisingly feels upset and mistreated. A preponderance of Passive Movement, especially Human Movement, alerts the clinician to the likelihood that the person withdraws from active interpersonal engagement into a passive stance about meeting her or his needs, retreating into an interpersonal world marked by fantasy. Such a person's personification of others is filled with emotional abuse and aggression. The predominate sense of self as "bad me," unworthy and damaged and lacking an ability for self-protection. The person withdraws into a passive way of being in which fantasizing about idealized relationships cuts off possible positive interpersonal experiences and growth.

Capacity for interpersonal cooperation and consensual validation are critical elements of interpersonal development for IPT. CS Rorschach variable of Cooperative Movement is a well-established measure, one common in protocols of heathy individuals. The COP variable is a valuable indication of an interest in cooperative social interchange and, where it is absent, there will likely be difficulty in living. Interestingly, Brand et al. (2009) found that Rorschach protocols of individuals with dissociative disorder often contained a COP, but a closer look at the response revealed COP responses confounded by interference of cognitive processes. While the desire for interpersonal cooperation was present, the dissociative disordered individual experiences anxiety-ridden cognitive distortion, signaling, considerable interpersonal trouble. Further, an elevated CS Hypervigilance Index can point to profound difficulty with interpersonal cooperation resulting from pervasive fear and suspicion of others. Where absent or distorted Cooperative Movement is found on the Rorschach, the capacity for interpersonal cooperation and for seeing real relationships as a source of cooperation and help is likely damaged and blocked and interferes with the possibility of interpersonal support and cooperation. The development of consensual validation is similarly impaired.

IPT emphasizes the experience of *anxiety* as a key element in understanding interpersonal connectedness. As suggested earlier in Chapter 3, this experiential characteristic of Sullivan's IPT later emerges in a more systematic and articulate form in Bowlby's attachment theory and concept of the internal working model (see Holmes, 1993). Bowlby and colleagues have found repeatedly that protracted and habitual *attachment disruption* sets up a pattern of chronic anxiety and interpersonal dysfunction. Berant et al.'s (2005) investigation of attachment dimensions on Rorschach provides a useful interpretative strategy for assessing such anxiety, in particular their *anxious attachment* facet. Diffuse Shading and Inanimate Movement provide useful variables for exploring pervasive anxiety and a sense of foreboding, while the Rorschach Oral Dependency Scale (see Bornstein & Masling, 2005) offers information about the dependence needs. The *avoidant attachment* dimension is assessed by looking CS scores such as Texture and Clothing responses. When both dimensions are elevated, a powerful conflict between interpersonal anxiety and avoidance on one hand and an intense yearning for a dependent relationship on the other hand can impair the capacity to tolerate distress.

In closing, the reconceptualization of the Rorschach as an interpersonal personality assessment measure can add considerable richness to its value in understanding others. The use of the CS provides empirically validated measures so valued by Hermann Rorschach and Sullivan, while careful participant observation of the interpersonal processes that emerge during administration provides a rich tapestry of structured information to inform the empirical elements.

## Notes

1   This case is an amalgam of several different clients seen by the author over his 45+ years practicing interpersonal psychotherapy.
2   This section is modified from a previous publication Evans, F. B. (2017). An interpersonal approach to Rorschach interpretation *Rorschachiana*, *38*(1), 33–48.

# Chapter 9

# Interpersonal Psychotherapy

> One sees that there is no essential difference between psychotherapeutic achieve-
> ment and the achievements in other forms of education ... There are several
> differences in technique required, but these are superficial rather than fundamental,
> and are to be regarded as determined by the early training of the patient, in the end
> reducible to the common denominator of experience incorporated into the self.
>
> (Sullivan, 1962: 281)

Sullivan's many extraordinary ideas about the nature and conduct of
psychotherapy were a crowning achievement. While Sullivan's major work on
psychotherapy, *The Psychiatric Interview*, is the most widely read and
accessible of Sullivan's books, the complexity and elegance of his thinking
about psychotherapy is perhaps the least understood of his many contributions to modern psychodynamic theory and practice. Starting with his
successful psychotherapy of the previously "untreatable" disorders of schizophrenia and paranoid states (see Freud, 1911b) and continuing with his
treatment of the highly related obsessional states, Sullivan was a psychotherapist whose clinical brilliance was renowned. His extraordinary success
with these clients gave credence to his conceptualizations about interpersonal
relations and psychotherapy. He developed an approach to psychotherapy
that grew directly out of his theories of personality and mental disorder, a
treatment approach which challenged, and deviated markedly from, basic
tenets of Freud's (1904, 1912b, 1912c, 1913, 1914a, 1915c) psychoanalytic
method. Historically, Sullivan's psychotherapeutic innovations came at a
time when "classical" psychoanalysts began to close ranks behind the Holy
Grail of Freud's technical suggestions. As Lipton (1977) pointed out, this
increased Freudian orthodoxy came largely in response to the controversy
over Alexander's (1961) concept of the corrective emotional experience. This
rigid adherence among U.S. psychoanalysts had the effect of making the
acceptance and integration of similar interpersonal psychotherapy concepts
difficult, lest the curious and creative be branded an infidel.

Like Alexander and Ferenczi before him, and his contemporary Fairbairn
(1952), Sullivan believed that wholesale application of Freud's psychoanalytic

DOI: 10.4324/9781003305712-12

method to all mental disorders was extremely problematic. His response to the problems of clinical psychoanalysis was to develop an intricate model of treatment, far more systematic than any of his predecessors or contemporaries, apart from Freud. As mentioned in Chapter One, many of his ideas and methods appear commonplace today, because others have appropriated and relabeled Sullivan's ideas over the years and because his widespread influence on psychotherapists passed along in the oral tradition of clinical supervision (Chapman, 1976). As Havens (1976) noted, Sullivan's interpersonal psychotherapy was a treatment approach which focused on the understanding of interpersonal relations (and the inner representation of these relations) from a participant-observer psychotherapeutic stance with learning as the key process for psychotherapeutic change. While Sullivan's formulation of the inherently interpersonal nature of all psychotherapy may appear to the modern reader so basic as to seem obvious, it must be remembered that before Sullivan the conceptual challenge to the ideal of the totally neutral and objective analyst was at best protean. Sullivan's early innovations in the hospital treatment of schizophrenics formed the foundation of what eventually developed into milieu therapy and group therapy, while his introduction of the use of collateral data from families and significant others in the treatment of schizophrenic clients was a well-spring for the future development of family therapy. Sullivan's sweeping conceptualization of personality and psychotherapy was so broad that careful reading reveals an approach which integrates the best of psychodynamic, client-centered, behavioral, cognitive, and existential approaches to treatment and can be seen as the earliest model for the important modern trend of integrative or systematic eclectic psychotherapy (e.g., Beutler, 1986; Beutler & Clarkin, 1990; Beutler & Consoli, 1992; Norcross, 1986).

The purpose of this chapter is to describe, elaborate, and extend some of Sullivan's most important ideas about psychotherapy. The first section will explain the author's perspective on Sullivan's basic stance on treatment. The second section will explore Sullivan's continuing influence on psychoanalytic psychotherapy and brief psychotherapy since the publication of the first edition of this book. The third section will briefly discuss Sullivan's largely unacknowledged influence on group psychotherapy, family therapy, and milieu therapy. Sullivan's important contributions to the field of psychotherapy could constitute a rather lengthy book in its own right, so a detailed explication is beyond the general purpose of this book. Readers interested in Sullivan's interpersonal psychotherapy are encouraged to explore primary sources, especially *The Psychiatric Interview*, as well as *Clinical Studies in Psychiatry*, *Schizophrenia as Human Process*, *Conceptions of Modern Psychiatry*, and the works of Frieda Fromm-Reichmann (1950), Otto Will (1961), Leon Salzman (1966, 1980), Leston Havens (1976, 1986, 1989), Edgar Levinson (1972, 1983), and the modern interpersonal psychotherapists (e.g., Achin & Kiesler, 1982; Carson, 1969; Chrzanowski, 1977).

## Sullivan's Basic Stance

While Sullivan was quite precise in detailing the operations of the psychiatric interview, his term for the psychotherapeutic endeavor, his fundamental principles about the nature of psychotherapy were less clearly stated. As Havens (1976) pointed out, much of Sullivan's approach to psychotherapy was spread throughout his writing, often expressed in anecdotes or through implication. The author will offer his perspective on Sullivan's basic psychotherapeutic stance as a background to understanding his more specific recommendations for conducting the psychiatric interview discussed in Chapter 8. From my perspective, Sullivan's *basic stance* was comprised of three elements – *the nature of the therapeutic relationship, the goals of psychotherapy*, and *treatment interventions tailored to fit the specific problem of living*. I choose the term *basic stance* over technique to emphasize the primary components of interpersonal psychotherapy, rather than the methods by which treatment is effectively achieved.

As has been repeatedly suggested throughout this book, Sullivan's conceptions of personality, mental disorder, and psychotherapy flowed from a single source – his fundamental assumption that psychiatry and human nature must be understood from the vantage point of interpersonal relations. He believed that personality and problems of living were formed from the development of the nature and quality of interpersonal relations. For Sullivan, psychotherapy was a special instance of an interpersonal relationship, one in which those seeking treatment from the psychotherapist required expert help in altering inadequate or inappropriate patterns of interpersonal relations, patterns shaped by underlying experiences of anxiety and interpersonal insecurity and irrational parental education and other such influences. As a result, because of the client's (and to some degree the therapist's) insecure attachment to others, the psychotherapist's engagement with the client was colored with anxiety and avoidance. In order for required interpersonal learning to occur, the patient or, as Sullivan often preferred, the client needed to be secure (not anxious) in the relationship with the psychotherapist. This secure therapeutic relationship was therefore necessary (though not sufficient) to achieve the goals of psychotherapy. What Sullivan called "modern dynamic psychiatry" involved establishing a therapeutic relationship which achieved a dynamic balance between therapeutic operations designed to maintain interpersonal security and those designed to facilitate interpersonal learning. Further, for Sullivan, the techniques for achieving these goals are determined by the goals themselves and not a priori assumptions about what comprised proper technique.

## The Therapeutic Relationship: Maintaining Interpersonal Security

The importance of establishing and maintaining an atmosphere of interpersonal security was a central tenet that guided Sullivan's psychotherapeutic work, a position which went well beyond Freud's (1910a) notion of the therapeutic positive transference. Whether in childrearing or psychotherapy, Sullivan believed that no productive interpersonal learning could occur in an atmosphere of severe or chronic anxiety, which would hamper access to the person's best cognitive abilities and would engender interpersonal avoidance. Throughout his clinical writings, Sullivan chastised psychotherapeutic practice which did not take into account this fundamental fact of interpersonal living. From Sullivan's perspective, interpersonal security could be achieved in psychotherapy through respectful, empathic listening to the details and specifics of the client's experience, informed by the psychotherapist's knowledge of human development and interpersonal processes and client's expectation of benefit. The client's experience of the psychotherapist's respect for, interest in, and knowledge of his or her problems in living provided a core security in which the client could elaborate and evaluate increasingly more anxiety-ridden interpersonal assumptions, confusions, and inadequacies as well as reveal and correct these difficulties in a here-and-now relationship. The basic attitude of the psychotherapist was what Sullivan termed "respectful seriousness" (1954: 56), with the psychotherapist as "an expert having expert knowledge in interpersonal relations" (1954: 12) whose expertise required an unceasing respect for the need for interpersonal security of the patient or client.

Sullivan's deep empathy for his clients arose in part from his philosophic view on how we come to know another person. Paradoxically, Sullivan started with an existential assumption about the general inaccessibility of any personality other than our own (see Yalom, 1980 on existential isolation for a comparison of Sullivan to other existential psychotherapists). Sullivan believed that the psychotherapist, through careful listening, questioning, and observing, could learn a great deal about the client. Yet, the psychotherapist could never have as direct a knowledge of the client as the psychotherapist had with his or her own experience. The tendency to see others' worlds through one's own particular vantage point was inescapable, but knowledge of this reality could provide a safeguard against assuming that the therapist's experience was identical to the client's experience. Even though Sullivan viewed the psychotherapist as an expert in interpersonal processes, he believed that no one could convey his or her unique personality *en toto* to another. Also, Sullivan recognized that each psychotherapist had his or her own limits of experience, suggesting that psychotherapists should be careful not to work with clients whose age, gender, or ethnicity were significantly foreign to the therapist. Sullivan believed strongly that it was more important to understand what an individual's actions and thoughts were actually intended for, rather than what the observer speculated them to mean. Sullivan emphasized that interpersonal communication and consensual validation provided the necessary bridge and connection between the experiences of the client and psychotherapist. As a result, the notion of the fully analyzed psychoanalyst who was free from transference and therefore a perfect receptor of the experience of the client was both incomprehensible and arrogant to Sullivan, inimical to his most basic beliefs about psychotherapy and human understanding. He believed that empathy was an interpersonal process worked out between the participants in treatment, based on the client's actual experience. Sullivan was highly intolerant of psychotherapists who were not careful to do so with their clients (see Kvarnes & Parloff, 1976 for excellent examples of Sullivan's impatience). His attitude of deep respect for the client and, especially, for inevitable differences in experiences between the psychotherapist and the client, was an ever-present corrective to the client being forced to take on the world view of others, which was all too common in the developmental experience of the client and in life in general.

Another aspect of Sullivan's careful attention to the processes of empathy and interpersonal communication was his awareness of the influence of the psychotherapist in the here-and-now social interaction with the client. As Sullivan stated ...

No two people have ever talked together in entire freedom of either one from effects of interaction of the other.

(1962: 292–293)

There is always interaction between interviewer and interviewed, between analyst and analysand, and from it, both must invariably learn if sound knowledge of the subject-personality is to result.

(1962: 297–298)

Sullivan understood, as did Freud, that the client's perceptions of psychotherapist strongly influenced the client's experience in psychotherapy and careful attention needed to be paid to these perceptions. Sullivan carried this idea beyond Freud's notion of transference to include the real relationship with the psychotherapist, including the psychotherapist's cultural role, anxieties, foibles, kindnesses, etc., as well as the effects of the psychotherapist's perception of the client. Sullivan saw the therapeutic relationship as intersubjective, leading him to formulate the psychotherapist's role as one of participant-observation. For Sullivan, the "objectivity" or "neutrality" of the psychotherapist was a fundamental misconception and fundamentally unempathic as it led to a perception of the client as an object to be studied, analyzed, and treated by a psychotherapist who lacked the same processes of the patient. Of particular importance to Sullivan was the psychotherapist's understanding and management of the client's anxiety, present in the form of the client's expectation and fear of the psychotherapist's disapproval and interpersonal operations designed to avoid this insecurity. The psychotherapist had an ongoing responsibility for, what Sullivan called, "integrating the situation," that is, joining with the client to assure, through skillful handling of the relationship, an atmosphere of interpersonal security. Additionally, the psychotherapist needed to understand what kinds of interpersonal stances could lead to a disintegration of the situation with the client, how to first protect the client from such situations and later to gradually educate the client to better understand these situations. While Sullivan did not believe the disintegration of situations could never inadvertently occur in treatment, he believed that the psychotherapist should be ever alert to this possibility and assist the client through these rocky waters in a skillful way. Sullivan spoke critically of psychoanalytic approaches such as Freud's, 1905 interpretation of aggressive impulses in the treatment of obsessional states and Freud's, 1911b "doctrine of homosexuality" in the treatment of paranoid states, in which the stance recommended for the analyst did not take into account his or her interpersonal impact on the client's specific dynamisms of difficulty. Lastly, Sullivan strongly believed that anxiety could arise from either side of the consulting room and the client's anxiety could lead to the therapist's counter-therapeutic security operations. Sullivan belief in the importance of the psychotherapist's reactions to the client as part of the data of treatment, presaged the work of Winnicott (1947) and Searles (1979) redefining the meaning of countertransference in psychoanalysis.

Additionally, the psychoanalytic technique (Freud, 1912b) of the blank screen, in which the analyst was impenetrable to the patient and served as a 'mirror' to the patient's processes, ran counter to Sullivan's basic ideas about the psychotherapeutic relationship. While Sullivan, like Freud, did not believe that the therapist should be chatty or use the client to meet social needs, his participant-observer stance alternated between respectful listening and skillful questioning. Sullivan believed that the psychotherapist should be empathic, respectful, interpersonally and engaged, a position similar to what Fairbairn (1952) called "genuine emotional contact," with all interpretations made by the client and the therapist being subjected to systematic inquiry and consensual validation. Naturally, Sullivan insisted on the use of common language in treatment, eschewing psychiatric jargon or theoretical formulations, which he called 'psychiatric banalities.' Additionally, Sullivan thought it a mistake for therapists to treat painful experiences or awful circumstances neutrally, avoiding, as Margaret Rioch (1960: 135) stated, "Years of listening to 'cases' ... mold(ing) their countenances into ducks' backs, from which the waters of woe and joy roll traceless." Unlike Freud (1910b) who believed in the elimination of countertransference reactions through personal analysis, Sullivan saw the strong feelings of the therapist toward the client as inevitable and part of the human dimension of treatment. Sullivan was undoubtedly influenced by his belief in the powerful need for human intimacy, applying what he saw developmentally in preadolescence to the establishment of a psychotherapy relationship which was respectful, empathic, and genuinely engaged, which in turn made it possible for the client to explore attitudes and habits that stood in the way of more effective interpersonal patterns.

There are striking parallels between Sullivan's position on the importance of interpersonal security in psychotherapy and similar ideas of Heinz Kohut and Carl Rogers. Sullivan, Kohut and Rogers believed that certain empathic relational qualities of the psychotherapist were necessary factors in treatment – for Sullivan, respectful, empathic engagement; for Kohut (1971, 1977), empathic sensitivity to the subjective experience of the client, especially the client's experience of the psychotherapist; and, for Rogers (1951, 1957, 1961), the psychotherapist's accurate empathy, warmth, and genuineness. For both Kohut and Rogers, the empathic connectedness of the psychotherapist constituted the fundamental element of therapeutic change, what Rogers (1957: 95) called "the necessary and sufficient conditions of therapeutic personality change." Yet, drawing his understanding of Sullivan's work, Havens' (1986) analysis of empathic statements provided a broader perspective. While simple empathic statements, so well represented in the work of Rogers, are a basic and necessary aspect of therapy, Havens' (1986: 53) remarked, "These stand helpless before the great mass of complex and contradictory feelings that are present in most cases," which he stated call for complex empathic statements. Such complex statements, which may seem even critical or sarcastic on their face, can be powerfully empathic and can be heard by damaged individuals who otherwise would reject direct warmth and empathy. It is clear that Havens believed Sullivan to be a master of complex empathy.

Additionally, the notion that simple empathic statements alone constitute the primary curative factor in psychotherapy has received serious challenges from the field of psychotherapy research. In reviewing the research literature of psychotherapist variables and psychotherapy outcome, Parloff et al. (1978), Mitchell et al. (1977) and Gurman (1977) all remarked that Rogers (1957) conception of the necessary and sufficient conditions for psychotherapeutic change was not adequately supported by the research literature. Instead, a complex relationship existed between therapist variables, patient variables (especially the patient's experience of the therapist), treatment modalities, and treatment outcome. Rogers' empathic variables on the whole appeared to be necessary, but not sufficient, conditions for therapeutic change, or, as Gurman (1977: 536) remarked, "not a few patients find warmth (or genuiness or empathy) highly aversive because of their interpersonal learning histories." With his vast experience treating individuals suffering from paranoid and schizophrenic dynamisms, and especially those having undergone significant malevolent transformation, Sullivan clearly understood that the important, but overly simple, therapeutic calculus proposed by Rogers and Kohut was inadequate. Rogers' et al.'s (1967) general lack of success in applying his method to schizophrenic clients and Kohut's (1971) position on the untreatability of borderline personality disorder and psychotic disorders provides further evidence for Gurman's observation and supports the perspective that Sullivan's ideas about psychotherapy are applicable to a broader range of human dilemmas.

A final divergence between Sullivan's and Rogers' and Kohut's approaches to the therapeutic relations is well illustrated by Yalom's (1980) discussion about the nature of empathy in treatment. Yalom expressed concern that empathy, as characterized in the works of Rogers and his followers, has been presented as a therapeutic technique. Similarly, Kohut's empathic sensitivity to the subjective experience of the patient was elaborated as a technical stance in treatment of narcissistic disorders which is a deviation from classic psychoanalytic technique. Yalom, recalling Buber (1965), believed that empathy, presented as a therapeutic technique (that is something the therapist does in treatment), lost the essence of the authentic relationship in which the therapist was fully invested out of his desire to understand the other. Sullivan never presented empathy as a technique or even discussed it much in his writings on psychotherapy. His empathic connectedness to his clients grew more from an existential position arising from his belief that we were simply more human than otherwise and that we shared the same existential conditions of anxiety and isolation in our interpersonal relations. For Sullivan, empathy was a state of being with the client, which could be seen indirectly, but powerfully, from his effort to truly and deeply understand the fundamental trouble of the person who sat across from him.

While seemingly obvious and deceptively simple, interpersonal psychotherapy practiced from the vantage of participant-observation remains difficult and challenging. While Sullivan believed that maintaining interpersonal security, through simple and complex empathic statements, was a necessary precondition in successful treatment change and itself an important corrective to earlier unfortunate interpersonal experience, he strongly emphasized that psychotherapy was fundamentally an educational enterprise of interpersonal learning.

### Building Interpersonal Security with the Hidden Ms. T

Sullivan's essential concern for establishing and maintaining interpersonal security is a key element of why interpersonal therapy works well with individuals with severe and profound problems in living. With regard to the case of The Hidden Ms. T, the maintenance of interpersonal security is better characterized as building of interpersonal security due to her psychological fragility. Frederickson's splendid *Co-creating safety* (2021) defines the fragile patient as someone whose past traumatic relationships so colour current relationships that they are readily flooded with overwhelming anxiety when interacting with others beyond superficial exchanges. They are unable to bear these intense emotions internally and rely on the dynamism of projection to ward off perilous anxiety. Examples of such projection including viewing others as the source of intolerable emotion, "not me" dissociation, and even pseudo-hallucinations, where intolerable thoughts are "heard" as separate from internal cognition. Building interpersonal security with fragile clients is *the* essential first step in establishing a meaningful therapeutic relationship, a step fraught with working through serious parataxic distortion and repairing treatment missteps and misalliances.

Based on her formal inception and reconnaissance, I hypothesized that Ms. T's submissive and remote (hidden) interpersonal stance was her primary dynamism in protecting herself from others' intrusions into her tenuous sense of personal agency and from their anticipated disparagement. It appeared to me that she was unable to tolerate having self-will, especially openly declaring a wish for help, without crushing anxiety. Additionally, Ms. T became frightened by clear expressions of warmth and empathy. My therapeutic stance mirrored her expectation of dominance by my taking the lead in our sessions for many months, using open-ended questions to elucidate an understanding of her situation and being ever alert to an upsurge in her anxiety during the interview. Throughout this process, I gently restructured Ms. T's overly entrenched dominant-submissive interpersonal paradigm by frequent invitation for her to declare what she wanted help with and withdrawing into guiding the session when her anxiety rose sharply.

I also took a concerned, but somewhat reserved therapeutic stance without much eye contact unless she initiated it, made easier by the ninety-degree chair arrangement in my office. For many months, when Ms. T became anxious, frightened, or disconnected, I subtly re-directed my interview questions to safer topics, without commenting on her rise in anxiety, to regulate her discomfort. As we established a tenuous security, Ms. T began to make more eye contact and appeared more curious, at which time I gradually began to query her about her discomfort about certain topics and invited her to notice and speak to it. As we approached discussing her first psychiatric hospitalization, Ms. T began to show overt indications of transient dissociative episodes, which I welcomed as her "safety valve" for when our work triggered severe anxiety. Reframing her experience allowed Ms. T to see dissociation as an important way she protected herself rather than a mental disorder symptom to be "treated." Additionally, going forward, "checking out" became for her an important way of noticing and regulating her distress, mitigating the involuntary nature of this protective measure. These early and continuing interventions to build and maintain interpersonal security laid the cornerstone to Ms. T's ability to find considerable benefit from interpersonal psychotherapy.

## Goals of Treatment: Facilitating Interpersonal Learning

While critical to the conduct of effective psychotherapy, establishing and maintaining an atmosphere of interpersonal security was for Sullivan a necessary pre-condition in treatment. As the second element of his basic stance, Sullivan made explicit the central role of interpersonal learning in his writings on treatment and established the goal of psychotherapy to be the facilitation of such learning. Rather than to embrace Freud's (1917) more meta-psychological language of treatment (e.g., enlargement of the ego and re-placing id energy with ego energy and so on), Sullivan chose to cast psychotherapy in terms of the processes of interpersonal learning. Sullivan's interpersonal psychotherapy was primarily psychodynamic in orientation, in that it had shared with other psychodynamic approaches an interest in the dynamic processes of the self, covert (mistakenly called unconscious) pro-cesses, the analysis of the relationship with the therapist, and a developmental approach. Yet, for Sullivan, all these factors served as a basis of under-standing what the client had learned about himself and others and how this learning history manifested itself in current ineffective and inappropriate interpersonal patterns. The evaluation of interpersonal patterns and pro-cesses was the precursor to formulating a treatment response in which new patterns could be learned, already existing effective patterns could be ac-cessed in new situations, and treatment could be fashioned to meet these learning goals.

As discussed earlier and further described by Havens (1973), Sullivan's ideas about learning and psychotherapeutic change bear a conspicuous sim-ilarity to behaviorism. Sullivan (1953) elucidated a model of learning that had striking parallels to Ferster and Skinner's (1957) core empirical findings of operant psychology, in which humans and other learning creatures act on the environment to increase positive, and decrease negative, consequences. For Sullivan, like modern social learning theorists (e.g., Bandura, 1977; Pratt et al., 2010), the human environment primarily involved transactions with other humans, hence his emphasis on interpersonal learning. Sullivan's belief in social learning and imitation can be best seen in his in-patient work with schizophrenics at Sheppard Pratt. Sullivan carefully selected and trained ward staff to work with schizophrenic individuals on the ward on how to engage in intimate relations. Staff members modeled appropriately warm and supportive interpersonal behavior, which served as a, to use Havens' (1976) term, counterprojection of and correction to the patients' prior unfortunate interpersonal learning. As a psychotherapist, i.e., an expert in interpersonal living, Sullivan conceptualized the work of psychotherapy in terms of the processes of change ...

> What major changes are to be had in mind, and what is the most promising ways of getting to them? In other words, what are to be regarded as the necessary achievements for great improvement? Note here I am avoiding the term "cure," since I do not think it applies in the realm of personality.
> (1956: 227–228)

Eschewing the medical concept of "therapeutic cure" (see M. Rioch's, 1970 paper which beautifully elaborated this position), Sullivan instead proposed that psychotherapy orient itself to correcting rigidities in the self-system, those avoidant interpersonal processes which served to protect the individual from interpersonal insecurity at the cost of self-knowledge and interpersonal effectiveness. Interpersonal psychotherapy addressed the continual interplay between working with conservative operations of self-system to minimize anxiety and the desire to learn which Sullivan called "the drive toward mental health" …

> There is a great deal of fairly subtle data to support the notion that every human being, if he is not too tediously demoralized by a long series of disasters, comes fairly readily to manifest processes which tend to improve his efficiency as a human being, his satisfactions, and his success in living.
>
> (1954: 100)

Clinical examples of Sullivan's therapeutic approach of the psychiatric interview amply illustrated his conviction about the importance of making sense of actual interpersonal experience and of subtly teaching more effective patterns of interpersonal relationships, a distinctly cognitive-behavioral orientation. Sullivan used skillful, open-ended questions to deftly and skillfully lead his clients to reveal their perceptions of themselves and others, to understand how they came to these perceptions, and to safely expose the inappropriate and ineffective aspects of the perceptions. As Sullivan stated (1940/1953: 207), "One achieves mental health to the extent that one becomes aware of one's interpersonal relationships" with the ultimate goal of "the expanding of the self to such a final effect that the client as known to himself is much the same person as the client behaving to others." Carson (1982) and Safran (1998; Safran & Segal, 1990) noted that Sullivan's concept of the self (including the self-system, security operations, personifications, and parataxic distortion) described social-cognitive processes that have been born out empirically and anticipated the development of cognitive behavior therapy.

Clearly, Sullivan accorded insight, in terms of increased awareness of interpersonal processes, center stage in the process of therapy. While perhaps Sullivan's goal of insight bore some similarity to Strachey's (1934) concept of the mutative interpretation, the process of interpretation in interpersonal psychotherapy was drastically different, in that it was an investigation directed toward mutual discovery. Instead of the detached, silent stance in psychoanalysis, Sullivan's actively shared impressions with the clients, conceptualizing them as hypotheses to be tested and worked out through consensual validation, a position similar to Beck et al. (1979) notion of collaborative empiricism in cognitive therapy. Sullivan's focus of interpretation, elucidating patterns of interpersonal living, was far broader than the assumption of interpreting intrapsychic conflict arising from the Oedipal complex found in Freudian psychoanalysis. As Lipton (1977) pointed out in his cogent critique of what he calls modern "classical" psychoanalytic technique, the overuse of silence and the limitation of the analyst's connection with the client to the interpretation of the transference result resulted in an overly restrictive, artificial, and dehumanized interpersonal approach which has iatrogenically increased the client's feelings of isolation and narcissistic injury. As Chapman (1976) commented, Sullivan maintained that unguided and unstructured introspection such as found in psychoanalysis actually increased the need for security operations in the patients and could contribute to distorted ideas about the self. The few interpretations made by the classical psychoanalyst were never fully tested out through inquiry but could easily be perceived by the client as truth coming from on high. As Havens (1986) discussed, Sullivan's notion of interpretations as hypotheses to be tested allowed details to be carefully explored and hypothetical statements were used to uncover covert aspects of interpersonal situations. In what Havens (1986: 107) termed "the democratization of psychotherapy," therapist dared to be wrong and thus corrected the imbalance between psychotherapist and client, setting an important example for the client about authority relationships.

To illustrate, a specific aspect of Sullivan's learning-based approach to interpersonal psychotherapy was his use of theorem of reciprocal emotion (which Leary, 1957 extended empirically as principle of reciprocal interpersonal relations). As a result of early anxiety-ridden experiences and inadequate interpersonal learning, the individual learned perceptions of self and others that were colored by these negative experiences (bad-me, bad-mother personifications) and anticipated similar interpersonal interactions in the future as a way of predicting and attempting to control the interpersonal environment to maintain interpersonal security. The individual's security operations, which functioned to avoid re-experiencing painful interactions, carried with them assumptions and expectations about others' behavior and attitudes based on past experience. In a process akin to the object relations psychoanalytic concept of projective identification (see Grotstein, 1981; Ogden, 1979, 1982), these interpersonal expectations become self-fulfilling prophecies (Carson, 1982) that influence the interpersonal environment by evoking in others expected behavior and attitudes similar to the person's prior experience. In his analysis of Sullivan's behavior in psychotherapy, Havens' (1976, 1986) uncovered techniques, which Havens' termed counter-assumptive statements, i.e., "comments made by therapists to unsettle assumptions they feel being made about them by their patients" (1986: 111) and counterprojective statements, i.e., "speaking about what is being projected onto the therapist and doing so with some of the feeling the patient has toward the projection" (1986: 125). Sullivan looked for ways to surprise, short-circuit, or otherwise render inoperative the client's projections and expectations, while at the same time maintaining the client's interpersonal security. By subtly challenging the client's expectational set, Sullivan opened the possibility of the client's reappraisal of interpersonal situations and development of more effective interpersonal behavior. In an atmosphere of interpersonal security and consensual validation, the client learned that language became primarily a way to communicate needs, rather than habitual, reflexive, and unthinking utterances to avoid anxiety and social disapproval. In many ways, Sullivan's basic stance of supplying interpersonal security through respectful, empathic engagement, in and of itself, provided a rich counterassumptive and counterprojective interpersonal learning experience, which increased the clients' freedom to act in their interpersonal world. Rather than to interpret or describe his patients' projections, parataxic distortions, or transference from a detached or objectified interpersonal stance, Sullivan, through techniques such as counterprojective and counterassumptive statements, demonstrated his willingness to lend his whole person to the goal of transforming the client's interpersonal experience.

Clearly, insight, in terms of increased awareness of interpersonal processes, was not the only level on which Sullivan intervened with clients. Sullivan was among the first (if not the first) psychotherapists to discuss and study in detail the non-verbal aspects of the interaction between the client and the therapist, an area which subsequently received significant psychotherapy research support (e.g., Mehrabian, 1972; Mahl, 1968; Matarazzo et al., 1968; Ekman & Friesen, 1968). Reminiscent of the great hypnotherapist Milton Erickson (see Haley, 1968), Sullivan explicitly noted disturbances in the "gestural components of communication" (1954: 179), e.g., body position and mannerisms, tonality and cadence of speech, and psychophysiological signs of discomfort, as critical information about the patient. Throughout his clinical examples, e. g. his positioning of the chairs in the session to allow the schizophrenic client to avoid eye contact and to have access to leaving the room without encumbrance, Sullivan demonstrated his willingness to utilize non-verbal interventions to circumvent security operations and to facilitate new learning. Additionally, his technique of counterassumptive and counterprojective statements revealed his understanding of the valuable social learning that went on at a non-verbal level. Whenever Sullivan took an interpersonal stance to neutralize anxiety and security operations, his manipulation of social behavior outside of the client's awareness was a powerful and effective intervention in the process of interpersonal learning which went above and beyond the cognitive components of his treatment model.

While the processes of learning form the underpinnings of all psychodynamic approaches (see Wachtel, 1979, 1982), Sullivan was the first psychodynamic psychotherapist to specifically declare *interpersonal learning* as the goal of treatment. His model of psychotherapy incorporated elements of what could be recognized today as social learning, behavioral, and cognitive approaches to treatment, within the context of a model which is fundamentally psychodynamic (and with existential-humanistic overtones). Overwhelming empirical evidence has demonstrated the efficacy of these learning-based approaches to treatment with a wide variety of clinical populations (see Kazdin, 1978; Mahoney & Arnkoff, 1978; Marks, 1978; Rosenthal & Bandura, 1978). Interpersonal therapy for depression (Klerman et al., 1984) is a brief treatment model for depression incorporated Sullivan's ideas about interpersonal learning and was shown to be effective for both moderate and severe depression in the landmark National Institute of Mental Health Collaborative study (Elkin et al., 1989). A systematic review of the literature by De Mello et al. (2005) demonstrated that interpersonal therapy for depression has continued to be effective and even superior to more popular cognitive behavioral therapy. Clearly, Sullivan's ideas about the important role of learning in the process of psychotherapy have received abundant support, demonstrating that his conceptualization of the appropriate goals for treatment was well ahead of his time.

### Facilitating Interpersonal Learning with Ms. T

The shift in psychotherapy from symptom identification and management to facilitating interpersonal learning is a key feature of Sullivan's approach to psychotherapy and an important corrective to the modern emphasis as seeing individuals primarily as mentally disordered and in need of symptom reduction. Because Ms. T had more than her share of the latter, she found the specialized form of education (see Rioch, 1970) quite suitable to her nascent, yet impressive capacity for learning about herself. In the course of her three years of interpersonal psychotherapy, Ms. T learned much about interpersonal living and herself. Her painful and terrifying experiences could be viewed with compassion and understanding rather than dehumanizing clinical distance. She could engage in relationships that were mutual and that honored her personal agency. Ms. T learned that previously mystifying and frightening experiences such as dissociation and pseudo-psychotic episodes mimicking auditory hallucinations (i.e., intrusive memories) were ways which many individuals coped with overwhelming horror. She learned that she did not have to hold a contemptuous and devaluative view of herself to remain connected to her family and that her anger about such parental insanity was a way to know she did not like something and to better protect herself. Ms. T learned to move beyond the terrible cost of her psychological trauma to a more satisfying life, freer from the images and constraints her oppressors had forced upon her.

### Tailoring the Intervention to Fit the Problem

The third element of Sullivan basic stance in interpersonal psychotherapy was that specific psychotherapy technique arose from the nature of the presenting difficulty and interpersonal learning required; in other words, *treatment intervention needed to be tailored to fit the problem.* As Will (1954: xviii) stated, Sullivan was "opposed to the casual prescription of courses of action without there being some idea of how such action is to be effected." The concept of psychotherapy technique, a central theme in other psychoanalytic psychotherapies, was not addressed directly by Sullivan. Instead, Sullivan focused on ways to conduct a detailed inquiry into the person's interpersonal relationships, in terms of the person's view of the self and others, problems in living, and the rest of the personality. Through careful assessment of interpersonal dynamisms and style by means of the psychiatric interview, Sullivan crafted specific responses to his client's dilemmas. Sullivan (1962: 281) saw psychotherapy as an educational enterprise in which there were "several differences in technique required," as dictated by the interpersonal learning necessary to modify ineffective patterns of interpersonal living. This idea implied that psychotherapy technique should be as variable as the circumstances of the client dictated. To achieve the ends for which the client sought benefit, the strategy of interventions and the psychotherapy techniques to effect these interventions needed to be fashioned in response to both the nature of the client's insecurity and the kinds of interpersonal learning which needed to occur. As a result, Sullivan's interpersonal psychotherapy was essentially a problem-based, rather than technique-based, model of treatment.

Sullivan's approach to tailoring the treatment to fit the problem included the assessment of the psychotherapeutic stance necessary to both maintain interpersonal security and engender specific learning necessary for more effective interpersonal relationships. The expertise of the psychotherapist in establishing the therapeutic alliance required knowledge of how to work collaboratively with the client, while having a sharp awareness of the kinds of interpersonal situations which would be especially disintegrating. As Sullivan stated ...

> But since no outline can possibly anticipate the variations that occur in a personal relationship with a stranger, it is not enough that the interviewer knows just what he expects to do; he must also be alert for any suggestion that something has happened which is unexpected, because the novelties which occur in an inconspicuously methodical investigation are the things that distinguish its results.
>
> (1954: 52–53)

Sullivan believed that the situations which integrated and disintegrated interpersonal relationships varied from dynamism to dynamism, person to person, and even situation to situation. No one specific technique to further communication and intimacy could be known or prescribed in advance of knowing the person's particular situation. Hence, psychotherapist was called upon to show interpersonal flexibility and creativity as an added dimension of interpersonal expertise.

Sullivan's perspective pointedly contrasted Freud's (1912b, c; 1913; 1914a; 1915c) recommendations on technique. Freud placed great emphasis on proper psychoanalytic technique such as free association, dream analysis, interpretation of transference, and blank screen, believing that these techniques were necessary to achieve therapeutic ends. While, as Lipton (1977) pointed out, Freud was not a slavishly devoted to his technique as are modern practitioners of "classical" psychoanalytic technique, nonetheless psychoanalysis started with technique, assuming it sufficient to respond to the universal nature of all neurotic conflict, resolving the Oedipal complex. Even with the introduction Eissler's (1953) concept of "parameters" (i.e., modifications) of technique within classical analytic circles, psychoanalysis has been a technique-based treatment model, in which more or less the same technique has been applied to a wide range of disorders. While Sullivan could see occasional usefulness of many of these techniques under certain circumstances (e.g., see Havens', 1989 brilliant analysis of the utility of "Freud's invention" for the treatment of hysteria), he mistrusted any model of treatment that purported to have the final answer, independent of research and experience that validated its methods. Sullivan saw clearly how psychoanalytic technique in the treatment of schizophrenic, paranoid, and obsessional dynamisms actually made it more difficult for the client to receive benefit. No single technical approach could possibly encompass the complexity, individual variation, and educational requirements of all disorders. For Sullivan, tailoring treatment interventions to fit the goals of treatment was the only rational course of action.

Naturally, within this more flexible model of treatment technique, the role of assessment was critical. As described in Chapter 8, Sullivan's concept of the psychiatric interview was an unfolding, guided dialogue between the therapist and client, which provided a method of systematic inquiry (assessment) into the nature of interpersonal difficulty. From this inquiry, treatment goals and technique could organically emerge, an approach to assessment later empirically elaborated by Leary's (1957) Interpersonal Circle, Peterson's (1982) functional analysis of interpersonal behavior, Benjamin's (1995) Structured Analysis of Social Behavior, and more recently Frederickson's model of intensive short term anxiety-provoking psychotherapy (ISTDP: 2013, 2021). Nowhere was Sullivan concerned that the psychotherapist be an expert in interpersonal living more clear than in his conception of the psychiatric interview. The psychotherapist gathered and explored information from the client's experience, interweaving data from past history, current interpersonal living, and the here-and-now interaction with the psychotherapist into a complex interpersonal tapestry, all the while maintaining the interpersonal security of the client. The psychotherapist might share hypotheses with the patient for further clarification and consensual validation or might use counterassumptive and counterprojective statements to neutralize and modify the client's distortions about the self or others.

Sullivan's approach required an interpersonal flexibility to strategically respond to and act towards the client that went well beyond the more limited requirements of maintaining an analytic blank screen and making the occasional interpretation during the relatively unguided introspection of the analysand. This flexibility by no means indicated that Sullivan was an unsystematic or wild analyst (see Freud, 1910c). While he believed that the psychiatric interview should not be a lock step methodology, Sullivan advocated a methodic procedure which demonstrated the psychotherapist's expertise and provided a systematic model for assessment and intervention. Ever skeptical of processes described under the penumbra of intuition, Sullivan strove to delineate and understand specific processes within the therapeutic relationship through an empirical approach to technique. He was one of the first psychiatrists to make use of wire and tape recordings of sessions for study and he speculated that film recordings could add a great deal as well. Today, the videotape recording of psychotherapy sessions is a standard for modern clinical training and research (see Barnett, 2011). While Sullivan did not have the benefit of modern learning theory-based psychotherapy techniques and modern psychotherapy research to validate effective treatment approaches, his concept of tailoring the intervention to the problems presaged modern eclectic assessment and treatment models.

Beginning with Lazarus' (1971, 1976) multimodal behavior therapy, a significant direction in modern psychotherapy has been the attempt to integrate the proliferation of effective treatment approaches and techniques in a systematic fashion. In an attempt offset the dilemmas inherent in the Sufi tale of the blind men and the elephant (Shah, 1970), integrative and systematic eclectic models of assessment (e.g., Beutler & Berren, 1995; Beutler & Clarkin, 1990) and treatment (e.g., Norcross & Goldfried, 2005; Norcross, 1986) have challenged psychotherapists to think beyond the narrow constraints of a particular model of treatment and to integrate what is known empirically to be effective approaches to treatment. Modern interpersonal theorists such as Kiesler (1996) and more recently Pincus et al. (2020) have suggested that an interpersonal model best synthesizes empirically effective treatment approaches under the rubric of a single integrated treatment model which is in turn founded on a specific theory of personality and psychopathology. Sullivan's interpersonal theory and psychotherapy provide the basis for such contemporary models, integrating significant elements of the best of psychodynamic, empathy-based (client-centered and self psychology approaches), learning theory (including operant, cognitive, and social learning approaches), and existential models of personality and psychotherapy.

### Tailoring Interventions for Ms. T

As stated above, interpersonal psychotherapy favors various treatment interventions and techniques in response to particular problems and is assessment oriented and not technique driven. Ms. T's treatment included a variety of approaches, several of which I will highlight below. The primary intervention in Ms. T's treatment was the extensive use of Sullivan's psychiatric interview approach where information about her experience was garnered and investigated, interlinking past history with her present functioning. As she was better able to tolerate person-to-person connection, we explored her experience with me in the here-and-now, focusing on her characteristic parataxic distortions, primarily projections, that interfered with her capacity to seek and use help from others. As stated above, because her capacity for accepting a helping relationship was damaged, building the interpersonal security and interpersonal collaboration was paramount for Ms. T throughout her three years in treatment.

Because of her deeply engrained expectation of exploitation and scorn in relationships, Ms. T's capacity for benefiting from empathy and positive regard on one hand, and direct interpretation on the other, was damaged. As a result, Haven's (1976, 1986) techniques of complex empathy were used to protect from the terror of engulfment, as well as counterprojective and counterassumptive statements, were employed to deactivate powerful parataxic distortions. Because Ms. T would find direct warmth and empathy too intrusive and frightening, I took a somewhat distant stance, looking for occasional opportunities to slip empathy through using statements that might otherwise appear sarcastic. For example, in response to her description of the various grim diagnoses she received, along with her obvious despair about them, I stated, "So through the many years process of diagnosis and treatment, you appear to have come away with a strong conviction of being rather terminally fucked up. We will see about that." Ms. T's response to intervention was to relax, engage eye contact, and become more open about her treatment experience. My statement was also counterassumptive to her expectation that I would favor "my profession, right or wrong" and counterprojective in that I named her fear that I would see her as hopeless. By challenging her set of expectations about me, a door could open for a reappraisal of what psychological treatment might offer her.

Another central influence on my treatment interventions with Ms. T was Judith Herman's (1992) three-stage model for trauma treatment and recovery. Paralleling both Sullivan's psychotherapy approach and Ms. T's treatment needs, Herman's first and foremost goal was the establishment of safety, both in the treatment relationship and in life when the client is in an abusive relationship. This approach can be easily seen in the establishing interpersonal security section above. Once there is sufficient safety, the next step is to actively bear witness to and explore traumatic experiences, especially to understand how the client protects herself from the awful awareness of what she had undergone, as well as the cost of her defenses. The preponderance of the work after the first year of Ms. T's treatment involved elucidating her trauma experience and looking at the impact it had on her life.

The final step in Herman's model was moving onto a life beyond having survived her the trauma. When Ms. T was nearing termination with me, she began to explore work possibilities and thoughts about moving back to her small house, which to my surprise, she had never sold.

## Conclusion

This section outlined Sullivan's intellectually sweeping ideas on his basic stance in psychotherapy. Respect, effectiveness, and expertise marked Sullivan's vision of treatment through maintaining interpersonal security, facilitating interpersonal learning, and tailoring treatment to fit the problems. The three elements of Sullivan's treatment model parallel factors, which Frank (1973, 1982) found to be the common features of effective psychotherapy – a trusting relationship with the psychotherapist, convincing rationale for treatment, the mastery of current interpersonal situations, and expectation or hope through the belief in the expertise of the therapist. Sullivan's interpersonal psychotherapy blended both insight and change-oriented approaches to treatment (see London, 1986) and embraced complexity over simplicity in formulating responses to human dilemmas. Integrating much of what has come to be recognized in modern times as core components of effective treatment, Sullivan's model of treatment remains vibrant and contemporary after nearly fifty years.

## Modern Interpersonal and Relational Psychoanalysis

An important branch of Sullivan's IPT actively practiced today is variously called interpersonal psychoanalysis (Lionells et al., 2014; Stern, 2017), relational psychoanalysis (Mitchell, 1988; Mitchell & Aron, 1999), and coparticipant psychoanalysis (Fiscalini, 2007). Under the auspices of the William Alanson White Foundation, in 1943 Clara Thompson, a close colleague and friend of Sullivan, established a New York City branch for clinical training of interpersonal psychotherapy called the William Alanson White Institute. Thompson (1964) remained closer to mainstream psychoanalysis than Sullivan, combining Sullivan's IPT with Sandor Ferenzi's emphasis on the importance of real relationships and with Fromm's humanistic perspective. Thompson's interpersonal psychoanalysis bred a rich tradition that remains more interpersonally focused today than any other psychodynamic training center. Important interpersonal thinkers from the interpersonal psychoanalysis tradition include Edgar Levenson (Levenson, 2013, Levenson & Slomowitz, 2016), Stephen Mitchell (Greenberg & Mitchell, 1983; Mitchell, 1988; Mitchell & Black, 1995), Darlene Ehrenberg (1992), John Fiscalini (2007), Irwin Hirsch (2014), Lewis Aron (2013), and Philip Bromberg (2012). This group emphasized that the detailed exploration of the nuances of patients' patterns of interacting with others begins with examination of the client-therapist interaction. I will briefly summarize the work of three of these authors with the hope that it will spur further reading on their extensions of interpersonal theory.

Perhaps the most influential of this group has been Edgar Levenson, who underscored Sullivan's central idea that problems in living, fundamental dysfunctional interpersonal patterns, are likely to be repeated in all principal areas of the person's life. Levenson focused on how the psychoanalytic relationship contained the elements necessary to elucidate the client's difficulties. Levenson emphasized that the process of change is a non-linear, "lived through" process within the context of the therapeutic relationship and that the client attempts to "pull" the therapist into acting as a participant in the client's habitual patterns. He viewed this dynamic as the continuous enacted process present in all relationships and that the therapist's job is decoding the signs of the process, including and perhaps especially the therapist's own reactions and behavior. Levenson is conceptually very similar to Sullivan's (1954, p.3) ideas of participant observation, such as "the psychiatrist cannot stand off to the side and apply his sense organs ... without becoming personally implicated in the process ... His primary instrument of observation is his self – his personality, him as a person." Yet, it was Levenson who elaborated more comprehensively the importance of the understanding therapist's participation or "pulls" in the process and moved this idea into the core of the psychoanalytic treatment.

Next, Stephen Mitchell's relational psychoanalysis began conceptually with his foundational book with Jay Greenberg (Greenberg & Mitchell, 1983) which provided a trenchant analysis of the two basic psychoanalytic paradigms: Freud's drive model, in which relations with others are generated and shaped by the need for drive gratifications, and relational models, exemplified by Sullivan's IPT, in which interpersonal relations are primary in human motivation. Mitchell (1988) then argued that psychoanalysis needed to move beyond attempts to harmonize modern relational theory with classic Freudian drive theory, instead positing that drive theory no longer was sufficient as either a viable theory of personality or model for treatment. Mitchell pulled together major approaches of relational-model traditions, melding British object relations theories such as Fairbairn, Bowlby, and Winnicott with Sullivan's interpersonal theory into an integrated framework for relational theory. Like other psychoanalytic theories, his model emphasized the impact of early experience, the importance of sexuality, the relationship between past experience and present behavior and beliefs, and the resulting tendency to develop personality patterns that repeat painful experiences. To this Mitchell added the centrality of the will as a core element in human personality along with ideas about the dynamic interplay between real experience and inner ideas about relationships based on past experience. In terms of the nature of the psychoanalytic situation, and the process of change, Mitchell focused on the transference and countertransference interplay in the here and now as a primary area of important understanding of dysfunctional patterns. Mitchell and Black (1995) noted that Sullivan tended to be more conservative in disclosing the therapist's experiences of the patient, while relational theorists tend to be less so. Mitchell died unexpectedly at age 54 but left behind an important legacy including the journal *Psychoanalytic Dialogues* and the Stephen Mitchell Relational Study Center, a training center for relational psychoanalysis.

Fiscalini's (2007) coparticipant psychoanalysis represents a more radical extension of modern interpersonal and relational models. Like Levenson and especially Mitchell, Fiscalini eschewed Freudian drive theory, seeing modern interpersonal and relational psychoanalysis as the future of theory and dynamic psychotherapy. Fiscalini was well steeped in interpersonal theory and offered a crucial challenge to Sullivan's (1940) rejection of the concept of will, also referred to as personal agency (Fiscalini, 2008). Sullivan believed that unique individuality was an illusion, stating "no such thing as the durable, unique, individual personality is ever clearly justified. For all I know, every human being has as many personalities as he has interpersonal relations" (Sullivan, 1956, 221). Clearly Sullivan was reacting to the one-person, "tempest in the teacup" model of personality central to Freud's thinking and expanded the basic unit of human understanding to the person in relationship to others and the society and culture in which they were embedded. The next step in his thinking was to eschew individual agency or will, in many ways an interesting contradiction from a man whose own personal agency helped him transcend the many obstacles of his early and later life. Fiscalini confronted this problem by transforming the issue of the multiple self by emphasizing the dialectic between the interpersonal (human similarity) and personal (human singularity). At no time does Fiscalini abandon the reality of interpersonal (communal) existence, but rather calls for the recognition of individuality and will (agentic) motives as key to understanding what it is to be human. He posited that this dialectic between the interpersonal self, the inherent and reflexive need to avoid anxiety based on interpersonal learning, and the personal self, the human striving for self-fulfillment and personal growth, was essential for psychotherapy.

The implications for dynamic psychotherapy, which Fiscalini (2007) calls coparticipant psychoanalytic inquiry, are many. He believed that interpersonal psychotherapists needed to go beyond understanding problematic dynamisms and early learning difficulties to incorporate the person's particular sources of motivation such as thought, emotion, desires, and wishes, which hold the person's striving for self-realization. Without considering these internal strivings, the psychotherapist cannot help clients activate their will to change. In coparticipant psychotherapy, the continuous dynamic tension between forward-moving needs for fulfillment, satisfaction, and love balances constraining needs for interpersonal security from anxiety. Fiscalini captures Sullivan's developmental idea of a striving for growth discussed in

Chapter 6 but moves beyond Sullivan's incomplete and not well-articulated notion to provide specific ways to activate the will to personal growth and greater interpersonal intimacy. Fiscalini's dual lens of self-protection and self-growth opens therapeutic inquiry, generating hypotheses about the client's behavior that may very well be multiply determined beyond a simple pathology focus. Fiscalini also expands Sullivan's concept of participant observer to a therapeutic frame of coparticipative inquiry, which is more open, less authoritarian and inviting of mutual exploration in which the client's agency is crucial. Included in this inquiry is the understanding that the client and psychotherapist both contribute to the relationship, which is part of the unfolding work. While the psychotherapist works hard to help activate the client's will to change, ultimately the responsibility for engaging in the work of psychotherapy, and for personal change, resides in the client. Such a position promotes a more respectful balance between the respective contributions of the client and psychotherapist.

## Psychodynamic Brief Psychotherapy and the Work of Jon Frederickson

Sullivan developed his approach to psychotherapy during an era when the psychoanalytic ideal encouraged longer and longer analyses, even ones that were seen ideally as interminable (Freud, 1937). The advent of brief psychotherapy in general and psychodynamic brief therapy was still years off (see Mann, 1973; Malan, 1976). It is of considerable interest that Sullivan (1972) was formulating ideas about the situations in which brief treatment could be useful as early as 1927. While Klerman and Weissman (Klerman et al., 1984) and Strupp and Binder (1984) acknowledged the importance of the interpersonal theory in the development of their models of brief treatment, Sullivan's conception of the psychiatric interview contained two elements of technique that are commonly recognized by all brief therapists as central to the conduct of effective brief therapy – a clear and focused goal and the awareness of time. With regard to the concept of clear and focused goals, Sullivan's psychiatric interview was highly problem-focused, stating that keeping the expected benefit in front of both the therapist and client sharpened the focus on the agreed upon goals of treatment. The formal inception culminated in the establishment of a therapeutic contract (see M. Rioch et al., 1976) and the beginning of highly focused collaboration.

Sullivan took an equally pragmatic (and existential) stance with regard to the importance of time in psychotherapy. As he stated ...

> if one is interested in a precisely defined, recurrent difficulty that people have in significant relations to others, it is quite possible that a good deal of work can be done in a rather short time ... the psychiatrist must follow events closely enough so that whenever a digression seems to be in

progress, or some subordinate problem seems to be in the center of things, he can inquire whether such is truly the case, or whether the topic actually does fit in with the business before them.

(1954: 76 footnote)

Reminiscent of Mann (1973), Sullivan commented (1954: 32), "If he sees the patient is repeating himself ... he may, without unkindness, discourage such moves, tolerating only a minimum of wasted time since he knows that there is plenty to do." The technical consideration of focused goals and an awareness of time so critical in the conduct of modern brief psychotherapy was simply an extension of what to Sullivan comprised good psychotherapy.

Forms of brief therapy have proliferated in modern times to treat a variety of different problems and diagnoses, using particular techniques and deriving from different theories of (Messer, Sanderson & Gurman 2013). Indeed, the way in which behavioral (e.g., cognitive behavior therapy [CBT, systems, and strategic therapies developed and are practiced predisposes them to be short term.

From an interpersonal psychodynamic perspective, few, if any, approaches rival the depth and complexity of Frederickson's method of intensive short-term dynamic psychotherapy (ISTDP: 2013, 2021).[1] In his seminal book *Cocreating Change*, Frederickson presents his revolutionary work on psychodynamic psychotherapy, which is a unique synthesis of the best of Sullivan, Freud, object relations theorists, and Habib Davanloo (1980, 2000) along with modern neuroscience and contemplative traditions. ISTDP utilizes an in-the-moment, emotional and interpersonally focused interventions that see psychoanalytic interpretation and exploration of the past over present suffering as a form of intellectualization, which is seen as reinforcing treatment resistance and projection rather than liberating patients from it. Frederickson views the nature of human suffering and its causes, not as psychiatric symptoms, but rather resistance to the reality of one's experience. The client resists the painful and inescapable experiences of life's losses, disappointments, and betrayals, actual and imagined, and feelings about these experiences are suppressed or denied due to interpersonal prohibitions. In turn, these patterns of denial become habitual problems in living called "symptoms." As Frederickson eloquently states, "We create our suffering and symptoms moment by moment all day long." (2020, p. 6). The task of psychotherapy becomes one of helping the client abandon this suffering by facing the reality of the moment and become more present to that reality. He states ...

To do this, the patient must relinquish his defenses and face the feelings he fears and has avoided. Through these two choices, the patient joins the therapist to co-create a relationship for change; the therapeutic alliance (p. 6)

Like Sullivan, Frederickson sees diagnosis as a highly dynamic process interwoven with intervention. Diagnosis is active throughout the therapeutic relationship – not a place of arrival, but a journey to be undertaken together with the patient. In every interaction with the client, the therapist acquires important diagnostic information, which, in turn, informs and guides the next intervention. This moment-to-moment focus in ISTPP is a core feature, observing and intervening in the client's characteristic ways of managing anxiety. The process of treatment for the therapist includes helping clients to maintain therapeutic focus, notice and regulate their anxiety, increase the clients' awareness of defensive patterns that contribute to their difficulties, deactivate their defenses, and cultivate greater self-observing capacity. Much the same as Sullivan's idea of therapist as expert in interpersonal living, therapists must have the psychological capabilities they are attempting to co-create with their patient: focus, emotional regulation, and self-reflection.

What sets Frederickson's work apart from the rest of psychotherapeutic teaching is his detailed and specific explication of *how and when* to help clients develop a focus and manage anxiety. With few exceptions, how to conduct psychotherapy in a moment-to-moment, issue-to-issue fashion is essentially absent from the writings of most important psychoanalytic thinkers. While Sullivan (1954) provided a more detailed road map for conducting inter-personal psychotherapy than most, the level of specificity was nowhere near what Frederickson provides. Additionally, instead of using prevalent psy-choanalytic levels of organization such as Kernberg's (1975) schema of neurotic, borderline and psychotic, Frederickson makes the distinction between highly resistant and fragile clients, along with embodied expressions of anxiety that allow the therapist to distinguish each. Because of differences in their particular defenses and their way of managing anxiety, the inter-ventions for each type are considerably different.

Highly resistant clients fear emotions and closeness in relationships and use a variety of defenses to keep feelings at bay and others at a distance. While self-protective, such defenses sap emotional vitality and prevent developing mutually satisfying, intimate relationships. This pattern makes it difficult for both the client and the therapist to form the collaboration to co-create change and relief from suffering. The focus of treatment is to provide challenges to emotional and relational distancing in a secure, compassionate relationship. Frederickson (2021) further describes fragile patients as having poorly developed capacity to tolerate closeness and anxiety because of insecure attachment from past relational trauma. Because of intense and unresolved feelings, such clients find themselves flooded by anxiety when stirred by strong emotions. As a result, their ability to tolerate emotions within themselves is easily overwhelmed by anxiety and they are vulnerable to confused and distorted thinking and physical distress as a result. Their way of managing is to locate the feeling or source of feeling outside themselves, a defense called projection. The focus of treatment is to provide a secure relationship in which clients' anxiety can be tolerated and regulated, and their thinking about the source of their distress understood. The conceptual clarity, theoretical breadth and therapeutic incisiveness of Frederickson's ISTDP is a revolutionary advance in interpersonal psychodynamic theory and practice that brings Sullivan's work to full fruition.

## Beyond Individual Psychotherapy

While Sullivan's psychiatric interview provides a comprehensive model for the conduct of interpersonal psychotherapy, his detailed writings on treatment were largely concentrated on individual, or more correctly, "two-group" interviews. While Sullivan's two papers (1930–31; 1931–32) on the inpatient treatment of schizophrenia contained many important innovations, his elaboration of the sociotherapeutic dimension of his inpatient treatment model was never as extensive as his writings on "two-group'" treatment. Similar to Freud's invention of the couch (he disliked being looked at all day), Sullivan's emphasis on one-on-one interaction was hardly surprising given his particular personality. His shyness and social awkwardness were legendary and, as can be seen in Kvarnes and Parloff's (1976) recorded supervisory seminar, his work in groups was marked with a high degree of control that was much less manifest in his individual work. Yet the logical extension of Sullivan's interpersonal model suggested treatment interventions that went well beyond the boundaries and constraints of individual treatment. Sullivan's emphases on both social learning and tailoring the intervention to meet the treatment, as well as the theoretical implications of interpersonal approach, forecasted the application of other social configurations to psychotherapy. Sullivan's interpersonal approach played a significant role in opening the door for milieu, group, family, and brief psychotherapy.

Sullivan's contributions to the development of milieu therapy are the most easily traced. Sullivan's papers (1930–31; 1931–32) about his in-patient ward for schizophrenic clients at Sheppard Pratt between 1929 to 1931 outlined key elements central to the conduct of milieu therapy. Sullivan's treatment goal on his special ward was to create an environment in which "schizophrenic patients were not schizophrenic when they were with me. That is, they did not do any of the things that schizophrenic patients are said to do" (Sullivan, quoted in Rioch and Stanton, 1953: 66). Sullivan's primary intervention was the modification of the treatment environment to facilitate more satisfactory interpersonal patterns and decrease the schizophrenic persons' need to use schizophrenic dynamisms. To achieve this end, Sullivan radically altered existing ward structure by establishing a small ward for first-break male schizophrenics utilizing carefully selected and specially trained male attendants. Sullivan believed the gender and authoritarian training of most hospital nurses placed an interpersonal overwhelming burden on the young schizophrenic men whose schizophrenic dynamisms existed in large part because of severe problems with early mothering and overwhelming anxiety about lust. While psychotherapy was conceptualized as part of the therapeutic milieu, Sullivan, the only psychiatrist on the ward, spent relatively little time conducting individual psychotherapy with schizophrenic clients on the ward. Instead he focused his energies on the training and ongoing supervision of his hand-picked male attendants, whom he taught to understand and respect the anxieties of patients and to create an atmosphere of a private, warm, accepting group of which the patient could be a part. Sullivan's innovation was so novel and counter to existing hospital norms that, in the brief time he ran the special ward, he upset many in the hospital staff (the nursing staff in particular) and generated wild rumors about overt homosexual activity (see Chatelaine, 1981). Additionally, Sullivan's approach directly challenged the prevailing psychiatric wisdom of Kraepelin and Freud that dementia praecox was an untreatable mental disorder. To compound the hospital administration's dilemma, Sullivan's ward had an here-to-fore unheard of recovery rate of better than 85 percent as measured by return to work or home, a rate of recovery that continued several years after Sullivan left Sheppard, under the direction of his hand-picked successor Dr. William Silverberg (Rioch & Stanton, 1953).

Sullivan's innovations were what Rioch and Stanton (1953) characterized as perhaps the earliest major example, and clearly one of the most significant studies, of milieu therapy in American psychiatry. Sullivan's later influence is readily traced to the important work on environmental treatment at The Chestnut Lodge (see Bullard, 1940; Fromm-Reichmann, 1950; Morse & Noble, 1942) as well as Chestnut Lodge and the Washington School of Psychiatry's sponsorship (Rioch, 1949) of the first major sociological study of mental hospitals (Stanton & Schwartz, 1949, 1954). Stanton and Schwartz's study persuasively demonstrated the power of the hospital social milieu to do both good and harm to patients, a finding that has confirmed and re-confirmed over and over again (e.g., Caudill, 1958; Goffman, 1961; Stotland and Kobler 1965; Levinson and Gallagher, 1964; Evans, 1976). In particular, the demonstration of deleterious effects of mental hospitalization has led to a modern emphasis on deinstitutionalization and community-based treatment of the severely mentally ill (see Harris & Bergman, 1993). While the rapid, intensive intervention of severe psychopathology has become standard practice (Dieterich et al., 2017) in the field of in-patient psychiatric treatment (though not so before Sullivan), it is a great tragedy that Sullivan's work of the positive effects of carefully designed environmental inpatient treatment has received so little acknowledgement in modern times. Without specific acknowledgement of Sullivan, the Therapeutic Community movement such as found at Cooper Riis Healing Community (see Loue, 2016) embodies many principles of IPT.

Sullivan's emphasis on the role of interpersonal learning in treatment, including the correction of inappropriate family and juvenile and adolescent social group patterns and resultant interpersonal distortions, has natural theoretical and clinical links to the practice of group psychotherapy. While Sullivan did not contribute any original thinking on group psychotherapy himself, he nonetheless had an important influence on its development. It is little known that the Jerome Frank, Morris Parloff, and Florence Powdermaker's original and groundbreaking study of group psychotherapy was conducted under a grant through the auspices of the Washington School of Psychiatry in 1947 (see D. Rioch, 1948). The proposal for the research study arose initially from Florence Powdermaker's Research Seminar on Group Psychotherapy which she taught at the Washington School of Psychiatry during the mid-1940s. The study developed into one of the first major books on group psychotherapy (Powdermaker and Frank, 1953). Frank and Parloff later significantly influenced the development of one of the most important figures in modern group psychotherapy, Irvin Yalom (1975). Obviously strongly influenced by Sullivan's interpersonal theory, Yalom (1975: 22) credited Sullivan's ideas about process and goals of psychotherapy as "clearly consistent with those of interactional group therapy."

Less well known and easily traced is Sullivan's influence on the field of family therapy. Sullivan (1954: 62) was among the first psychodynamic theorists and therapists to suggest that "collateral information should not be refused without good reason." He was well aware of the hidden agenda of the sources of this collateral information and of the potential dangers to the confidentiality of the therapeutic relationship. He still believed that valuable information not available from the client could be obtained from the collateral parties and that contact with significant others in the client's life provided him a special opportunity to directly observe interpersonal transactions and distortions in the family unit. Sullivan's interest in collateral data by itself does not represent the beginning of the development of family therapy. Indeed, Fromm-Reichmann (1950), a close colleague of Sullivan, was far more explicit about the need for including the family in the course of treatment.

A discussion with Jay Haley (1979), the noted American family therapist, afforded an unusual opportunity to understand an important connection between Sullivan and the development of family therapy. Haley acknowledged Sullivan as one of his two major models for his development of strategic family therapy, through the influence on another family psychotherapy pioneer and supervisee of Sullivan, Don D. Jackson (Jackson, 1968; Watzlawick et al., 1967). Jackson played an important role in developing the double bind theory of schizophrenia (Bateson et al., 1956) which expanded Sullivan's ideas about schizophrenic communication into the study of disturbed communications and interactional patterns of the families of schizophrenics. Jackson's clinical work focused on the correction of inappropriate family patterns within schizophrenic families, which was the beginning of systems-oriented or communication model of family therapy, an approach thoroughly consistent with interpersonal theory.

Having traversed Sullivan's penetrating approach to psychopathology, psychodiagnosis and psychotherapy and its modern influence on theory and clinical practice, we will last turn toward his remarkable contributions to understanding social problems.

## Note

1   Adapted in part from Evans, F. B., & Maris, J. A. (2016). Book review: *Co-creating change: Effective psychodynamic therapy techniques* by Jon Frederickson, *Psychiatry, 79(4),* 335–338.

# Chapter 10

# Social Psychiatry and the Problems of Society

During his productive lifetime Sullivan, perhaps more than any other person, labored to bring about the fusion of psychiatry and social science.

(Allport in Cantril, 1950: 135)

Harry Stack Sullivan was a social scientist whose specialty was psychiatry.

Dorothy Blitstein (1953)

Having sampled the breadth and depth of Sullivan's thinking on developmental theory, psychopathology, psychological assessment, and psychotherapy and established his impact historically on the development of treatment approaches beyond individual treatment, it would be easy for this book on this important contributor in the field of psychodynamic theory and practice to end here. Yet, Sullivan made one more important contribution that should not go unacknowledged – his application of interpersonal theory and social psychiatry to the problems of society. While Sullivan eloquently elaborated his concerns about the role of society in the causation of mental illness and social problems throughout his career, the last years of his life were passionately, and almost exclusively, devoted to the problem of international conflict and world peace. His decision not to rest on his prior accomplishments and to take up the invitation of Brock Chisholm, the first head of the World Health Organization, to serve as a consultant to the post-World War II International Congress on Mental Health almost certainly brought his life to an early end. As Perry (1964: xi) stated, Sullivan was reluctant "to set schizophrenia apart from living itself; in part, also, he came to feel, increasingly over the last ten years of his life, that the main implication of his work was in the area of social psychology – in the wide spectrum of preventive measures within society itself."

In this final chapter, it is only appropriate to come full circle back to the theme which runs throughout this book and throughout Sullivan's work – the relationship between the problems of the person and the problems of society. Along with Fromm (1941, 1947, 1955), Sullivan's theory of personality was

DOI: 10.4324/9781003305712-13

fundamentally social psychological, elucidating how the forces of society affected the person and how the processes of the person (e.g., anxiety and parataxic distortion) were manifested in the problems of society. Sullivan's deep understanding of the impact of social forces, down the minute interactions between the mother and the child, was interwoven throughout his ideas about personality, psychopathology, and psychotherapy.

Sullivan's achievements were remarkable and almost incomprehensible from his background and, at his time, history. This quintessential loner and social outsider grew up in a parochial rural community with a very troubled adolescence and young adulthood and an undistinguished academic and early work career, only emerge at age 30 as a psychiatrist with revolutionary ideas about the relation between the person and society. Rather than to be crushed by the circumstances of his early life, Sullivan transformed his unfortunate personal experiences by becoming a penetrating observer and social critic who dared to explore taboo and destructive social forces of repressive sexual attitudes, anti-Semitism, racism, and international conflict.

## Sullivan as Social Scientist

Sullivan's works on social psychiatry are found in the collection of articles published as a book, *The Fusion of Psychiatry and Social Sciences* (1964) containing 17 previously published pieces on such topics as racism, anti-Semitism, the causes of international tensions, and world peace. Sullivan was surprisingly optimistic, and had creative ideas about how psychiatry, which he defined as the "science of interpersonal living," could make important contributions about easing international tensions and other social problems. While the vast majority of early psychodynamic/psychoanalytic theorists' ideas were rooted in their medical training, Sullivan's roving mind took him further afield, likely spurred by the seminal influence of William Alanson White. Dating back to his earliest professional days, Sullivan's interest in the social sciences blossomed, including collaborations with some of the finest minds in sociology and anthropology of the famous University of Chicago School. His later alliance with anthropologist/linguist Edward Sapir and political scientist Harold Lasswell was essential in the founding of the William Alanson White Foundation. Sapir's untimely death in 1939 interrupted what could have formed a potent research initiative combining interpersonal psychiatry and social sciences. As it was, throughout his editorship, Sullivan's journal *Psychiatry* was a model for interdisciplinary scholarship, aspects of which are still coming to light as will be discussed in this influence on the clinical pastoral movement (see Lawrence, 2022).

Sullivan's (1926, 1930) first contribution to social psychiatry was his analysis of the impact of cultural values on the patterning of male sexual needs. Like Freud, Sullivan took a strong position regarding the destructive effects of cultural sexual prohibitions, which impeded sexual development. As stated earlier, his clear-minded, though incomplete, analysis of the psychogenesis of homosexuality was especially radical for his time in history. As Sullivan (1953: 294) stated, "to talk about homosexuality's being a problem really means about as much as to talk about humanity's being a problem." He believed that homosexuality was a comprehensible human process, arising from specific problematic parental sexual attitudes and child-rearing practices. No doubt his understanding and acceptance of homosexuality at a time when the topic was never openly discussed, and his belief that the taboo against it constituted a virulent and irrational prejudice, contributed to the dismissal of his ideas by the psychiatric community. While Sullivan focused primarily on male sexuality, his observations on the effect of cultural sexual attitudes on female development were often incisive. Sullivan (1953) believed that the culturally based double standard had an especially deleterious impact on the development of women's sexuality and intimacy Sullivan's views on sex role stereotyping were exceptionally lucid and compassionate, raising questions still to be answered even today.

Quite likely spurred by the events in Nazi Germany, Sullivan wrote one of the earliest psychiatric articles on the age-old problem of anti-Semitism (1938b). He believed that the crude classification of people found in religious prejudice impeded the development of a rational view of others and was a significant source of difficulty for the recipient, as well as the holder, of the stereotype. Sullivan stated that anti-Semitism was deeply ingrained in Christian tradition and present in all Christian societies. He compared anti-Semitism to other prejudices, including one of his own experience, the strong anti-Catholic sentiment found a largely Protestant communities. He characterized prejudice and stereotyping, the attribution of inferred differences in personality based on a variety of factors such as religion, gender, race, and social status, as a way of displacing feelings of inferiority and resentment toward authority arising from irrationally punitive parenting processes onto external, devalued social groups. It is also important to note that Sullivan published his article on anti-Semitism before the United States entered World War II at a time when the U.S. government was well aware of, and unresponsive to, the atrocities of Nazi Germany (Dinnerstein, 1995).

In 1938, Sullivan collaborated in field research with black sociologists Charles S. Johnson and E. Franklin Frazier as part of a study on the personality development and difficulties in Southern rural black youth. This study led to Sullivan's (1940a, 1941) formulations on the effects of racism on black youth and the cost that racial prejudice has on American society. He found that black youth in the South had a ubiquitous fear of whites, an experience which he found completely understandable considering the virulent and dangerous racial prejudice and diminished economic opportunity that these youth faced. Interestingly, Sullivan found black youths' predominant experience of whites changed from fear to rage, as they were geographically closer to the border between the south and north. Sullivan movingly described the depth of these experiences, which persisted even in the face of contrary evidence, and foresaw the continuation of racial conflict resulting of these deep cultural wounds. Instead of taking the commonly held position that there were significant differences in personality between blacks and whites, he found nothing distinct except which could be accounted for by social factors. Sullivan was well ahead of his time in challenging genetic inferiority model such as Jansen's (Jensen & Johnson, 1994), instead anticipating the now well-established relationship between social class on intellectual development (Sternberg et al., 2005) and personality (Hollingshead & Redlich, 1958). As Sullivan (1940/1962: 107) stated, "If we are to develop ... a national solidarity, we must ... cultivate a humanistic, rather than a paternalistic, and exploiting, or indifferent attitude to these numerous citizens."

No discussion of Sullivan's contributions to social science would be complete without an examination of his ideas regarding international conflict and peace. Based on his close relationship with Lasswell (1930), father of the field of political psychology, Sullivan became interested early in his career in the application of psychiatry to political science. Sullivan (1940b) spoke out against about censorship and propaganda as ultimately an ultimately divisive interpersonal influence, which served short-range political goals, but which had the long-term effects of continuing international tensions. Anticipating the world after World War II, Sullivan (1942) turned his attention to the ways in which psychiatry could be useful in helping what he called opinion leadership to correct damaging stereotypes of others from different cultures. He maintained that it was a responsibility of national leadership to seek ways to integrate communities and nations as a means to decreasing international conflict. In particular, he believed that comprehension of the process of consensual validation could be used productively for greater international understanding, an important process utilized heavily in international negotiation today (see Fisher & Ury, 1981; Shapiro, 2010). On the other side of the coin, Sullivan's work on selective inattention spurred White's (1988) subsequent examination of motivated resistance to the change about war, to the horror of nuclear danger and possible ideas about how to prevent it, and to blocking realistic empathy toward real or perceived international enemies.

Following World War II, Sullivan became active in the work of the new World Health Organization. Perhaps Sullivan's (1950b) best statement of the role of psychiatry in international peace was his seminal paper given at the UNESCO International Tensions Conference in 1948. Sullivan envisioned that the reduction of stereotypes of other cultures, which were often promoted for political ends, was the path to achieve international peace. He believed that it was necessary to reduce cultural isolation through education about different patterns of living around the world. To this end, Sullivan thought it imperative to have face-to-face contact with persons of different societies. Additionally, he promoted the idea that sane child-rearing techniques led to better-adjusted citizens who were more immune to political manipulation and the cancer of societal insecurity. Tragically, Sullivan died shortly after this work was completed, preventing from developing his exceptional ideas further. Though nearly fifty years old, his ideas about the promotion of international understanding through cross-cultural education are remarkably contemporary. Sullivan's ideas about international peace stand as a final testament to his vast personal vision, one which clearly and compassionately integrates the mother-infant relationship, the complexities of juvenile and adolescent development, psychotherapy with schizophrenic persons, the problems of prejudice, and the need for global understanding.

## Contemporary Applications of Interpersonal Theory and Society

Though Sullivan's influence largely has been forgotten in mainstream mental health, throughout this book, I have pointed out some remarkable exceptions where his IPT is alive and thriving. Sullivan may have had a similar influence on important figures in the social sciences. For example, one is tempted to give Sullivan credit for influencing the work of renowned scholar Herbert Kelman's work on the sociopsychological analysis of international behavior, who subsequently mentored Daniel Shapiro, another eminent scholar in relational identity theory and international negotiation. Kelman was a member of Harvard University's Social Relations Department at the time Timothy Leary used Sullivan's IPT to develop the interpersonal circumplex. Earlier, Kelman collaborated with Morris Parloff and Jerome Frank (Kelman & Parloff, 1957; Parloff, Kelman & Frank, 1954) on the early development of group psychotherapy which was originally sponsored by Sullivan (see Chapter 9). Kelman's (1965) book on international behavior featured chapters from Harold Lasswell, who collaborated with Sullivan in the founding of the William Alanson White Foundation, and Ralph White, who adapted elements of Sullivan's interpersonal theory to international conflict. Unfortunately, no definitive link has been established. To close this chapter, I will review the modern application of Sullivan IPT has had on two disparate areas involving social issues – the influence on the development of clinical pastoral care and the development of an interpersonally based approach to forensic assessment, especially in determinations of child custody in family court and asylum in U.S. Immigration Court.

Due to the recent scholarship of the Reverend Doctor Raymond Lawrence (2022), we now have a window into the heretofore unexplored collaboration and friendship between Sullivan and the founder of the clinical pastoral movement, Reverend Dr. Anton Boisen. While Sullivan has a well-deserved reputation for bringing a greater scientific emphasis to the field of psychodynamic theory and practice, Lawrence's book introduces a different side of Sullivan, one in which he explored links between mental disorder and religious beliefs with Boisen. Unlike Freud's (1927) view of religion as a culture-wide form of irrationality and neurosis in opposition to science, Sullivan welcomed and encouraged Boisen's explorations of religious experience as a legitimate area of psychiatric study. Based on his research, including long misplaced letters between Boisen and Sullivan, Lawrence discovered that Boisen and Sullivan began their relationship when Sullivan was doing cutting-edge treatment of schizophrenic individuals at the Sheppard Pratt Hospital, a collaboration that would continue throughout the rest of Sullivan's life. Boisen (1936) believed that the problem of mental illness is fundamentally rooted in the individual's experiences, beliefs, and philosophy about life, particularly occasioned by the sense of personal failure. He also wrote persuasively about the similarity of certain religious experiences and severe psychopathology, laying groundwork for the importance of an individual's religious beliefs as one aspect of a comprehensive understanding of the whole person. He took the unprecedented step of training religious workers, especially in mental hospital chaplaincies, in the treatment of the problems of mental disease and enlisted Sullivan to teach in his clinical pastoral training programs. With Sullivan's encouragement, Boisen published eight articles on religion and mental health in Sullivan's journal *Psychiatry*, a rare inclusion for a psychiatric journal. Much the same as Sullivan, Boisen was a groundbreaking thinker whose modern influence is not widely understood.

Another modern inspiration of Sullivan's IPT is found in the area of forensic psychological assessment, specifically in child custody and Immigration Court matters. Evans (2012) proposed an adaptation of IPT-influenced Therapeutic Assessment (see Chapter 8) as an alternative method in lieu of child custody and parenting plan evaluations to help resolve antagonistic legal situations by working directly with the parent litigants and their attorneys. By assisting litigants to resolve their own parenting plan disputes through the use of interpersonally focused Therapeutic Assessment intervention, children may be shielded from the crushing emotional impact of high conflict custody litigation (see Garrity & Baris, 1997). Additionally, parents can learn to model cooperation in the midst of deep personal conflict and attorneys can find these high-stress legal representations to be more satisfying.

This method was subsequently developed into a broad model of collaborative/therapeutic assessment called Building Empathy through Assessment (BETA: Smith & Evans, 2017) with greater applicability to other forensic settings, including civil litigation in personal injury and disability determinations as well as child custody and immigration matters. By conceptualizing forensic neutrality as incorporating both compassion and skepticism as dual lenses of observation, BETA allows for a deeper, and ultimately more objective, personal engagement in matters which typically are dealt only with cold, impersonal, and heavily skeptical detachment. BETA utilizes Sullivan's participant-observer approach and the psychiatric interview to forensic psychological assessment combined with the IPT one genus hypothesis that we are all simply more human than otherwise.

Another area in which Sullivan's IPT is well suited to social issues is in forensic psychological assessment in Immigration Court (IC). Evans and Hass (2018) point out that these assessments require a more complex approach. because they encompass issues well beyond individual concerns and must take into consideration social and cultural context. Many of these evaluations require an understanding of the family as well in matters involving deportation. Any conceptual model for conducting forensic psychological assessment in Immigration Court must provide integration of individual, social group, culture, political, and cross-cultural concerns along with issues of psychological trauma and an often-hostile societal attitude towards immigrants. As such, Sullivan's IPT is ideally suited to the task. While it is beyond the scope of this book to go into detail, the forensic psychological assessment of torture in asylum claims provides a strong illustrative example. Readers wanting to explore this area of practice in more depth are referred to Evans and Hass (2018), Mercado et al. (2022), and Evans (2000).

Perhaps no area of psychological practice is more fraught than working with victims of torture (see Evans, 2005, 2011, 2016). The forensic psychological assessor enters the interpersonal world of women and men who must share horrific experiences beyond ordinary comprehension if their claim of persecution and torture is to be seen as credible before an immigration judge. The role of the independent forensic psychological assessment is to provide psychological evidence to claims of torture as part of their petitions for asylum in the U.S. In such work, the devastating impact of political terrorism on these individuals' view of themselves, their relationships, and the world around them is a deeply disturbing, but unavoidable reality. These individuals have much to teach us about our own reactions to terrorism, something about terrorists, and a great deal about the evil that exists in the world around us. We share with victims of torture what Jeffrey Jay (1991) calls "Terrible Knowledge," the palpable and undeniable awareness that evil exists, has existed, and will always exist in the world around us and that without warning can affect us in ways that are incomprehensible, whether or not we are good people living good lives. Much in our current Western culture attempts to insulate us from this truth, providing caricatures of evil defeated by the forces of good, for example, so common in our media. Unfortunately, this denial of reality can leave policy makers, immigration officials, and to some degree even immigration judges, deaf to the reality of terrible knowledge, or what Arendt (1963) called the "banality of evil."

Neo-Kraepelinian mental disorder diagnosis and individual models of personality functioning fall far short of being useful in such settings. To properly address the complexity of persecution and asylum, forensic psychological assessment must include a broad cultural and political perspective as well as an understanding of psychological trauma. Cross-cultural, gender, and legal issues must be taken into account in an informed and compassionate assessment of an individual seeking asylum after an especially brutal experience of torture. As Evans (2012) stated, Sullivan's interpersonal theory provides the framework for integrating these complex interactions by integrating the complex multiple levels of influence into a comprehensible whole. Also, Sullivan's participant observer approach necessitates the assessor to pay careful attention to the social and cultural relationship between the assessor and the client if a full understanding of the assessment is to be gained. For example, many female victims of sexual torture have strong cultural prohibitions about revealing their experiences to a male assessor, even though withholding such information can be detrimental to their claim of persecution and asylum. As such, the forensic assessor must offer a secure place for such overwhelming and culturally prohibited information to emerge.

As such, Evans (2005) called into question so-called neutral forensic assessment seen as the standard of practice (Greenberg & Shuman, 1997, 2007). This standard model is by nature skeptical and doubting like most science and seen as ideally conducted with a detached stance. This perspective fails to account for the forensic examiner's impact interpersonally and that such relationship of skepticism and doubt by itself is actually not neutral. A lack of understanding of the impact of skepticism and disbelief in the interpersonal realm can potentially and substantially skew information gathered in a forensic assessment. For example, Mollica et al. (1992; 1987) and Herman (1992) found such skepticism is extremely toxic to torture victims and others who have suffered from interpersonal violence, leading them to shut down emotionally and withhold crucial information. From an interpersonal perspective, to be fully neutral, skepticism must be balanced with an openness to the experience of the other person.

As such, forensic psychology should be reconsidered as a human process with specific goals and methods, rather than a purely scientific one. Although forensic assessment by its nature requires a more explicitly factual basis and concern for malingering and deception than clinical work (see Jacobs et al., 2001a, b), it does not follow that forensic assessment should be practiced with greater human detachment. An interpersonal approach to forensic assessment requires that the assessor to enter what Martin Buber (1957) called the "realm of the interhuman," where the examiner is comfortable with, or can at least tolerate, nearness of human experience, however terrible.

In closing this section and this book, it is hopefully now clear that Harry Stack Sullivan was a true visionary comparable to Freud and arguably beyond. The scope of Sullivan's interpersonal theory of personality was fundamentally social psychological, illuminating how the forces of society affect the person and how the processes within the person are manifested in the problems of society. Along with his deep understanding of the impact of social forces, Sullivan also described the intricate interactions between the mother and the child (and in therapy the psychotherapist and client) which were intertwined throughout his revolutionary ideas about personality, mental illness, and psychotherapy. On a personal level, Sullivan transformed his own unfortunate personal history to become an astute observer of the human condition and a social critic who dared to explore taboo and destructive social forces. In the 25 years since this book was first published, it has been a great pleasure to see his ideas alive and well, furthered by modern thinkers who explicitly acknowledge his influence.

# Glossary of Terms for Interpersonal Theory

**ANXIETY** The experience of interpersonal insecurity, which for Sullivan was the primary cause of inadequate or inappropriate patterns of interpersonal relations. Sullivan's postulate of a tension of anxiety as one of two important motivational systems (see TENSION OF NEED) is perhaps the most unique and central motivational postulate within his interpersonal theory and clinical practice and is closely related to Bowlby's concept of attachment. The tension of anxiety is the first purely interpersonal motivation system in the history of psychodynamic theory. Sullivan believed that anxiety in the infant was induced by anxiety in the mothering one by a process which he called empathy. Mild forms of anxiety such as disapproval and forbidding gestures, which he called the gradient of anxiety, were important in the learning of socially appropriate behavior beginning in early childhood. Sullivan saw severe anxiety, the experience of intense and overwhelming insecurity in response to anxiety in the mothering one, to be an interruptive influence in the development of healthy interpersonal relationships. The sense of self is made up of reflected appraisals of others and is formed through interpersonal interaction involving reward, gradients of anxiety, and severe anxiety (see SELF).

**CONSENSUAL VALIDATION** The interpersonal process by which the person develops common understanding with another about the signs, signals, and meaning of experience through language and communication. Consensual validation is the primary activity in the syntaxic mode of experience.

**DISSOCIATION** The underlying process by which a person deals with needs that are met with severe anxiety. It involves a complete inhibition of motivation toward satisfying certain needs with the total exclusion of any recognition of their existence to prevent the experience of uncanny emotion. The person is blithely unaware of dissociated behavior and its impact on others. Sullivan saw dissociation as a process that was overutilized in severe mental disorders. The failure of dissociation was attended by overwhelming, unbearable anxiety, the kind found primarily in psychotic decompensations. Sullivan later conceptualized dissociation as the part of the self-system, the primary operation of the not-me personification (see PERSONIFICAT-ION), in which experiences and motivations that were so anxiety-ridden that they needed to be excluded from all awareness of the self.

**DYNAMISM** A relatively enduring pattern of interpersonal transactions that characterize the person. In concept of the dynamism, Sullivan stressed that, while human behavior was a dynamic process of ever-unfolding flux and change within the interpersonal field, it became organized into characteristic patterns of interpersonal transaction directed toward the satisfaction of needs and the avoidance of distress. Sullivan emphasized that the common principles of interpersonal behavior were more critical than the relatively insignificant, particular differences between people.

**DYNAMISMS OF DIFFICULTY** Patterns of inadequate or inappropriate patterns of interpersonal relations. Dynamisms of difficulty are problematic patterns of interpersonal relations arising from experience with intense anxiety. These dynamisms arise from the serious and relatively unresolvable conflict between the satisfaction of physical and interpersonal needs and the expectations and requirements of significant others that restricted the expression or satisfaction of these needs. Sullivan used the terms dynamisms of difficulty or inadequate and inappropriate patterns of interpersonal relations instead of mental disorder. Sullivan believed that it was more accurate and effective to focus on problematic interpersonal processes rather than to describe clinical entities. EUPHORIA The experience of a state of well-being arising from the reduction or elimination of tensions regarding human biological and psychosocial requirements of living. Unlike Freud's pleasure principle in which euphoria came as the result of gratifying psychosexual (oral, anal, phallic, and genital) needs, Sullivan defined two distinct categories of tensions, tension of needs (physical) and tension of anxiety (interpersonal), the reduction of which led respectively to the experiences of satisfaction and interpersonal security.

**EXPERIENCE** The internal component of events of the person's interpersonal world. Experience was the primary element of the person's cognitive-perceptual world, the way in which the person came to know the interpersonal world. Because all knowledge of the world is subjective, experience is never the same as the event in which the organism participates. Because of this fact, the psychotherapist could never assume to know the person's inner life and must depend on consensual validation to understanding the meaning of the person's experience. In this regard, Sullivan shared a philosophical base with phenomenology (see Husserl 1965 and Merleau-Ponty 1963).

**FORESIGHT** The anticipation of certain consequences associated with experiences and actions taken to modify these experiences. Sullivan saw the cognitive capacity of foresight as the process by which persons formulated ways to meet needs and avoid anxiety and anticipated the interpersonal consequences of taking particular actions. Foresight is necessary for successful interpersonal living. and is interrupted by severe anxiety.

**INTERPERSONAL SECURITY** The absence of the tension of anxiety. The need for interpersonal security was especially critical from Sullivan's perspective. Interpersonal tension could only be relaxed through the removal of anxiety which leads to the experience of interpersonal security. JUVENILE ERA The years between entrance to school and the time when one forms a relationship with a chum (see PREADOLESCENCE). The importance of the juvenile era and peer relations in human development was one of Sullivan's signature contributions. New social influences provided in the juvenile era offered the opportunity, through comparisons with teachers and other juveniles' parents, to more clearly evaluate parental behaviors, values and expectations. More importantly opened the juvenile to world of peer relationships which involved a critical shift in the role of playmates from the more egocentric patterns of play in childhood to more cooperative and competitive patterns of interaction in the juvenile era. In addition to the kind of unilateral, top-down authority the juvenile experiences with adults, peer relations offered the juvenile the opportunity and requirement to interact with peers with direct or symmetrical reciprocity. Through the give and take of concession, while maintaining their own positions, peers in the juvenile era learned the critical social processes of compromise and cooperation, through which juveniles develop patterns of friendship. LONELINESS The experience of the failure to achieve an intimate relationship. Loneliness, though difficult to describe, was a very important motivation in interpersonal development. Sullivan believed the actual experience of loneliness was a phenomenon which came only in preadolescence and afterward. While Sullivan's observations on how loneliness contributed to interpersonal development and psychopathology were penetrating, he had difficulty, similar to his earlier formulations about anxiety, with the underlying cause of the phenomenon, which Bowlby achieved more successfully in his formulation of attachment theory.

**LUST** The experiential component of the genital need culminating in genital activity leading to orgasm. The last of the truly zonal tensions of need, lust, like all tensions of need, required interpersonal cooperation around which the dynamisms of lust developed. The internal physical maturational changes of puberty lead to genital interest which served as the transition from preadolescence into early adolescence, whether the person was ready or not. Due in part to the advent of lust, there is a shift in the need for intimacy from the isophilic (same sex intimacy) to the heterophilic (same sex intimacy) relationships. Sullivan believed that the eruption of the need for lustful satisfaction in early adolescence collided with the developing interpersonal needs for personal security (freedom from anxiety) and for interpersonal intimacy (collaboration with at least one other person leading to freedom from loneliness). Failure to find a satisfactory integration of these three powerful motivations lead to mental disorder.

**MALEVOLENT TRANSFORMATION** The anticipation that the need for tenderness will bring anxiety and pain which leads to the transformation of the frustrated need for tenderness into an attitude of exploitation of others. Sullivan looked directly at the effects of parental cruelty. He reasoned that, when the child of cruel parents experienced and expressed his or her need for tenderness, the child received anxiety or pain. When malevolent parents took advantage of their position of authority to ridicule, ignore, lie to, and hurt the child, the child would soon come to anticipate that his or her need for tenderness will bring anxiety and pain. Malevolent transformation is a dynamism utilizing security operations to reduce this extreme distress, in child transformed his or her experience of weakness and helplessness into an attitude of exploitation of the needs and vulnerabilities of others.

**MODES OF REPRESENTATION** Sullivan's attempt to conceptualize a model of cognitive-social development (unique among the early psychoanalysts) which included the prototaxic, the parataxic, and the syntaxic modes. The prototaxic mode is the earliest and most primitive, described as the infant's limited awareness of himself or herself as separate from the environment. The overall experience is a flowing, undifferentiated, and cosmic sense of the world. As experiences and percepts accumulate in the young infant and actions become attached to relatively reliable consequences, the sense of undifferentiated wholeness is broken, and the infant begins to develop experience in the parataxic mode. Experiences become associated with consequences as the infant develops recall, memories of prior consequences attach to certain experiences, and foresight, the anticipation of certain consequences associated with experiences and actions taken to modify these experiences. In the parataxic mode, experiences are linked by association, not by logic. As certain events in the inner and outer world become consistently associated with certain experiences and consequences of these experiences, through recall and foresight these events become signs and signals for the satisfactions, frustrations, security, or insecurity which follows. A particular meaning becomes attached to each sign. Since all satisfactions and security for the infant require interpersonal cooperation, signs and their meanings are representations of interpersonal transaction as well. As these experiences become represented through language, signs, signals, and meanings can be spoken and the child person can begin to consensually validate his or her experience with others, developing common understanding about the signs, signals, and meaning of experience. Communicative behavior (both speech and gesture) and its potential for greater logical differentiation and precision become the primary ways of knowing, which is experience in the syntaxic mode, the third and most advanced mode of experience.

**ONE GENUS HYPOTHESIS** Sullivan's most elegant postulate in which he stated, "everyone is much more simply human than otherwise." Sullivan utilized this principle to draw attention to universality of interpersonal processes for all humans, challenging Kraepelin's perspective regarding the fundamental differences between mentally health and the mentally disorder. Sullivan believed that, for the vast majority of people, interpersonal learning accounted for the variation in personality, not their underlying biological or constitutional makeup.

**ORIENTATION IN LIVING** A recurrent set of patterns or tendencies of interpersonal relations that were manifest in all spheres of life. The extensive social experiences of the juvenile, with the complex of relationships with parents, peers, and adult authorities beyond the family, were required to establish an orientation to living. Sullivan described someone as adequately oriented if they developed a good grasp generally of their own needs and motives; insight into how to adequately meet these needs, while avoiding undue anxiety; had the capacity to set medium and long range goals, foregoing momentary impulsive satisfaction; and the ability to enhance the opportunity for prestige.

**PARATAXIC DISTORTION** The misunderstandings and misconceptions of others that characterize all human relations. Sullivan defined this concept in the two ways. In the more narrow sense of the term, Sullivan used parataxic distortion to describe when the client unwittingly perceived and treated another person as if the other person was similar to a problematic early interpersonal relationship from the past. In this sense, parataxic distortion bears a similarity with Freud's concept of transference. In the broader definition of parataxic distortion, Sullivan saw this process as a variant of the ubiquitous human tendency toward misconception or incorrect interpersonal attribution.

**PARTICIPANT OBSERVATION** The basic role of the psychotherapist in interpersonal psychotherapy. Sullivan believed that the psychotherapist can never be a purely objective observer, but also participates in the interpersonal interaction within the treatment setting. The psychotherapist needs to be aware that much of what the client does and says is addressed to and influenced by the therapist in the here-and-now interaction. Because of this inevitable interpersonal influence, the psychotherapist needed to be ever-alert to the meaning of his or her participation in the psychiatric interview. The psychotherapist as an expert in interpersonal relations must be able to observe both the processes in the patient and him or her self as well.

**PERSONALITY** The relatively stable and ongoing pattern of interpersonal situations which characterize a person. Sullivan did not see personality as a fixed entity residing in an individual, but relatively stable patterns of relatedness. The stability of this pattern is determined by the relative regularity of the interpersonal environment. Dramatic shifts in environment will heavily impact on the stability of the patterns which make up the personality. The idea that the personality resides more in the nature of relationships than in an individual is a dramatic difference from most psychodynamic theories.

**PERSONIFICATION** The central set of internal assumptions, ideas, and fantasies about people and the self, based on interpersonal experience, which constitutes that way a person interprets the interpersonal world. A personification is a cognitive representation of learned experiences of transactional relatedness, i.e. the transactions of interpersonal cooperation and of the concurrent experiences of interpersonal security. There are two kinds of personifications – self and others. Personifications are based on the person's experience of him or her self and others and should not be confused with the "real" other person. The earliest form of personification, the good mothering one and the bad mothering one, does not differentiate into an object (the "real" mother) or a subject (the self). These two concepts are actually representations of good and bad mothering, i.e. representations of the flow of experience where the distinction between self and other is a primitive and vaguely differentiated sense of satisfying, unsatisfying, or seriously anxiety-ridden interpersonal transaction.

As the infant becomes more aware of his or her body, three personifications of "me" or self personifications develop in relationship to interpersonal experience. Satisfactory, tender, and secure interpersonal experiences are organized into the self personification which Sullivan called good-me. Interpersonal experiences associated with disapproval, forbidding gestures, and general tension in the other are organized into the personification of bad-me. The not-me personification arises from interpersonal experiences of severe anxiety. When the mothering one responds to the behavior of the infant with severe and overwhelming anxiety, the infant cannot escape and can only engage in dissociative reactions to avoid intensely dysphoric experience.

**PREADOLESCENCE** A significant transformation in peer relationships and interpersonal relatedness from the need for compeers to the need for intimacy. The appearance of a different kind of peer relationship than the playmates in the juvenile era is marked by a new, more specific relationship to a particular member of the same sex who becomes a chum or a close friend. Forming the relationship with a chum represented the first step in the maturation of interpersonal relations in which the chum's needs were keenly felt as relatively as important as one's own, the first step in the development of the collaboration. Unlike the more impersonal or self-centered juvenile social operations, collaboration involved making sure each others' satisfactions and security were met and taking satisfaction in the success of each other as part of the maintenance of prestige, status, and freedom from anxiety. Preadolescence is the first stage in the development of the capacity for intimacy.

**PSYCHIATRIC INTERVIEW** Sullivan's structure for the conduct of what is more commonly called psychotherapy. The psychiatric interview involves communication between a client and an expert in interpersonal living for the purpose of understanding the client's characteristic interpersonal relationships. The client expects to derive benefit from the interview to better understand patterns of relationship that are troublesome or beneficial. The psychiatric interview is structured into four stages – the formal inception, the reconnaissance, the detailed inquiry, and the termination.

**PSYCHIATRY** Sullivan's most distinguishing contribution is the revision of psychiatry as science of interpersonal relations, including the events or processes in which the psychiatrist participates while being an observant psychiatrist. Interpersonal theory is a significant critique and reworking of Freud's individualistic, psychoanalytic approach and a major departure from Kraepelin's descriptive psychiatry.

**SECURITY OPERATIONS** Interpersonal psychological and behavioral maneuvers of the self-system organized primarily to reduce and avoid anxiety. These more primitive avoidant operations conflicted with the development of a more advanced comprehension of interpersonal situations through recall and foresight. The self-system is not readily open to later educative influences, as later learning is hampered by the imperfect observation and definite inventions which comprise the self-system. Security operations are difficult to modify, as anxiety and its inner experienced component, the self personification of bad-me, lead the person to adapt to social expectations at the cost of the avoidance of new experience and the distortion of the experience of need.

**SELF** The representation of those experiences about what one takes oneself to be. The process by which one develops this sense of self comes through interpersonal interaction. As Sullivan stated (1940/1947: 22), "The self may be said to be made up of reflected appraisals of others." The sense of self begins in the infant first by learning about "my body" (see PERSONIFICATION).

**SELF-SYSTEM** The anti-anxiety dynamism which lead operationally to the maintenance of interpersonal security and the avoidance of interpersonal situations likely to produce anxiety. The self-system is the part of the personality that controls awareness, particularly as a means of avoiding anxiety (see SECURITY OPERATIONS).

**TENSION OF NEEDS** The experienced component of various specific biological requirements of the human organism. Conceptually close to Freud's psychosexual needs found in his theory of the libido, Sullivan's concept included such needs as hunger, thirst, warmth, dermal physiochemical regulation (e.g., removal of urine and feces from the skin), and oxygen requirements, as well as general biological requirements such as the need to sleep and the need for touch and human contact. Sullivan's tension of needs were either in experienced through specific zones of interaction or experienced in general.

**THEOREM OF TENDERNESS** The shared experience between the mother and the infant in which the mother feels tenderness in response to the need-driven tension in the infant. The critical interpersonal process links the satisfaction of specific zonal needs and general need for interaction with others. The child experiences the mother's behavior towards the relief of his or her needs, not only as a zonal satisfaction, but also as a tender act. The relaxing effect of the satisfaction of the need is associated with the tenderness of the mother, creating a general need for tenderness as well. The need for tenderness, as well as the need for contact (such as touch and later emotional contact), are "the very genuine beginnings of purely interpersonal or human needs" (Sullivan, 1953: 40).

# Chronology of Sullivan's Life and Beyond

1892   Born, Harry Stack Sullivan on February 21 in Norwich, New York. The only child Timothy Sullivan and Ella Stack Sullivan, first generation Irish-American immigrants. The Sullivan's had lost two sons prior, both born in February.

1894   Moves to the Stack family farm in Smyrna, NY after his mother disappears for several months. Sullivan's father unhappily moves to Smyrna where he farms the Stack farm until his death.

1897   Enters school one-room school in Smyrna as the only Irish-Catholic student in an anti-Catholic town.

1908   Enters Cornell University on a scholarship.

1909   Suspended from Cornell University for involvement in mail fraud. Disappears for two years.

1911   Matriculates to medical school at the Chicago College of Medicine and Surgery.
Awarded his medical degree in 1917.

1918   Commission as a Captain in U. S. Officers Reserve Medical Corps.

1921   Liaison officer for the Veterans Bureau at St. Elizabeth's Hospital in Washington, DC.

1922   Psychiatrist at Sheppard Pratt Hospital in Towson, MD, where he establishes special in-patient ward for schizophrenics.

1925   Publishes his first two papers on schizophrenia.

1926   Ella Stack Sullivan dies in Smyrna, New York.
Meets Edward Sapir, beginning his collaboration with the University of Chicago School of Sociology.

1927   Dr. Clara Thompson travels to Budapest to be analyzed by Sandor Ferenczi and later provides training analysis to Sullivan for admission to American Psychoanalytic Society.

1928   Participates in First Colloquium on Personality Investigation, landmark interdisciplinary conference of top social science and psychiatry scholars.

1930 Leaves Sheppard Pratt for a private practice in New York City and collaboration with Sapir at Yale University.
"Zodiac" group begins with Erich Fromm and Karen Horney.

1931 Timothy Sullivan dies in Smyrna, New York.

1933 Founds the William Alanson White Foundation.

1936 The Washington School of Psychiatry is incorporated.

1938 Founds the journal *Psychiatry*.

1939 Moves to Bethesda, MD, near Washington, DC.

1940 *Conceptions of modern psychiatry* published.
Psychiatric consultant to U.S. Selective Service.

1942 Consultantship at Chestnut Lodge

1943 Washington School of Psychiatry separates from the Washington-Baltimore Psychoanalytic Institute and establishes curriculum in interpersonal psychiatry.

1945 Becomes seriously ill and is under medical pressure to retire due to his seriously weakened heart
Begins collaboration with Brock Chisholm, first director of the World Health Organization as consultant to International Congress on Mental Health.

1948 Consultant to UNESCO International Tensions Project

1949 Dies January 14 in Paris returning from a meeting of the World Health Organization.
Committee on the Publication of Sullivan's writings formed.

1953 Interpersonal theory of psychiatry published.
*Conceptions of modern psychiatry* re-published.

1954 *The psychiatric interview* published.

1956 *Clinical studies in psychiatry* published.

1962 *Schizophrenia as a human process* published.

1964 *The fusion of psychiatry and social science* published.

1972 *Personal psychopathology* published.

# Bibliography

## PUBLICATIONS OF HARRY STACK SULLIVAN

*Books*

Sullivan, H. S. (1940/1953). *Conceptions of modern psychiatry, 2nd ed.* New York, NY: W.W. Norton & Company.

Sullivan, H. S. (1953). *The interpersonal theory of psychiatry.* New York, NY: Norton.

Sullivan, H. S. (1954). *The psychiatric interview.* New York, NY: Norton.

Sullivan, H. S. (1956). *Clinical studies in psychiatry.* New York, NY: Norton.

Sullivan, H. S. (1962). *Schizophrenia as a human process.* New York, NY: Norton.

Sullivan, H. S. (1964). *Fusion of psychiatry and social sciences.* New York, NY: Norton.

Sullivan, H. S. (1972). *Personal psychopathology.* New York, NY: Norton.

*Articles*

Sullivan, H. S. (1924–1925). Schizophrenia: Its conservative and malignant features. *American Journal of Psychiatry, 81,* 77–91. In *Schizophrenia as a human process.* New York, NY: W.W. Norton & Co.

Sullivan, H. S. (1925). The oral complex. *Psychoanalytic Review, 12,* 31–38.

Sullivan, H. S. (1926). Erogenous maturation. *Psychoanalytic Review, 13,* 1–15.

Sullivan, H. S. (1927–1928). Medical education. *American Journal of Psychiatry. 83,* 837–839.

Sullivan, H. S. (1930/1962). Archaic sexual culture and schizophrenia. In N. Haire (Ed.), *Sexual reform congress.* London, UK: Kegan Paul, Trench, Trubner & Co., Ltd. (In *Schizophrenia as a human process.* New York, NY: W.W. Norton & Co.).

Sullivan, H. S. (1930–1931). Socio-psychiatric research: Its implications for the schizophrenia problem and for mental hygiene. *American Journal of Psychiatry, 87,* 977–991. (In *Schizophrenia as a human process.* New York, NY: W.W. Norton & Co.).

Sullivan, H. S. (1931–1932). The modified psychoanalytic treatment of schizophrenia. *American Journal of Psychiatry, 88,* 519–540. (In *Schizophrenia as a human process.* New York, NY: W.W. Norton & Co.).

Sullivan, H. S. (1938a). Antisemitism. *Psychiatry, 1,* 593–598. (In *Fusion of psychiatry and social science.* New York, NY: W.W. Norton & Co.).

Sullivan, H. S. (1938b). Psychiatry: Introduction to the study of interpersonal relations: The data of psychiatry. *Psychiatry, 1,* 121–134. (In *Fusion of psychiatry and social science.* New York, NY: W.W. Norton & Co.).

Sullivan, H. S. (1940a). Censorship and propaganda. *Psychiatry, 3,* 628–632. (In *Fusion of psychiatry and social science.* New York, NY: W.W. Norton & Co.).

Sullivan, H. S. (1940b). Discussion of the case of Warren Wall. In E. Franklin Frazier (Ed.), *Negro youth at the crossroads: Their development in the middle states* (pp. 228–234). Washington, DC: American Council on Education. (In *Fusion of psychiatry and social science.* New York, NY: W.W. Norton & Co.).

Sullivan, H. S. (1941). Memorandum on a psychiatric reconnaissance. In Charles Johnson (Ed.), *Growing up in the Black Belt: Negro youth in the rural south* (pp. 328–333). Washington, DC: American Council on Education. (In *Fusion of psychiatry and social science.* New York, NY: W.W. Norton & Co.).

Sullivan, H. S. (1942). Leadership, mobilization, and postwar change. *Psychiatry, 5,* 263–282. (In *Fusion of psychiatry and social science.* New York, NY: W.W. Norton & Co.).

Sullivan, H. S. (1943). How sweet are the uses of adversity? *Psychiatry, 6,* 217–240.

Sullivan, H. S. (1944). The language of schizophrenia. In J. S. Kasanin (Ed.), *Language and thought in schizophrenia: Collected papers* (pp. 4–15). Los Angeles, CA: University of California Press.

Sullivan, H. S. (1947a). Remobilization for enduring peace and social progress. *Psychiatry, 10,* 239–245.

Sullivan, H. S. (1947b). Therapeutic investigations in schizophrenia. *Psychiatry, 10,* 121–125.

Sullivan, H. S. (1947). Notes on investigation, therapy, and education in psychiatry and their relations to schizophrenia. *Psychiatry, 10,* 271–280.

Sullivan, H. S. (1948). Towards a psychiatry of peoples. *Psychiatry, 11,* 105–116.

Sullivan, H. S. (1949). The theory of anxiety and the nature of psychotherapy. *Psychiatry, 12,* 3–12.

Sullivan, H. S. (1950a). The illusion of individuality. *Psychiatry, 13,* 317–332. (In *Fusion of psychiatry and social science.* New York, NY: W.W. Norton & Co.).

Sullivan, H. S. (1950b). Tensions interpersonal and international. In H. Cantril (Ed.), *Tensions that cause wars.* Urbana, IL:University of Illinois Press. (In *Fusion of psychiatry and social science.* New York, NY: W.W. Norton & Co.).

*Editorials*

References to Sullivan's many unsigned editorials in the journal *Psychiatry* can be found in *Thirty-year index 1938–1967* (pp. 103–104). New York, NY: William Alanson White Psychiatric Foundation.

**GENERAL WORKS**

Achin, J. C., & Kiesler, D. J. (Eds.) (1982). *Handbook of interpersonal psychotherapy.* New York, NY: Pergamon Press.

Ainsworth, M. D. S. (1969). Object relations, dependency, and attachment: A theoretical review of the infant-mother relationship. *Child Development, 40*(4), 969–1025.

Ainsworth, M. D. S. (1979). Infant–mother attachment. *American Psychologist, 34*(10), 932.

Ainsworth, M. D. S. (1982). Attachment: Retrospect and prospect. In C. M. Parkes & J. Stevenson-Hinde (Eds.), *The place of attachment in human behavior* (pp. 3–30). New York, NY: Basic Books.

Ainsworth M. D. S., Blehar, M. C., Waters, E., & Wall, S. (1978). *Patterns of attachment: A psychological study of the Strange Situation.* Hillsdale, NJ: Erlbaum.

Akavia, N. (2013). *Subjectivity in motion. Life, art and movement in the work of Hermann Rorschach.* New York, NY: Routledge.

Alden, L. E., Wiggins, J. S., & Pincus, A. L. (1990). Construction of circumplex scales for the Inventory of Interpersonal Problems. *Journal of Personality Assessment, 55*(3–4), 521–536.

Alexander, F. (1961). *The scope of psychoanalysis, 1921–1961: The selected papers of Franz Alexander.* New York, NY: Basic Books.

Allen, M. S. (1995). Sullivan's closet: A reappraisal of Harry Stack Sullivan's life and his pioneering role in American psychiatry. *Journal of Homosexuality, 29*(1), 1–18.

American Psychiatric Association. (1994). *Diagnostic and statistical manual of mental disorders, 4th ed.* Washington, DC: Author.

American Psychiatric Association. (2013). *Diagnostic and statistical manual of mental disorders, 5th ed.* Washington, DC: Author.

American Psychiatric Association. (1980). *Diagnostic and statistical manual of mental disorders.* 3rd ed. Washington, DC: Author.

American Psychiatric Association, Committee on Relations with the Social Sciences. (1929). *Proceedings: First colloquium on personality investigation.* Baltimore, MD: Lord Baltimore Press.

American Psychiatric Association, Committee on Relations with the Social Sciences. (1930). *Proceedings: Second colloquium on personality investigation.* Baltimore, MD: Johns Hopkins Press.

Andreasen, N. C. (2007). DSM and the death of phenomenology in America: An example of unintended consequences. *Schizophrenia Bulletin, 33*(1), 108–112.

Ansell, E. B., Kurtz, J. E., DeMoor, R. M., & Markey, P. M. (2011). Validity of the PAI interpersonal scales for measuring the dimensions of the interpersonal circumplex. *Journal of Personality Assessment, 93*(1), 33–39.

Arendt, H. (1963). *Eichmann in Jerusalem: A report on the banality of evil.* New York, NY: Viking.

Aron, L. (2013). *A meeting of minds: Mutuality in psychoanalysis.* New York, NY: Routledge.

Aschieri, F., Emmerik, A., Wibbelink, C., & Kamphuis, J. H. (in press). A systemic review of collaborative assessment methods. In C. E. Hill & J. C. Norcross (Eds.), *Psychotherapy skills and methods that work.* Oxford, UK: Oxford University Press.

Atkinson, L., & Zucker, K. J. (Eds.). (1997). *Attachment and psychopathology.* Guilford Press.

Bakermans-Kranenburg, M. J., & Van IJzendoorn, M. H. (1993). A psychometric study of the Adult Attachment Interview: Reliability and discriminant validity. *Developmental Psychology, 29*(5), 870–879.

Bandura, A. (1977). *Social learning theory.* Englewood Cliffs, NJ: Prentice Hall.

Barnett, J. (1980). Interpersonal processes, cognition, and the analysis of character. *Contemporary Psychoanalysis, 16*, 397–416.

Barnett, J. E. (2011). Utilizing technological innovations to enhance psychotherapy supervision, training, and outcomes. *Psychotherapy*, *48*(2), 103–108.

Bateman, A. W., & Fonagy, P. (2004). *Psychotherapy of borderline personality disorder: Metallization-based treatment*. Oxford, UK: Oxford University Press.

Bateson, G., Jackson, D. D., Haley, J., & Weakland, J. (1956). Toward a theory of schizophrenia. *Behavioral Science*, *1*, 251–264.

Baumrind, D. (1978). Parental disciplinary patterns and social competence in children. *Youth & Society*, *9*(3), 239–276.

Beck, A. T., & Emory, G. (1985). *Anxiety disorders and phobias: A cognitive perspective*. New York, NY: Basic Books.

Beck, A. T., & Freeman, A. (1990). *Cognitive therapy of personality disorders*. New York, NY: Guilford Press.

Beck, A. T., Rush, A., Shaw, B., & Emory, G. (1979). *Cognitive therapy of depression*. New York, NY: Guilford Press.

Benedict. R. (1934). *Patterns of culture*. New York, NY: Houghton Mifflin.

Benjamin, L. S. (1995). *Interpersonal diagnosis and treatment of personality disorders*. New York, NY: Guilford Press.

Berant, E., Mikulincer, M., Shaver, P. R., & Segal, Y. (2005). Rorschach correlates of self-reported attachment dimensions: Dynamic manifestations of hyperactivating and deactivating strategies. *Journal of Personality Assessment*, *84*(1), 70–81.

Berger, P., & Luckman, T. (1966). *The social construction of reality*. Garden City, NY: Anchor Books.

Berndt, T. J. (1982). The features and effects of friendship in early adolescence. *Child Development*, *53*, 1447–1460.

Bérubé, A. (1990). *Coming out under fire: The history of gay men and women in World War Two*. New York, NY: Free Press.

Beutler, L. E. (1986). Systemic eclectic psychotherapy. In J. C. Norcross (Ed.), *Handbook of eclectic psychotherapy* (pp. 94–131). New York, NY: Brunner/Mazel.

Beutler, L. E., & Berren, M. R. (1995). *Integrative assessment of adult personality*. New York, NY: Guilford Press.

Beutler, L. E., & Clarkin, J. F. (1990). *Systemic treatment selection: Toward targeted therapeutic interventions*. New York, NY: Brunner/Mazel.

Beutler, L. E. & Consoli, A. J. (1992). Systemic eclectic psychotherapy. In J. C. Norcross & M. R. Goldfried (Eds.), *Handbook of psychotherapy integration* (pp. 268–299). New York, NY: Basic Books.

Bigelow, B. J. (1977). Children's friendship expectations: A cognitive developmental study. *Child Development*, *48*, 246–253.

Bigelow, B. J., & LaGaipa, J. J. (1975). Children's written descriptions of friendship: A multidimensional analysis. *Developmental Psychology*, *11*, 857–858.

Bion, W. R. (1957). Differentiation of the psychotic from the non-psychotic parts of the personality. In W. R. Bion (Ed.), *Second thoughts*. New York, NY: Jason Aronson.

Bion, W. R. (1976). Personal communication. West Los Angeles, CA.

Blechner, M. J. (2005). The gay Harry Stack Sullivan: Interactions between his life, clinical work, and theory. *Contemporary Psychoanalysis*, *41*(1), 1–19.

Blechner, M. J. (2013). Psychoanalysis in and out of the closet. In B. Gerson (Ed.), *The therapist as a person: Life crises, life choices, life experiences, and their effects on treatment* (pp. 223–240). The Analytic Press.

Blitstein, D. R. (1953). *The social theories of Harry Stack Sullivan.* New York, NY: William Frederick Press.

Blos, P. (1962). *On adolescence: A psychoanalytic interpretation.* New York, NY: Simon and Schuster.

Boisen, A. T. (1936). *The exploration of the inner world: A study of mental disorder and religious experience.* Philadelphia, PA: University of Pennsylvania Press.

Bornstein, R. F., & Masling, J. M. (2005). The Rorschach Oral Dependency Scale. In R. F. Bornstein & J. M. Masling (Eds.), *The LEA series in personality and clinical psychology. Scoring the Rorschach: Seven validated systems* (pp. 135–157). Mahwah, NJ: Lawrence Erlbaum Associates.

Bowlby, J. (1958). The nature of the child's tie to the mother. *International Journal of Psychoanalysis, 39,* 350–373.

Bowlby, J. (1960). Grief and mourning in infancy and early childhood. *The Psychoanalytic Study of the Child, 15,* 9–52.

Bowlby, J. (1961). Separation anxiety: A critical review of the literature. *Journal of Child Psychology and Psychiatry, 1,* 251–269.

Bowlby, J. (1969). *Attachment and loss: Vol. I. Attachment.* New York, NY: Basic Books.

Bowlby, J. (1973). *Attachment and Loss: Vol. 2. Separation: Anxiety and anger.* New York, NY: Basic Books.

Bowlby, J. (1979). *The making and breaking of affectional ties.* London, UK: Tavistock Publications.

Bowlby, J. (1980). *Attachment and loss: Vol. 3. Loss: Sadness and depression.* New York, NY: Basic Books.

Bowlby, J. (1988). *A secure base: Parent–child attachment and healthy human development.* New York, NY: Basic Books.

Bowlby, J., Robertson, J., & Rosenbluth, D. (1952). The two-year-old goes to the hospital. *The Psychoanalytic Study of the Child, 7,* 82–94.

Brand, B. L., Armstrong, J. G., Loewenstein, R. J., & McNary, S. W. (2009). Personality differences on the Rorschach of dissociative identity disorder, borderline personality disorder, and psychotic inpatients. *Psychological Trauma: Theory, Research, Practice, and Policy, 1*(3), 188–205.

Brazelton, T. B., & Cramer, B. (1990). *The earliest relationship: Parents, infants, and the drama of early attachment.* Reading, MA: Addison-Wesley.

Bretherton, I., & Munholland, K. A. (2016). The Internal Working Model Construct in light of contemporary neuroimaging research. In J. Cassidy & P. R. Shaver (Eds.), *Handbook of attachment: Theory, research, and clinical applications, 3rd ed.* (pp. 330–348). New York, NY: Guilford Press.

Brewin, C. R., Cloitre, M., Hyland, P., Shevlin, M., Maercker, A., Bryant, R. A., … Reed, G. M. (2017). A review of current evidence regarding the ICD-11 proposals for diagnosing PTSD and complex PTSD. *Clinical Psychology Review, 58,* 1–15.

Bridgman, P.W. (1945). Some general principles of operational analysis. *Psychological Review, 52,* 246–249.

Bromberg, P. M. (2012). *The shadow of the tsunami: And the growth of the relational mind.* New York, NY: Routledge.

Buber, M. (1957). Three elements of the interhuman: The William Alanson White Memorial lectures, fourth series. *Psychiatry, 20,* 95–129.

Buber, M. (1965). *Between man and man.* New York, NY: MacMillan.

Buhrmester, D., & Furman, W. (1987). The development of companionship and intimacy. *Child Development, 58,* 1101–1113.

Bullard, D. M. (1940). The organization of psychoanalytic procedure in the hospital. *Journal of Nervous and Mental Diseases, 91,* 697–703.

Byrne, J. G., O'Connor, T. G., Marvin, R. S., & Whelan, W. F. (2005). Practitioner review: The contribution of attachment theory to child custody assessments. *Journal of Child Psychology and Psychiatry, 46*(2), 115–127.

Cain, N. M., De Panfilis, C., Meehan, K. B., & Clarkin, J. F. (2017). A multisurface interpersonal circumplex assessment of rejection sensitivity. *Journal of Personality Assessment, 99*(1), 35–45.

Cantril, H. (Ed.). (1950). *Tensions that cause wars.* Urbana, IL: University of Illinois Press.

Carson, R. C. (1969). *Interactional concepts of personality.* Chicago, IL: Aldine.

Carson, R. C. (1982). Self-fulfilling prophecy, maladaptive behavior, and psychotherapy. In J. C. Achin & D. J. Kiesler (Eds.), *Handbook of interpersonal psychotherapy* (pp. 64–77). New York, NY: Pergamon Press.

Cassidy, J., & Shaver, P. R. (Eds.). (2016). *Handbook of attachment: Theory, research, and clinical applications* (pp. 997–1011). New York, NY: Guilford Press.

Caudill, W. (1958). *The psychiatric hospital as a small society.* Cambridge, MA: Harvard University Press.

Chapman, A. (1976). *Harry Stack Sullivan: The man and his work.* New York, NY: Putnam & Sons.

Chatelaine, K. (1981). *Harry Stack Sullivan: The formative years.* Washington, DC: University Press of America.

Chatelaine, K. (1992). *Good me, bad me, not me: Harry Stack Sullivan: An introduction to his thought.* Dubuque, IA: Kendall/Hunt Publishing Company.

Chrzanowski, G. (1977). *Interpersonal approach to psychoanalysis: A contemporary view of Harry Stack Sullivan.* New York, NY: Gardner Press.

Chrzanowski, G. (1982). Interpersonal formulations of psychotherapy: A contemporary model. In J. C. Achin & D. J. Kiesler (Eds.), *Handbook of interpersonal psychotherapy* (pp. 25–45). New York, NY: Pergamon Press.

Clark, L. A., Livesley, W. J., & Morey, L. (1997). Personality disorder assessment: The challenge of construct validity. *Journal of Personality Disorders, 11*(3), 205–231.

Cloitre, M., Koenen, K. C., & Cohen, L. R. (2006). *Treating survivors of childhood abuse: Psychotherapy for the interrupted life.* New York, NY: Guilford Press.

Cohen, M. B. (1952). Countertransference and anxiety. *Psychiatry, 15,* 231–243.

Cohen, M. B. (Ed.). (1959). *Advances in psychiatry: Recent developments in interpersonal relations.* New York, NY: W.W. Norton & Company.

Coleman, J. C. (1988). *Intimate relationships, marriage, and family,* 2nd ed. New York, NY: Macmillan Publishing Co.

Collins, W. A., Maccoby, E. E., Steinberg, L., Hetherington, E. M., & Bornstein, M. H. (2000). Contemporary research on parenting: The case for nature and nurture. *American Psychologist, 55*(2), 218–232.

Cooley, C. H. (1937). *Social organization.* New York, NY: Charles Scribner.

Cooley, C. H. (1964). *Human nature and the social order.* New York, NY: Charles Scribner.

Cooley, C. H. (1966). *Social process*. Carbondale, IL: Southern Illinois University Press.

Coopersmith, S. (1967). *The antecedents of self-esteem*. San Francisco: W. H. Freeman.

Cozolino, L. (2014). *The neuroscience of human relationships: Attachment and the developing social brain, 2nd ed. (Norton Series on Interpersonal Neurobiology)*. New York, NY: W.W. Norton & Company.

Crowell, J. A., Fraley, C., & Roisman, G. I. (2016). Measurement of individual differences in adult attachment. In J. Cassidy & P. R. Shaver (Eds.), *Handbook of attachment: Theory, research, and clinical applications, 3rd ed.* (pp. 598–637). New York, NY: Guilford Press.

Dalenberg, C. J., Brand, B. L., Gleaves, D. H., Dorahy, M. J., Loewenstein, R. J., Cardeña E., ... Spiegel, D. (2012) Evaluation of the evidence for the trauma and fantasy models of dissociation. *Psychological Bulletin, 138*(3), 550–588.

Davanloo, H. (1980). *Basic principles and technique in short-term dynamic psychotherapy*. Lanham, MD: Jason Aronson.

Davies, R. (1992). *Reading and writing*. Salt Lake City, UT: University of Utah Press.

Davies, R. (1995). *The cunning man*. New York, NY: Viking Penguin.

DeGangi, G. A., Breinbauer, C., Roosevelt, J. D., Porges, S., & Greenspan, S. (2000). Prediction of childhood problems at three years in children experiencing disorders of regulation during infancy. *Infant Mental Health Journal: Official Publication of The World Association for Infant Mental Health, 21*(3), 156–175.

De Mello, M. F., de Jesus Mari, J., Bacaltchuk, J., Verdeli, H., & Neugebauer, R. (2005). A systematic review of research findings on the efficacy of interpersonal therapy for depressive disorders. *European Archives of Psychiatry and Clinical Neuroscience, 255*(2), 75–82.

de Saeger, H. (2019). *Therapeutic assessment in patients with personality disorders*. Psychologische Methodenleer (Psychologie, FMG).

Deutsch, H. (1942). Some forms of emotional disturbance and their relationship to schizophrenia. *Psychoanalytic Quarterly, 11*, 301–321.

de Villemor-Amaral, A. E., & Finn, S. E. (2020). The Rorschach as a window into past traumas during therapeutic assessment. *Rorschachiana, 41*(2), 93–106.

Dewey, J. (1922). *Human nature and conduct*. New York, NY: Henry Hold and Company.

Dewey, J. (1929). *Experience and nature*. New York, NY: The Open Court Publishing Company.

DeYoung, P. A. (2015). *Understanding and treating chronic shame: A relationall neurobiological approach*. New York, NY: Routledge.

Diamond, G., Russon, J., & Levy, S. (2016). Attachment-based family therapy: A review of the empirical support. *Family Process, 55*(3), 595–610.

Dieterich, M., Irving, C. B., Bergman, H., Khokhar, M. A., Park, B., & Marshall, M. (2017). Intensive case management for severe mental illness. *Cochrane Database of Systematic Reviews, 1*, 1–268.

DiMauro, J., Carter, S., Folk, J. B., & Kashdan, T. B. (2014). A historical review of trauma-related diagnoses to reconsider the heterogeneity of PTSD. *Journal of Anxiety Disorders, 28*(8), 774–786.

Dinnerstein, L. (1995). *Antisemitism in America*. Oxford, UK: Oxford University Press.

Dixon, N. F. (1981). *Preconscious processing*. New York, NY: John Wiley & Sons.

Dodge, K. A. (1986). A social information processing model of social cognition in children. In M. Perlmutter (Ed.), *Cognitive perspectives on children's social and behavioral development* (pp. 77–126). Hillsdale, NJ: Russell Erlbaum Associates.

Dodge, K. A., & Frame, C. L. (1982). Social cognitive biases and deficits in aggressive boys. *Child Development, 53*, 620–635.

Dodge, K. A., Pettit, G., McClasky, C., & Brown, M. (1986). Social competence in children. *Monographs of the Society for Research in Child Development: Volume 51*.

Dollard, J., Doob, L. W., Miller, N. E., Mowrer, O. H., & Sears, R.R. (1939). *Frustration and aggression*. New Haven, CT: Yale University Press.

Driver, J. (2001). A selective review of selective attention research from the past century. *British Journal of Psychology, 92*(1), 53–78.

Durosini, I., & Aschieri, F. (2021). Therapeutic Assessment efficacy: A meta-analysis. *Psychological Assessment, 33*(10), 962–972.

Eckardt, M. H. (1978). Organizational schisms of American psychoanalysis. In J. M. Quen & E. T. Carlson (Eds.), *American psychoanalysis: Origins and development* (pp. 141–161). New York, NY: Brunner/Mazel.

Ehrenberg, D. B. (1992). *The intimate edge: Extending the reach of psychoanalytic interaction*. New York, NY: W.W. Norton & Co.

Eissler, K. R. (1953). The effect of the structure of the ego on psychoanalytic technique. *Journal of the American Psychoanalytic Association, 1*, 104–143.

Ekman, P., & Friesen, W. V. (1968). Nonverbal behavior in psychotherapy research. In J. M. Shlien (Ed.), *Research in psychotherapy* (Vol. 3, pp. 179–217). Washington, DC: American Psychological Association.

Eliason, M. (2000). Bi-negativity: The stigma facing bisexual men. *Journal of Bisexuality, 1*(2–3), 137–154.

Elkin, I., Shea, M. T., Watkins, J. T., & Imber, S. T. (1989). National Institute of Mental Health Treatment of Depression Collaborative Research Program: General effectiveness of treatments. *Archives of General Psychiatry, 46*, 971–982.

Erdberg, P. & Exner, J. (1990). Rorschach assessment. In G. Goldstein & M. Hersen (Eds.), *Handbook of psychological assessment* (pp 387–399). Oxford, UK: Pergamon.

Erdelyi, M. H. (1985). *Psychoanalysis: Freud's cognitive psychology*. New York, NY: Freeman.

Erdelyi, M. H. (1990). Repression, reconstruction, and defenses: History and integration of psychoanalytic and experimental frameworks. In J. L. Singer (Ed.), *Repression and dissociation* (pp. 1–32). Chicago, IL: University of Chicago Press.

Erikson, E. H. (1950). *Childhood and society*. New York, NY: Norton.

Erikson, E. H. (1959). *Identity and the life cycle*. New York, NY: International Universities Press.

Eskridge, W. N. (2008). *Dishonorable passions: Sodomy laws in America, 1861–2003*. New York, NY: Penguin.

Evans, F. B. III. (1976). An attempt to reorganize a Veterans Administration Hospital ward and unit: Its effects on ward atmosphere. *Dissertation Abstracts International*.

Evans, F. B. III. (1991). *Why has Sullivan been forgotten?* Paper presented at the Harry Stack Sullivan Centennial Conference., Washington School of Psychiatry, Washington, DC.

Evans, F. B. III. (1992). *Beyond the borderline: Abuse, trauma, and the borderline state.* Workshop presented at the District of Columbia Psychological Association Annual Meeting, Washington, DC.

Evans, F. B. III. (1993). *Beyond the borderline personality: Abuse, trauma, and the borderline state.* Workshop presented at the Maryland Psychological Association Annual Meeting. Columbia, MD.

Evans III, F. B. (1996). *Harry Stack Sullivan: Interpersonal theory and psychotherapy.* Routledge.

Evans, F. B. III. (2000). Forensic psychology and immigration court: An introduction. In R. Auberbach (Ed.), *Handbook of immigration and nationality law* (Vol. 2, pp. 446–458). Washington, DC: American Immigration Lawyers Association.

Evans, F. B. III. (2005). Trauma, torture, and transformation in the forensic assessor. *Journal of Personality Assessment, 84*(1), 25–28.

Evans, F. B. (2011). Harry Stack Sullivan, intergroup conflict, and world peace. *Society for Interpersonal Theory and Research Newsletter, 11*(3), 5–16.

Evans, F. B. (2011, October). Integrating security, lust & intimacy: Sullivan's view of interpersonal relatedness and mature sexuality. Paper presented at *Sexuality and Intimacy in Society at Large and in the Therapist's Office; Remembering Harry Stack Sullivan.* Washington School of Psychiatry, Washington, DC.

Evans, F. B. (2012). Therapeutic assessment alternative to custody evaluation: An adolescent whose parents could not stop fighting. In S. E. Finn, C. T. Fischer, & L. Handler (Eds.), *Collaborative/therapeutic assessment: A casebook and guide* (pp. 357–378). New York, NY: John Wiley & Sons Inc.

Evans, F. B. (2014). PTSD: An experiential approach. *The North Carolina Psychologist, 66*(4), 10–11, 23.

Evans, F. B. (2015). PTSD as a human experience: An interpersonal approach. *The TA Connection. 3*(1), 11–16.

Evans, F. B. (2016). What torture survivors teach assessors about being more fully human. *Journal of Personality Assessment, 98*(6), 590–593.

Evans, F. B. (2017). An interpersonal approach to Rorschach interpretation. *Rorschachiana, 38*(1), 33–48.

Evans, F. B., Brand, B. L., & Kaser-Boyd, N. (2023). Differentiating bipolar spectrum and psychological trauma spectrum disorders. In J. H. Kleiger & I. B. Weiner (Eds.), *Psychological assessment of bipolar spectrum disorders.* (pp. 233–252), Washington, DC: American Psychological Association Press.

Evans III, B. F. , & Hass, G. A. (2018). *Forensic psychological assessment in immigration court: A guidebook for evidence-based and ethical practice.* Routledge.

Evans, F. B., & Maris, J. A. (2016). Book review. [Review of the book *Co-creating change: Effective psychodynamic therapy techniques,* by Jon Frederickson]. *Psychiatry, 79*(4), 335–338.

Exner, J. E., Jr. (2003). *Basic foundations and principles of interpretation. The Rorschach: A comprehensive system, 4th ed.* New York, NY: John Wiley.

Exner, J. E., Andronikof, A., & Fontan, P. (2022). *The Rorschach: A Comprehensive system ®- Revised administration and coding manual.* Rorschach Workshops.

Fairbairn, W. R. D. (1952). *An object relations theory of personality.* Boston, MA: Routledge and Kegan Paul.

Fairbairn, W. R. D. (1958). On the nature and aims of psychoanalytic treatment. *International Journal of Psychoanalysis*, *39*, 374–385.

Fairbairn, W. R. D. (1963). A synopsis of an object relation theory of the personality. *International Journal of Psychoanalysis*, *44*, 224–225.

Fantini, F., Aschieri, F., David, R. M., Martin, H., & Finn, S. E. (2022). *Therapeutic Assessment with adults: Using psychological testing to help clients change*. New York, NY: Routledge.

Farrington, D. P., & Bergstrøm, H. (2018). Family background and psychopathy. In C. J. Patrick (Ed.), *Handbook of psychopathy* (2nd ed., pp. 354–379). New York, NY: Guilford Press.

Feeny, N. C., Zoellner, L. A., Fitzgibbons, L. A., & Foa. E. B. (2000) Exploring the roles of emotional numbing, depression, and dissociation in PTSD. *Journal of Traumatic Stress. 13*: 489–498.

Ferenczi, S. (1933). Confusion of tongues between adults and the child: The language of tenderness and the language of passion. In S. Ferenczi (Ed.), *Collected papers Volume 3: Final contributions*. New York, NY: Basic Books.

Ferenczi, S. (1952). *First contributions to psychoanalysis*. London, UK: Hogarth Press.

Ferster, C. B., & Skinner. B. F. (1957). *Schedules of reinforcement*. New York, NY: Appleton-Century-Crofts.

Field, T. M., Woodson, R., Greenberg, R., & Cohen, D. (1982). Discrimination and imitation of facial expressions by neonates. *Science*, *218*, 179–181.

Finkelhor, D. (1984). *Child sexual abuse: New theory and research*. New York, NY: The Free Press.

Finn, S. E. (2007a). *In our clients' shoes: Theory and techniques of therapeutic assessment*. New York, NY: Routledge.

Finn, S. E. (2007b). Therapeutic assessment: Would Harry approve? In S. E. Finn (Ed.), *In our clients' shoes: Theory and techniques of therapeutic assessment*. (pp. 23–31). New York, NY: Routledge.

Finn, S. E. (2012a). Implications of recent research in neurobiology for psychological assessment. *Journal of Personality Assessment*, *94*(5), 440–449.

Finn, S. E. (2012b). Therapeutic assessment with a couple in crisis: Undoing problematic projective identification via the Consensus Rorschach. In S. E. Finn, C. T. Fischer, & L. Handler (Eds.), *Collaborative/therapeutic assessment: A casebook and guide* (pp. 379–400). New York, NY: John Wiley & Sons Inc.

Finn, S. E., & Kamphuis, J. H. (2006). Therapeutic Assessment with the MMPI-2. In J. N. Butcher (Ed.), *MMPI-2: A practitioner's guide* (pp. 165–191). Washington, DC: American Psychological Association.

Finn, S. E., & Martin, H. (1997). Therapeutic Assessment with the MMPI-2 in managed health care. In J. N. Butcher (Ed.), *Personality assessment in managed health care: Using the MMPI-2 in treatment planning* (pp. 131–152). Oxford, UK: Oxford University Press.

Finn, S. E., & Tonsager, M. E. (1992). Therapeutic effects of providing MMPI-2 test feedback to college students awaiting therapy. *Psychological Assessment*, *4*(3), 278–287.

Finn, S. E., & Tonsager, M. E. (1997). Information-gathering and therapeutic models of assessment: Complementary paradigms. *Psychological Assessment*, *9*(4), 374–385.

Finn, S. E., & Tonsager, M. E. (2002). How Therapeutic Assessment became humanistic. *The Humanistic Psychologist, 30*(1–2), 10–22.

Fiscalini, J. (2007). *Coparticipant psychoanalysis; Toward a new theory of clinical inquiry.* New York, NY: Columbia University Press.

Fiscalini, J. (2008). Dimensions of agency and the process of co-participant inquiry. In R. Frie, (Ed.), *Psychological agency: Theory, practice, and culture.* (pp. 155–174). Cambridge, MA: The MIT Press.

Fischer, C. T. (1994). *Individualizing psychological assessment, 2nd ed.* New York, NY: Routledge.

Fisher, R., & Ury, W. (1981). *Getting to yes.* New York, NY: Penguin Books.

Fiske, S. T., & Taylor, S. E. (1991). *Social cognition, 2nd ed.* New York, NY: McGraw-Hill Publishers.

Flavell, J. H. (1963). *The developmental psychology of Jean Piaget.* New York, NY: D. Van Nostrand Company.

Fonagy, P. (2018). *Attachment theory and psychoanalysis.* New York, NY: Routledge.

Fonagy, P., Luyten, P., & Allison, E. (2015). Epistemic petrification and the restoration of epistemic trust: A new conceptualization of borderline personality disorder and its psychosocial treatment. *Journal of Personality Disorders, 29,* 575–609.

Frances, A. (2014). *Saving normal: An insider's revolt against out-of-control psychiatric diagnosis, DSM-5, big pharma, and the medicalization of ordinary life.* New York, NY: William Morrow.

Frank, J. D. (1973). *Persuasion and healing.* Baltimore, MD: Johns Hopkins University Press.

Frank, J. D. (1982). Therapeutic components shared by all psychotherapies. In J. H. Harvey & M. M. Parks (Eds.), *Psychotherapy research and behavioral change* (pp. 5–37). Washington, DC: American Psychological Association.

Frederickson, J. (2014). *Co-creating change: Effective dynamic therapy.* Kensington, MD: Seven Leaves Press.

Frederickson, J. (2021). *Co-creating safety: Healing the fragile patient.* Kensington, MD: Seven Leaves Press.

Freud, S. (1900). *The interpretation of dreams.* In J. Strachey, A. Freud, A. Strachey, & A. Tyson (Eds., Trans.) (1953–1974), *The standard edition of the complete psychological works of Sigmund Freud* (Vols. 4–5). London, UK: Hogarth Press.

Freud, S. (1901). *Psychopathology of everyday life.* In J. Strachey, A. Freud, A. Strachey, & A. Tyson (Eds., Trans.), (1953–1974), *The standard edition of the complete psychological works of Sigmund Freud* (Vol. 6). London, UK: Hogarth Press.

Freud, S. (1904). *Freud's psycho-analytic procedure.* In J. Strachey, A. Freud, A. Strachey, & A. Tyson (Eds., Trans.), (1953–1974), *The standard edition of the complete psychological works of Sigmund Freud* (Vol. 7, pp. 249–256). London, UK: Hogarth Press.

Freud, S. (1905). *Three essays on a theory of sexuality.* In J. Strachey, A. Freud, A. Strachey, & A. Tyson (Eds., Trans.), (1953–1974), *The standard edition of the complete psychological works of Sigmund Freud* (Vol. 7, pp. 125–145). London, UK: Hogarth Press.

Freud, S. (1910a). *Five lectures on psychoanalysis.* In J. Strachey, A. Freud, A. Strachey, & A. Tyson (Eds., Trans.), (1953–1974), *The standard edition of the complete psychological works of Sigmund Freud* (Vol. 11, pp. 7–55). London, UK: Hogarth Press.

Freud, S. (1910b). *The future prospects of psycho-analytic therapy.* In J. Strachey, A. Freud, A. Strachey, & A. Tyson (Eds., Trans.), (1953–1974), *The standard edition of the complete psychological works of Sigmund Freud* (Vol. 11, pp. 139–152). London, UK: Hogarth Press.

Freud, S. (1910c). *Observations on "wild" psychoanalysis.* In J. Strachey, A. Freud, A. Strachey, & A. Tyson (Eds., Trans.), (1953–1974), *The standard edition of the complete psychological works of Sigmund Freud* (Vol. 11, pp. 221–227). London, UK: Hogarth Press.

Freud. S. (1910d). *A special type of choice of object made by men.* In J. Strachey, A. Freud, A. Strachey, & A. Tyson (Eds., Trans.), (1953–1974), *The standard edition of the complete psychological works of Sigmund Freud* (Vol. 11, pp. 163–175). London, UK: Hogarth Press.

Freud, S. (1911a). *Formulations on the two principles of mental functioning.* In J. Strachey, A. Freud, A. Strachey, & A. Tyson (Eds., Trans.), (1953–1974), *The standard edition of the complete psychological works of Sigmund Freud* (Vol. 12, pp. 218–226). London, UK: Hogarth Press.

Freud, S. (1911b). *Psychoanalytic notes upon an autobiographical account of a case of paranoia.* In J. Strachey, A. Freud, A. Strachey, & A. Tyson (Eds., Trans.), (1953–1974), *The standard edition of the complete psychological works of Sigmund Freud* (Vol. 12, pp. 9–82). London, UK: Hogarth Press.

Freud, S. (1912a). *The dynamics of transference.* In J. Strachey, A. Freud, A. Strachey, & A. Tyson (Eds., Trans.), (1953–1974), *The standard edition of the complete psychological works of Sigmund Freud* (Vol. 12, pp. 99–108). London, UK: Hogarth Press.

Freud, S. (1912b). *A note on the unconscious in psycho-analysis.* In J. Strachey, A. Freud, A. Strachey, & A. Tyson (Eds., Trans.), (1953–1974), *The standard edition of the complete psychological works of Sigmund Freud* (Vol. 12, pp. 255–266). London, UK: Hogarth Press.

Freud, S. (1912c). *Recommendations to physicians practicing psycho-analysis.* In J. Strachey, A. Freud, A. Strachey, & A. Tyson (Eds., Trans.), (1953–1974), *The standard edition of the complete psychological works of Sigmund Freud* (Vol. 12, pp. 109–120). London, UK: Hogarth Press.

Freud, S. (1913). *Further recommendations in the technique of psychoanalysis: On beginning the treatment.* In J. Strachey, A. Freud, A. Strachey, & A. Tyson (Eds., Trans.), (1953–1974), *The standard edition of the complete psychological works of Sigmund Freud* (Vol. 12, pp. 123–144). London, UK: Hogarth Press.

Freud, S. (1914a). *Further recommendations in the technique of psychoanalysis: Recollection, repetition and working through.* In J. Strachey, A. Freud, A. Strachey, & A. Tyson (Eds., Trans.), (1953–1974), *The standard edition of the complete psychological works of Sigmund Freud* (Vol. 12). London, UK: Hogarth Press.

Freud, S. (1914b). *On narcissism: An introduction.* In J. Strachey, A. Freud, A. Strachey, & A. Tyson (Eds., Trans.), (1953–1974), *The standard edition of the complete psychological works of Sigmund Freud* (Vol. 14, pp. 67–102). London, UK: Hogarth Press.

Freud, S. (1915a). *Further recommendations in the technique of psychoanalysis: Observations on transference love.* In J. Strachey, A. Freud, A. Strachey, & A. Tyson (Eds., Trans.), (1953–1974), *The standard edition of the complete psychological works of Sigmund Freud* (Vol. 12). London, UK: Hogarth Press.

Freud, S. (1915b). *Repression.* In J. Strachey, A. Freud, A. Strachey, & A. Tyson (Eds., Trans.), (1953–1974), *The standard edition of the complete psychological works of Sigmund Freud* (Vol. 14, pp. 141–158). London, UK: Hogarth Press.

Freud, S. (1915c). *The unconscious.* In J. Strachey, A. Freud, A. Strachey, & A. Tyson (Eds., Trans.), (1953–1974), *The standard edition of the complete psychological works of Sigmund Freud* (Vol. 14, pp. 159–215). London, UK: Hogarth Press.

Freud, S. (1917). *Introductory lectures on psychoanalysis.* In J. Strachey, A. Freud, A. Strachey, & A. Tyson (Eds., Trans.), (1953–1974), *The standard edition of the complete psychological works of Sigmund Freud* (Vol. 16, pp. 243–448). London, UK: Hogarth Press.

Freud, S. (1920). *Beyond the pleasure principle.* In J. Strachey, A. Freud, A. Strachey, & A. Tyson (Eds., Trans.), (1953–1974), *The standard edition of the complete psychological works of Sigmund Freud* (Vol. 18, pp. 3–64). London, UK: Hogarth Press.

Freud, S. (1923a). *The ego and the id.* In J. Strachey, A. Freud, A. Strachey, & A. Tyson (Eds., Trans.), (1953–1974), *The standard edition of the complete psychological works of Sigmund Freud* (Vol. 19, pp. 1–66). London, UK: Hogarth Press.

Freud, S. (1923b). *The infantile genital organization of the libido: An interpolation into the theory of sexuality.* In J. Strachey, A. Freud, A. Strachey, & A. Tyson (Eds., Trans.), (1953–1974), *The standard edition of the complete psychological works of Sigmund Freud* (Vol. 19, pp. 139–145). London, UK: Hogarth Press.

Freud, S. (1925). *Some psychical consequences of the anatomical distinction between the sexes.* In J. Strachey, A. Freud, A. Strachey, & A. Tyson (Eds., Trans.), (1953–1974), *The standard edition of the complete psychological works of Sigmund Freud* (Vol. 19, pp. 241–258). London, UK: Hogarth Press.

Freud, S. (1926). *The question of lay analysis.* In J. Strachey, A. Freud, A. Strachey, & A. Tyson (Eds., Trans.), (1953–1974), *The standard edition of the complete psychological works of Sigmund Freud* (Vol. 20, pp. 177–258). London, UK: Hogarth Press.

Freud. S. (1927). *The future of an illusion.* In J. Strachey, A. Freud, A. Strachey, & A. Tyson (Eds., Trans.), (1953–1974), *The standard edition of the complete psychological works of Sigmund Freud* (Vol. 21, pp. 59–145). London, UK: Hogarth Press.

Freud, S. (1930). *Civilizations and its discontents.* In J. Strachey, A. Freud, A. Strachey, & A. Tyson (Eds., Trans.), (1953–1974), *The standard edition of the complete psychological works of Sigmund Freud* (Vol. 21, pp. 59–145). London, UK: Hogarth Press.

Freud, S. (1933). *New introductory lectures on psychoanalysis.* In J. Strachey, A. Freud, A. Strachey, & A. Tyson (Eds., Trans.), (1953–1974), *The standard edition of the complete psychological works of Sigmund Freud* (Vol. 22, pp. 1–182). London, UK: Hogarth Press.

Freud, S. (1937). *Analysis terminable and interminable.* In J. Strachey, A. Freud, A. Strachey, & A. Tyson (Eds., Trans.), (1953–1974), *The standard edition of the complete psychological works of Sigmund Freud* (Vol. 23, pp. 209–253). London, UK: Hogarth Press.

Freud, A. (1936). *The ego and the mechanisms of defense*. New York: International Universities Press.

Freud, S. (1940). *An outline of psychoanalysis*. In J. Strachey, A. Freud, A. Strachey, & A. Tyson (Eds., Trans.), (1953–1974), *The standard edition of the complete psychological works of Sigmund Freud* (Vol. 23, pp. 139–207). London, UK: Hogarth Press.

Freyd, J. J. (1996). *Betrayal trauma: The logic of forgetting childhood abuse*. Cambridge, MA: Harvard University Press.

Fromm, E. (1939). The social philosophy of "will therapy." *Psychiatry, 2*, 229–237.

Fromm, E. (1941). *Escape from freedom*. New York, NY: Avon.

Fromm, E. (1947). *Man for himself*. Greenwich, CT: Fawcett.

Fromm, E. (1955). *The sane society*. Greenwich, CT: Fawcett.

Fromm-Reichmann, F. (1949). Notes on the personal and professional requirements of a psychotherapist. *Psychiatry, 12*(4), 361–378.

Fromm-Reichmann, F. (1950). *Principles of intensive psychotherapy*. Chicago, IL: University of Chicago Press.

Fromm-Reichmann, F. (1959). Loneliness. *Psychiatry, 22*, 1–15.

Furman, W., & Buhrmester, D. (1985). Children's perceptions of the personal relations of their social networks. *Developmental Psychology, 21*, 1016–1024.

Gabbard, G. O. (2000). Disguise or consent: problems and recommendations concerning the publication and presentation of clinical material. *Int. J. Psychoanal., 81*, 1071–1086.

Garfield, D. A. S. (1995). *Unbearable affect: A guide to the psychotherapy of psychosis*. New York, NY: John Wiley & Sons.

Garfield, D. A. S. (2018). *Unbearable affect: A guide to the psychotherapy of psychosis*. New York, NY: Routledge.

Garrity, C. B., & Baris, M. A. (1997). *Caught in the middle: Protecting the children of high-conflict divorce*. San Francisco, CA: Jossey Bass.

Gaw, K. F., & Beutler, L. E. (1995). Integrating treatment recommendations. In L. E. Beutler & M. R. Berren (Eds), *Integrative assessment of adult personality* (pp. 280–319). New York, NY: The Guilford Press.

George, C., Kaplan, N., & Main, M. (1985). Attachment interview for adults. *Unpublished manuscript, University of California, Berkeley*.

George, C., & West, M. (2001). The development and preliminary validation of a new measure of adult attachment: The Adult Attachment Projective. *Attachment and Human Development, 3*, 30–61.

George, C., & West, M. (2012). *The Adult Attachment Projective Picture System: Attachment theory and assessment in adults*. New York, NY: Guilford Press.

Gergen, K. J. (1971). *The concept of self*. New York, NY: Holt.

Goffman, E. (1961). *Asylums*. Garden City, NY: Anchor Books.

Golding, W. (1962). *Lord of the flies*. New York, NY: Coward-McCann.

Goldring, S. L. (1978). Toward a more adequate theory of personality: Psychological organizing principles. In H. London & N. Hirschberg (Eds.), *Personality: A new look at metatheories*. Washington, DC: Hemisphere Press.

Gottman, J. M. (1983). How children become friends. *Monographs of the Society for Research in Child Development, 48*(201).

Greenberg, J. R., & Mitchell, S. A. (1983). *Object relations in psychoanalytic theory*. Cambridge, MA: Harvard.

Greenberg, S. A., & Shuman, D. W. (1997). Irreconcilable conflict between therapeutic and forensic roles. *Professional Psychology: Research and Practice, 28*(1), 50.

Greenberg, S. A., & Shuman, D. W. (2007). When worlds collide: Therapeutic and forensic roles. *Professional Psychology: Research and Practice, 38*(2), 129–132.

Greenspan, S. I. (1983). *Clinical infant reports: No. 3: Infants in multi-risk families.* New York, NY: International Universities Press.

Greenspan, S., & Shanker, S. (2007). The developmental pathways leading to pattern recognition, joint attention, language and cognition. *New Ideas in Psychology, 25*(2), 128–142.

Griffin, B. J., Purcell, N., Burkman, K., Litz, B. T., Bryan, C. J., Schmitz, M., ... Maguen, S. (2019). Moral injury: An integrative review. *Journal of Traumatic Stress, 32*(3), 350–362.

Groth, A. N. (1979). *Men who rape: The psychology of the offender.* New York, NY: Plenum Press.

Grotstein, J. (1981). The significance of Kleinian contributions to psychoanalysis I: Kleinian instinct theory. *International Journal of Psychoanalytic Psychotherapy, 8,* 375–392.

Guntrip, H. (1969a). My experience of analysis with Fairbairn and Winnicott. *International Review of Psychoanalysis, 2,* 145–156.

Guntrip, H. (1969b). *Schizoid phenomena, object relations, and the self.* New York, NY: International Universities Press.

Guntrip, H. (1971). *Psychoanalytic theory, therapy, and the self.* New York, NY: Basic Books.

Guntrip, H. (1975). My experience of analysis with Fairbairn and Winnicott: How complete a result does psycho-analytic therapy achieve. *International Review of Psycho-Analysis, 2*(2), 145–156.

Gurman, A. S. (1977). The patient's perception of the therapeutic relationship. In A. S. Gurman & A. M. Razin (Eds.). (1977). *Effective psychotherapy: A handbook of research* (pp. 503–543). New York, NY: Pergamon Press.

Gurtman, M. B. (2009). Exploring personality with the interpersonal circumplex. *Social and Personality Psychology Compass, 3*(4), 601–619.

Haith, M. M. (1980). *Rules that babies look by.* Hillsdale, NJ: Lawrence Erlbaum Associates.

Haley, J. (1968). *Uncommon therapy: The therapeutic techniques of Milton Erickson.* New York, NY: Grune & Stratton.

Haley, J. (1979). Personal communication. Washington, DC.

Hamblin, R. J., & Gross, A. M. (2014). Religious faith, homosexuality, and psychological well-being: A theoretical and empirical review. *Journal of Gay & Lesbian Mental Health, 18*(1), 67–82.

Handler, L. (2006). The use of therapeutic assessment with children and adolescents. In S. R. Smith & L. Handler (Eds.), *The clinical assessment of children and adolescents: A practitioner's handbook* (pp. 53–72). New York, NY: Erlbaum.

Hare, R. D. (1993). *Without conscience: The disturbing world of the psychopaths among us.* New York, NY: Simon & Schuster.

Hare, R. D., & Neumann, C. S. (2008). Psychopathy as a clinical and empirical constriuct. *Annual Review of Clinical Psychology, 4,* 217–246.

Harlow, H. F. (1962). The heterosexual affectional systems in monkeys. *American Psychologist, 17*, 1–13.

Harlow, H. F., & Harlow, M. K. (1971). Psychopathology in monkeys. In H. D. Kimmel (Ed.), *Experimental psychopathology; Recent research and theory* (pp. 203–229). New York, NY: Academic Press.

Harris, G. T., & Rice, M. E. (2006). Treatment of psychopathy: A review of empirical findings. In C. J. Patrick (Ed.), *Handbook of psychopathy* (pp. 555–572). New York, NY: Guilford.

Harris, M., & Bergman, H. E. (Eds.). (1993). *Case management of mentally ill patients: Theory and practice.* Langhorne, PA: Harwood Academic Publishers.

Hartmann, H. (1939). *Ego psychology and the problem of adaptation.* New York, NY: International Universities Press.

Hartup, W. W. (1979). The social worlds of childhood. *American Psychologist, 34*, 944–950.

Hartup, W. W. (1989). Social relationships and their developmental significance. *American Psychologist, 44*, 120–126.

Hartup, W. W. (1992). Friendship and their developmental significance. In H. McGurk (Ed.), *Child social development: Current perspectives* (pp. 175–205). Hilldale, NJ: Lawrence Erlbaum Associates.

Hartup, W. W. (1993). Adolescents and their friends. In B. Laursen (Ed.), *New directions in child development* (pp. 3–22). San Francisco, CA: Jossey-Bass Publishers.

Havens, L. L. (1968). Main currents of psychiatric development. *International Journal of Psychiatry, 5*, 288–310.

Havens, L. L. (1973). *Approaches to the mind.* Boston, MA: Little, Brown.

Havens, L. L. (1976). *Participant observation.* New York, NY: Jason Aronson.

Havens, L. L. (1986). *Making contact: Uses of language in psychotherapy.* Cambridge, MA: Harvard University Press.

Havens, L. L. (1989). *A safe place.* New York, NY: Ballantine Books.

Havens, L. L., & Frank, J. (1971). Review of P. Mullahy, "psychoanalysis and interpersonal psychiatry." *American Journal of Psychiatry, 127*, 1704–1705.

Heimann, P. (1952a). Certain functions of introjection and projection in early infancy. In M. Klein, P. Heimann, & J. Riviere (Eds.), *Developments in psychoanalysis.* London, UK: Hogarth Press.

Heimann, P. (1952b). Notes on the theory of the life and death instincts. In M. Klein, P. Heimann, & J. Riviere (Eds.), *Developments in psychoanalysis.* London, UK: Hogarth Press.

Heisenberg, W. (1958). *Physics and philosophy.* New York, NY: Harper and Row.

Henriques, F. (1959). *Love in action: The sociology of sex.* New York, NY: Dell Books.

Herman, J. L. (1992). *Trauma and recovery.* New York, NY: Basic Books.

Hesse, E. (2016). The Adult Attachment Interview: Protocol, method of analysis, and selected empirical studies: 1985–2015. In J. Cassidy & P. R. Shaver (Eds.), *Handbook of attachment: Theory, research, and clinical applications, 3rd ed.* (pp. 553–597). New York, NY: Guilford Press.

Hinde, R. A. (1982). *Ethology: Its nature and relation to other sciences.* New York, NY: Oxford University Press.

Hirsch, I. (2014). *The interpersonal tradition: The origins of psychoanalytic subjectivity.* New York, NY: Routledge.

Hodges, A. (2014). *Alan Turing: The enigma*. Princeton, NJ: Princeton University Press.

Hogg, M. A., & Abrams, D. (1988). *Social identifications: A social psychology of intergroup relations and group process*. New York, NY: Routledge, Chapman, and Hall.

Hollingshead, A. B., & Redlich, F. C. (1958). *Social class and mental illness*. New York, NY: John Wiley & Sons.

Holmes, J. (1993). *John Bowlby and attachment theory*. New York, NY: Routledge.

Holowka, D. W., Marx, B. P., Kaloupek, D. G., & Keane, T. M. (2012). PTSD symptoms among male Vietnam veterans: Prevalence and associations with diagnostic status. *Psychological Trauma: Theory, Research, Practice, and Policy, 4*(3), 285–292.

Hopwood, C. J. (2023). Personal communication. email correspondence.

Hopwood, C. J., Ansell, E. B., Pincus, A. L., Wright, A. G., Lukowitsky, M. R., & Roche, M. J. (2011). The circumplex structure of interpersonal sensitivities. *Journal of Personality, 79*(4), 707–740.

Hopwood, C. J., Pincus, A. L., & Wright, A. G. (2019). The interpersonal situation: Integrating personality assessment, case formulation, and intervention. In D. B. Samuel & D. Lynam (Eds.), *Using basic personality research to inform personality pathology* (pp. 94–121). Oxford, UK: Oxford University Press.

Hopwood, C. J., Thomas, K. M., Luo, X., Bernard, N., Lin, Y., & Levendosky, A. A. (2016). Implementing dynamic assessments in psychotherapy. *Assessment, 23*(4), 507–517.

Horney, K. (1939). *New ways in psychoanalysis*. New York, NY: W.W. Norton & Company.

Horney, K. (1967). *Feminine psychology*. New York, NY: W.W. Norton & Company.

Horowitz, L. M., Rosenberg, S. E., Baer, B. A., Ureño, G., & Villaseñor, V. S. (1988). Inventory of interpersonal problems: Psychometric properties and clinical applications. *Journal of Consulting and Clinical Psychology, 56*(6), 885.

Horváth, S., & Mirnics, K. (2015). Schizophrenia as a disorder of molecular pathways. *Biological Psychiatry, 77*(1), 22–28.

Hunter, M. (Ed.). (1990). *The sexually abused male*. Lexington, MA: Lexington Books.

Husserl, E. (1965). *Phenomonology and the crisis of philosophy*. New York, NY: Harper & Row Torchbooks.

Jackson, D. D. (1968). *Communication, family and marriage*. Palo Alto, CA: Science and Behavioral Books, Inc.

Jacobs, U., Evans, F. B., & Patsilides, B. (2001a). Forensic psychology and documentation of torture. Part I. *Torture, 11*(3), 85–89.

Jacobs, U., Evans, F. B., & Patsilides, B. (2001b). Forensic psychology and documentation of torture. Part II. *Torture, 11*(4), 100–102.

Jacobson, E. (1955). Review of Sullivan's "Interpersonal theory of psychiatry." *Journal of the American Psychoanalytic Association, 3*, 149–156.

Jacobson. E. (1964). *The self and the object world*. New York, NY: International Universities Press.

Janoff-Bulman, R. (1992). *Shattered assumptions: Toward a new psychology of trauma*. New York, NY: Free Press.

Jay, J. A. (1991). Terrible knowledge. *Family Therapy* Networker, *15*, 18–29.

Jensen, A. R., & Johnson, F. W. (1994). Race and sex differences in head size and IQ. *Intelligence, 18*(3), 309–333.

Johnson, C. (1941). *Growing up in the Black Belt: Negro youth in the rural south.* Washington, DC: American Council on Education.

Johnstone, L. & Boyle, M., withCromby, J., Dillon, J., Harper, D., Kinderman, P., Longden, E., Pilgrim, D. & Read, J. (2018a). *The power threat meaning framework: Overview.* Leicester, UK: British Psychological Society.

Johnstone, L., & Boyle, M., withCromby, J., Dillon, J., Harper, D., Kinderman, P., Longden, E., Pilgrim, D., & Read, J. (2018b). *The Power Threat Meaning Framework: Towards the identification of patterns in emotional distress, unusual experiences and troubled or troubling behavior, as an alternative to functional psychiatric diagnosis.* Leicester, England: British Psychological Society.

Jones, E., Kanhouse, D., Kelley, H., Nisbett, R., Valins, S., & Weiner, B. (1971). *Attribution theory.* Morristown, NJ: General Learning Press.

Jones, M. (1958). *Social psychiatry in practice.* Baltimore, MD: Penguin Books.

Kagan, J. (1984). *The nature of the child.* New York, NY: Basic Books.

Kahneman, D. (2011). *Thinking, fast and slow.* New York, NY: Macmillan.

Kahneman, D., Slovic, P., & Tversky, A. (Eds.). (1982). *Judgment under uncertainty: Heuristics and biases.* Cambridge, UK: Cambridge University Press.

Kamphuis, J. H., & Finn, S. E. (2019). Therapeutic Assessment in personality disorders: Toward the restoration of epistemic trust. *Journal of Personality Assessment, 101*(6), 662–674.

Kardiner, A., & Spiegel, A. (1947). *War, stress, and neurotic illness.* New York, NY: Hoeber.

Kazdin, A. E. (1978). The application of operant techniques in treatment, rehabilitation, and education. In S. L. Garfield & A. E. Bergin (Eds.), *Handbook of psychotherapy and behavior change: An empirical analysis* (2nd ed., pp. 549–590). New York, NY: John Wiley & Sons.

Kelman, H. C., & Parloff, M. B. (1957). Interrelations among three criteria of improvement in group therapy: Comfort, effectiveness, and self-awareness. *The Journal of Abnormal and Social Psychology, 54*(3), 281–288.

Kelman, H. C. (Ed.). (1965). *International behavior: A sociopsychological analysis.* New York: Holt, Rinehart and Winston.

Kempf, E. (1921). *Psychopathology.* St. Louis, MO: C.V. Mosby.

Kernberg, O. (1967). Borderline personality organization. *Journal of the American Psychoanalytic Association, 15*, 641–685.

Kernberg, O. (1975). *Borderline conditions and pathological narcissism.* New York, NY: Jason Aronson.

Kernberg, O. (1976). *Object relations theory and clinical psychoanalysis.* New York, NY: Jason Aronson.

Kiesler, D. J. (1996). *Contemporary interpersonal theory and research: Personality, psychopathology, and psychotherapy.* New York, NY: John Wiley & Sons.

Klein, M. (1964). *Contributions to psychoanalysis, 1921–1945.* New York, NY: McGraw-Hill.

Klein, M. (1975). *Envy and gratitude, 1946–1963.* New York, NY: Delacorte Press.

Klein, M., & Riviere, J. (1964). *Love, hate and reparation.* New York, NY: W.W. Norton & Company.

Klerman, G., Weissman, M., Rounsaville, B., & Chevron, E. (1984). *Interpersonal therapy for depression*. New York, NY: Basic Books.

Klopfer, B., & Kelley, D. M. (1942). *The Rorschach technique*. Chicago, IL: World Book.

Kluft, R. P. (1985). *Childhood antecedents of multiple personality*. Washington, DC: American Psychiatric Press, Inc.

Kluft, R. P. (1990). *Incest-related syndromes of adult psychopathology*. Washington, DC: American Psychiatric Press, Inc.

Knight, R. P. (1953). Borderline states. *Bulletin of the Menninger Clinic, 17*, 1–12.

Kohut, H. (1971). *The analysis of the self*. New York, NY: International Universities Press.

Kohut, H. (1977). *The restoration of the self*. New York, NY: International Universities Press.

Kotov, R., Krueger, R. F., Watson, D., Achenbach, T. M., Althoff, R. R., Bagby, R. M., ... Zimmerman, M. (2017). The hierarchical taxonomy of psychopathology (HiTOP): A dimensional alternative to traditional nosologies. *Journal of Abnormal Psychology, 126*(4), 454.

Kotov, R., Jonas, K. G., Carpenter, W. T., Dretsch, M. N., Eaton, N. R., Forbes, M. K., ... & HiTOP Utility Workgroup. (2020). Validity and utility of Hierarchical Taxonomy of Psychopathology (HiTOP): I. Psychosis superspectrum. *World Psychiatry, 19*(2), 151–172.

Kraepelin, E. (1918). *Dementia praecox*. London, UK: Livingstone.

Kraepelin, E. (1968). *Lectures on clinical psychiatry*. New York, NY: Hafner.

Kuhn, T. (1962). *The structure of scientific revolutions, 2nd ed*. Chicago, IL: University of Chicago Press.

Kurtz, R., & Prestera, H. (1977). *The body reveals*. New York, NY: Bantam Books.

Kvarnes, R., & Parloff, G. (1976). *A Harry Stack Sullivan case seminar*. New York, NY: W.W. Norton & Company.

LaGaipa, J. J. (1979). A developmental study of the meaning of friendship in adolescence. *Journal of Adolescence, 2*, 201–213.

Laing, R. D. (1965). *The divided self: The study of sanity and madness*. Baltimore, MD: Penguin Books.

Laing, R. D. (1967). *Politics of experience*. New York, NY: Pantheon.

Laing, R. D., & Estreson, A. (1964). *Sanity, madness, and the family*. London, UK: Tavistock Publications.

Lambert, M. J., & Barley, D. E. (2001). Research summary on the therapeutic relationship and psychotherapy outcome. *Psychotherapy: Theory, Research, Practice, Training, 38*(4), 357–361.

Landers, M. S., & Sullivan, R. M. (2012). The development and neurobiology of infant attachment and fear. *Developmental Neuroscience, 34*(2–3), 101–114.

Lasswell, H. (1930). *Psychopathology and politics*. Chicago, IL: University of Chicago Press.

*Lawrence v Texas*, 123 S.Ct. 2472 (2003). Lawrence v Texas 539 US 558.

Lawrence, R. L. (2022). *Harry Stack Sullivan and Anton T. Boisen: Comrades and revolutionaries in psychotherapy*. London, UK: International Psychoanalytic Books.

Lazare, A., Cohen, F., Jacobson, A. M., Williams, M. W., Mignone, R. J. & Zisook, S. (1972). The walk-in patient as a customer: A key dimension of evaluation and treatment. *American Journal of Orthopsychiatry, 42*, 872–883.

Lazare, A., Eisenthal, S., & Wasserman, L. (1975). The customer approach to pa-tienthood: Attending to patient requests in a walk-in clinic. *Archives of General Psychiatry*, *32*, 553–559.

Lazarus, A. A. (1971). *Behavior therapy and beyond*. New York, NY: McGraw-Hill.

Lazarus, A. A. (Ed.). (1976). *Multimodal behavior therapy*. New York, NY: Springer.

Leary, T. (1957). *Interpersonal diagnosis of personality*. New York, NY: Ronald Press.

Leichsenring, F., & Rabung, S. (2008). Effectiveness of long-term psychodynamic psychotherapy: A meta-analysis. *JAMA*, *300*(13), 1551–1565.

Lekka, D., Madoglou, A., Karamanoli, V., Yotsidi, V., Alexias, G., Karakasidou, E., ... Stalikas, A. (2022). Mental disorders and dehumanization: A systematic review. *Psychology*, *13*, 1343–1352.

Levinson, D. J. (1978). *The seasons of a man's life*. New York, NY: A.A. Knopf.

Levinson, D. J. (1996). *The seasons of a woman's life*. New York, NY: A.A. Knopf.

Levinson, D. J., & Gallagher, E. (1964). *Patienthood in the mental hospital*. Boston, MA: Houghton-Mifflin.

Levinson, D. J., Merrifield, J., & Berg, K. (1967). Becoming a patient. *Archives of General Psychiatry*, *17*, 385–406.

Levinson, E. A. (1972). *The fallacy of understanding: An inquiry into the changing structure of psychoanalysis*. New York, NY: New York Basic Books.

Levinson, E. A. (1983). *The ambiguity of change: An inquiry into the nature of psy-choanalytic reality*. New York, NY: New York Basic Books.

Levenson, E. A. (2013). *The fallacy of understanding & the ambiguity of change*. New York, NY: Routledge.

Levenson, E. A., & Slomowitz, A. (2016). *The purloined self: Interpersonal perspectives in psychoanalysis*. New York, NY: Routledge.

Lichtenberg, J. D. (1981). Implications for psychoanalytic theory of research on the neonate. *International Review of Psychoanalysis*, *8*, 35–52.

Lichtenberg, J. D. (1983). *Psychoanalysis and infant research*. Hillsdale, NJ: Lawrence Erlbaum Associates.

Lingiardi, V., & McWilliams, N. (Eds.). (2017). *Psychodynamic diagnostic manual: PDM-2*. New York, NY: Guilford Publications.

Lingiardi, V., McWilliams, N., Bornstein, R. F., Gazzillo, F., & Gordon, R. M. (2015). The Psychodynamic Diagnostic Manual Version 2 (PDM-2): Assessing patients for improved clinical practice and research. *Psychoanalytic Psychology*, *32*(1), 94.

Lionells, M., Fiscalini, J., Mann, C., & Stern, D. B. (2014). *Handbook of interpersonal psychoanalysis*. New York, NY: Routledge.

Lipton, S. D. (1977). The advantage of Freud's technique as shown in his analysis of the Rat Man. *International Journal of Psychoanalysis*, *58*, 255–273.

Litz, B. T. (1992). Emotional numbing in combat-related post-traumatic stress dis-order: A critical review and reformulation. *Clinical Psychology Review*, *12*, 417–432.

Locke, K. D. (2010). Circumplex measures of interpersonal constructs. In L. M. Horowitz & S. Strack (Eds.), *Handbook of interpersonal psychology* (pp. 313–324). New York, NY: Wiley.

London, P. (1986). *Modes and morals of psychotherapy, 2nd ed*. New York, NY: Hemisphere Publishing Corp.

Lorenz, K. (1952). *King Solomon's ring*. New York, NY: Crowell.

Loue, S. (2016). CooperRiis healing community. In S. Loue (Ed.), *Therapeutic farms* (pp. 69–78). New York, NY: Springer.

Mahl, G. F. (1968). Gestures and body movements in interviews. In J. M. Shlien (Ed.), *Research in psychotherapy* (Vol. 3, pp. 245–346). Washington, DC: American Psychological Association.

Mahler, M. S. (1968). *On human symbiosis and the vicissitudes of individuation.* New York, NY: International Universities Press.

Mahler, M. S., Pine, F., & Bergman, A. (1975). *The psychological birth of the child.* New York, NY: Basic Books.

Mahoney, M. J., & Arnkoff, D. (1978). Cognitive and self-control therapies. In S. L. Garfield & A. E. Bergin (Eds.), *Handbook of psychotherapy and behavior change: An empirical analysis* (2nd ed., pp. 689–721). New York, NY: John Wiley & Sons.

Malan, D. H. (1976). *The frontiers of brief psychotherapy.* New York, NY: Plenum Press.

Malle, B. F. (2011). Attribution theories: How people make sense of behavior. *Theories in social psychology, 23,* 72–95.

Mann, J. (1973). *Time-limited psychotherapy.* Cambridge, MA: Harvard University Press.

Marks, I. (1978). Behavioral psychotherapy of adult neurosis. In S. L. Garfield & A. E. Bergin (Eds.), *Handbook of psychotherapy and behavior change: An empirical analysis* (2nd ed., pp. 493–548). New York, NY: John Wiley & Sons.

Marvin, R. S., Britner, P. A., & Russell, B. S. (2016). Normative development: The ontogeny of attachment in childhood. In J. Cassidy & P. R. Shaver (Eds.), *Handbook of attachment: Theory, research, and clinical applications* (pp. 273–289). New York, NY: Guilford Press.

Marvin, R. S., Cooper, G., Hoffman, K., & Powell, B. (2002). The Circle of Security project: Attachment-based intervention with caregiver-pre-school child dyads. *Attachment & Human Development, 4*(1), 107–124.

Maslow, A. H. (1962). *Toward a psychology of being.* Princeton, NJ: D. Van Nostrand.

Masters, W., & Johnson, V. (1966). *Human sexual response.* Boston, MA: Little, Brown and Company.

Matarazzo, J. D., Wiens, A. N., Matarazzo, R. G., & Saslow, G. (1968). Speech and silence in clinical psychotherapy and its laboratory correlates. In J. M. Shlien (Ed.), *Research in psychotherapy,* (Vol. 3, pp. 347–394). Washington, DC: American Psychological Association.

McAdams, D. P., Trzesniewski, K., Lilgendahl, J., Benet-Martinez, V., & Robins, R. W. (2021). Self and identity in personality psychology. *Personality Science, 2,* 1–20.

McClelland, D. (1961). *The achieving society.* Princeton, NJ: D. Van Nostrand.

McCrae, R. R., & Costa Jr., P. T. (2008). The five-factor theory of personality. In O. P. John, R. W. Robins, & L. A. Pervin (Eds.), *Handbook of personality: Theory and research* (pp. 159–181). New York, NY: The Guilford Press.

Mead, G. H. (1934). *Mind, self, and society.* Chicago, IL: University of Chicago Press.

Mead, G. H. (1952). *Selected writings.* Chicago, IL: University of Chicago Press.

Mead, G. H. (1956). *On social psychology: Selected papers.* Chicago, IL: University of Chicago Press.

Mehrabian, A. (1972). *Nonverbal behavior.* Chicago, IL: Aldine.

Mercado, A., Antuña, C. S., Bailey, C., Garcini, L., Hass, G. A., Henderson, C., ... Venta, A. (2022). Professional guidelines for psychological evaluations in immigration proceedings. *Journal of Latinx Psychology*, *10*(4), 253–276.

Merleau-Ponty, M. (1963). *The structure of behavior*. Boston, MA: Beacon Press.

Messer, S. B., Sanderson, W. C., & Gurman, A. S. (2013). Brief psychotherapies. In G. Stricker, T. A. Widiger, & I. B. Weiner (Eds.), *Handbook of psychology: Clinical psychology* (pp. 431–453). New York, NY: John Wiley & Sons, Inc.

Meyer, A. (1957). *Psychobiology: A science of man*. Springfield, IL: Charles C. Thomas.

Mihura, J. L., Meyer, G. J., Dumitrascu, N., & Bombel, G. (2013). The validity of individual Rorschach variables: Systematic reviews and meta-analyses of the comprehensive system. *Psychological Bulletin*, *139*(3), 548.

Miller, A. G. (Ed.). (1982). *In the eye of the beholder: Contemporary issues in stereotyping*. New York, NY: Praeger.

Millon, T. (1969). *Modern psychopathology: A biosocial approach to maladaptive learning and functioning*. Philadelphia, PA: W.B. Saunders.

Millon, T. (1981) *Disorders of personality: DSM-III: Axis II*. New York, NY: John Wiley & Sons.

Millon, T., & Everly. G. S. (1985). *Personality and its disorders: A biosocial learning approach*. New York, NY: John Wiley & Sons.

Mischel, W. (1974). Processes in the delay of gratification. In L. Berkowitz (Ed.), *Advances in experimental social psychology* (Vol. 7, pp. 249–292). New York, NY: Academic Press.

Mischel, W., & Patterson, C. J. (1976). Substantive and structural elements in effective plans for self-control. *Journal of Personality and Social Psychology*, *34*, 942–950.

Mitchell, K. M., Bozarth, J. D., & Krauft, C. C. (1977). A reappraisal of the therapeutic effectiveness of accurate empathy, nonpossessive warmth, and genuiness. In A. S. Gurman & A. M. Razin (Eds.), *Effective psychotherapy: A handbook of research* (pp. 482–502). New York, NY: Pergamon Press.

Mitchell, S. (1988). *Relational concepts in psychoanalysis*. Cambridge, MA: Harvard University Press.

Mitchell, S. A. , & Aron, L. E. (1999). *Relational psychoanalysis: The emergence of a tradition*. Analytic Press.

Mitchell, S. A. & Black, M. J. (1995). *Freud and beyond: A history of modern psychoanalytic thought*. New York, NY: Basic Books.

Mitchell, S. A., & Black, M. J. (2016). *Freud and beyond: A history of modern psychoanalytic thought, 2nd ed*. New York, NY: Basic Books.

Mollica, R. F., Caspi-Yavin, Y., Bollini, P., Truong, T., Tor, S., & Lavelle, J. (1992). The Harvard Trauma Questionnaire: Validating a cross-cultural instrument for measuring torture, trauma, and posttraumatic stress disorder in Indochinese refugees. *Journal of Nervous and Mental Disease*, *180*, 111–116.

Mollica, R. F., Wyshak, G., & Lavelle, J. (1987). The psychosocial impact of war trauma and torture among Southeast Asian refugees. *American Journal of Psychiatry*, *144*, 1567–1572.

Money, J. (1986). *Venuses penises: Sexology, sexosophy, and exigency theory*. Totowa, NJ: Prometheus Books/Rowman & Littlefield.

Money, J. (1988). *Gay, straight, and in-between: The sexology of erotic orientation*. New York, NY: Oxford University Press.

Money, J. (2012). *Lovemaps: Clinical concepts of sexual/erotic health and pathology, paraphilia, and gender transposition in childhood, adolescence, and maturity.* Totowa, NJ: Prometheus Books.

Morey, L. C. (2007). *Personality Assessment Inventory professional manual, 2nd ed.* Lutz, FL: Psychological Assessment Resources.

Morse, R. T., & Noble, D. (1942). Joint endeavors of the administrative physician and psychotherapist. *Psychiatric Quarterly, 16,* 578–585.

Mullahy, P. (1948). *Oedipus: Myth and complex.* New York, NY: Hermitage Press.

Mullahy, P. (1970). *Psychoanalysis and interpersonal psychiatry: The contributions of Harry Stack Sullivan.* New York, NY: Science House.

Nathanson, D. L. (2014). Affect theory and the compass of shame. In M. R. Lansky & A. T. Morrison (Eds.), *The widening scope of shame* (pp. 339–354). New York, NY: Routledge.

Neiderland, W. (1974). *The Schreber case.* New York, NY: Quadrangle.

Nelson, C. A. (2001). The development and neural bases of face recognition. *Infant and Child Development: An International Journal of Research and Practice, 10*(1–2), 3–18.

Norcross, J. C. (Ed.). (1986). *Handbook of eclectic psychotherapy.* New York, NY: Brunner/Mazel.

Norcross, J. C., & Goldfried, M. R. (Eds.). (1992). *Handbook of psychotherapy integration.* New York, NY: Basic Books.

Norcross, J. C., & Goldfried, M. R. (2005). *Handbook of psychotherapy integration, 2nd ed.* Oxford, UK: Oxford University Press.

Ogden, T. H. (1979). On projective identification. *International Journal of Psychoanalysis, 60,* 357–372.

Ogden, T. H. (1982). *Projective identification and psychotherapeutic technique.* New York, NY: Jason Aronson.

Ogloff, J. R., & Wood, M. (2010). The treatment of psychopathy: Clinical nihilism or steps in the right direction. In L. Malatesti & J. McMillan (Eds.), *Responsibility and psychopathy: Interfacing law, psychiatry and philosophy* (pp 155–181). Oxford, UK: Oxford University Press.

Parker, J. G., Rubin, K. H., Erath, S. A., Wojslawowicz, J. C., & Buskirk, A. A. (2006). Peer relationships, child development, and adjustment: A developmental psychopathology perspective. In D. Cicchetti & D. J. Cohen (Eds.), *Developmental psychopathology: Theory and method* (pp. 419–493). New York, NY: John Wiley & Sons, Inc.

Parloff, M. B. (1980). Psychotherapy and research: An anaclitic depression. *Psychiatry, 43,* 279–293.

Parloff, M. B. (1994). Personal communication. Bethesda, MD.

Parloff, M. B., Kelman, H. C., & Frank, J. D. (1954). Comfort, effectiveness, and self-awareness as criteria of improvement in psychotherapy. *American Journal of Psychiatry, 111*(5), 343–352.

Parloff, M. B., Waskow, I. E., & Wolfe, B. E. (1978). Research on therapist variables in relation to process and outcome. In S. L. Garfield & A. E. Bergin (Eds.), *Handbook of psychotherapy and behavior change: An empirical analysis* (2nd ed., pp. 233–282). New York, NY: John Wiley & Sons.

Patterson, C. J., & Mischel, W. (1976). Effects of temptation-inhibiting and task facilitating plans on self-control. *Journal of Personality and Social Psychology, 33,* 207–217.

PDM Task Force. (2006). *Psychodynamic diagnostic manual (PDM)*. Alliance of Psychoanalytic Organizations.

Peña-Vargas, C., Armaiz-Peña, G., & Castro-Figueroa, E. (2021). A biopsychosocial approach to grief, depression, and the role of emotional regulation. *Behavioral Sciences, 11*(8), 110.

Perry, H. S. (1964). Introduction. In H. S. Sullivan (Ed.), *Fusion of psychiatry and social sciences*. New York, NY: W.W. Norton & Company.

Perry, H. S. (1982). *Psychiatrist of America: The life of Harry Stack Sullivan*. New York, NY: W.W. Norton & Company.

Peterson, D. R. (1982). Functional analysis of interpersonal behavior. In J. C. Achin & D. J. Kiesler (Eds.), *Handbook of interpersonal psychotherapy* (pp. 149–167). New York, NY: Pergamon Press.

Piaget, J. (1965). *The moral judgement of the child*. New York, NY: Free Press.

Pincus, A. L. (2005). A contemporary integrative interpersonal theory of personality disorders. In M. Lenzenweger & J. F. Clarkin (Eds.), *Major theories of personality disorder* (2nd ed., pp. 282–331). New York, NY: Guilford.

Pincus, A. L., & Hopwood, C. J. (2012). A contemporary interpersonal model of personality pathology and personality disorder. In T. A. Widiger (Ed.), *Oxford handbook of personality disorders* (pp. 372–398). Oxford, UK: Oxford University Press.

Pincus, A. L., Hopwood, C. J., & Wright, A. G. C. (2020). The interpersonal situation: An integrative framework for the study of personality, psychopathology, and psychotherapy. In D. Funder, J. F. Rauthmann, & R. Sherman (Eds.), *Oxford handbook of psychological situations* (pp. 124–142). Oxford, UK: Oxford University Press.

Plato. (1929). Apology. In I. Edman (Ed.), *The works of Plato*. New York, NY: Modern Library.

Poston, J. M., & Hanson, W. E. (2010). Meta-analysis of psychological assessment as a therapeutic intervention *Psychological Assessment, 22*(2), 203–212.

Powdermaker, F., & Frank, J. (1953). *Group psychotherapy*. Cambridge, MA: Harvard University Press.

Powell, B., Cooper, G., Hoffman, K., & Marvin, B. (2013). *The Circle of Security intervention: Enhancing attachment in early parent–child relationships*. New York, NY: Guilford.

Pratt, T. C., Cullen, F. T., Sellers, C. S., Winfree, L. T., Jr., Madensen, T. D., Daigle, L. E., … Gau, J. M. (2010). The empirical status of social learning theory: A meta-analysis. *Justice Quarterly, 27*(6), 765–802.

Putnam, F. W. (1985). Dissociation as a response to extreme trauma. In R. P. Kluft (Ed.), *Childhood antecedents of multiple personality* (pp. 65–97). Washington, DC: American Psychiatric Press, Inc.

Putnam, F. W. (1997). *Dissociation in children and adolescents: A developmental perspective*. New York, NY: Guilford.

Putnam, F. W. (2003). Ten-year research update review: Child sexual abuse. *Journal of the American Academy of Child & Adolescent Psychiatry, 42*(3), 269–278.

Putnam, F. W. (2016). *The way we are: How states of mind influence our identities, personality and potential for change*. London, UK: International Psychoanalytic Books.

Regier, D. A., Narrow, W. E., Kuhl, E. A., & Kupfer, D. J. (2009). The conceptual development of DSM-V. *American Journal of Psychiatry, 166*(6), 645–650.

Reich, W. (1945). *Character analysis*. New York, NY: Simon and Schuster.

Richard, B. A., & Dodge, K. A. (1982). Social maladjustment and problem solving in school-age children. *Journal of Clinical and Consulting Psychology, 50*(2), 226–233.

Rieff, P. (1959). *Freud: The mind of the moralist*. Garden City, NY: Anchor Books.

Rioch, D. M. (1938). Certain aspects of the behavior of decorticate cats. *Psychiatry, 1*(3), 339–345.

Rioch, D. M. (1940). Neurophysiology of the corpus striatum and globus pallidus. *Psychiatry, 3*, 119–139.

Rioch, D. M. (1948). Editorial notes: The Washington School of Psychiatry. *Psychiatry, 11*, 203–205.

Rioch, D. M. (1949). Editorial notes: The Program of the Washington School of Psychiatry. *Psychiatry, 12*, 87–88.

Rioch, D. M. (1950). Editorial notes: The Washington School of Psychiatry. *Psychiatry, 13*, 259–263.

Rioch, D. M. (1985). Reflections of Harry Stack Sullivan and of the development of his interpersonal psychiatry. *Psychiatry, 48*, 141–158.

Rioch, D. M., & Stanton, A. H. (1953). Milieu therapy. *Psychiatry, 16*, 65–72.

Rioch, M. J. (1960). The meaning of Martin Buber's "Elements of the Interhuman" for the practice of psychotherapy. *Psychiatry, 23*, 133–140.

Rioch, M. J. (1970). Should psychotherapists do therapy? *Professional Psychology, 1*, 139–142.

Rioch, M. J. (1989). Personal communication. Chevy Chase, MD.

Rioch, M. J., Coulter, W., & Weinberger, D. (1976). *Dialogues for therapists*. San Francisco, CA: Jossey-Bass.

Riviere, J. (1936a). A contribution to the analysis of the negative therapeutic reaction. *International Journal of Psychoanalysis, 17*, 304–320.

Riviere, J. (1936b). On the genesis of psychical conflicts in early infancy. *International Journal of Psychoanalysis, 55*, 397–404.

Rogers, C. R. (1951). *Client-centered therapy*. Boston, MA: Houghton Mifflin.

Rogers, C. R. (1957). The necessary and sufficient conditions of therapeutic personality change. *Journal of Consulting Psychology, 21*, 95–103.

Rogers, C. R. (1961). *On becoming a person: A therapist's view of psychotherapy*. Boston, MA: Houghton Mifflin.

Rogers, C. R., Gendlin, G. T., Kiesler, D. V., & Truax, C. B. (1967). *The therapeutic relationship and its impact: A study of psychotherapy with schizophrenics*. Madison, WI: University of Wisconsin Press.

Rosenthal, T., & Bandura, A. (1978). Psychological modeling: Theory and practice. In S. L. Garfield & A. E. Bergin (Eds.), *Handbook of psychotherapy and behavior change: An empirical analysis* (2nd ed., pp. 621–658). New York, NY: John Wiley & Sons.

Rothschild, B. (2000). *Body remembers: The psychophysiology of trauma and trauma treatment*: Vol. 1. New York, NY: W.W. Norton & Company.

Rubin, K. H., Coplan, R., Chen, X., Bowker, J., & McDonald, K. L. (2013). Peer relationships in childhood. In M. E. Lamb & M. H. Bornstein (Eds.), *Social and personality development* (pp. 317–368). New York, NY: Psychology Press.

Ruggero, C. J., Kotov, R., Hopwood, C. J., First, M., Clark, L. A., Skodol, A. E., ... Zimmermann, J. (2019). Integrating the hierarchical taxonomy of psychopathology (HiTOP) into clinical practice. *Journal of Consulting and Clinical Psychology*, *87*(12), 1069–1084.

Rychlak, J. (1973). *An introduction to personality and psychotherapy*. Boston, MA: Houghton-Mifflin.

Safran, J. D. (1998). *Widening the scope of cognitive therapy: The therapeutic relationship, emotion, and the process of change*. Lanham, MD: Jason Aronson Incorporated.

Safran, J. D., & Segal, Z. V. (1990). *Interpersonal processes in cognitive therapy*. New York, NY: Basic Books.

Salzman, L. (1966). *Treatment of the obsessive personality*. New York, NY: Jason Aronson.

Salzman, L. (1980). Sullivan's views on the obsessional states. *Contemporary Psychoanalysis*, *16*, 271–286.

Salzman, L. (1992). Personal communication. Washington, DC.

Sapir, E. (1936–1937). The contribution of psychiatry to an understanding of behavior in society. *American Journal of Sociology*, *42*, 862–870.

Sarbin T., & Mancuso, J. (1980). *Schizophrenia: Diagnosis or moral verdict*. New York, NY: Pegamon.

Schafer, R. (1953). Content analysis in the Rorschach test. *Journal of Projective Techniques*, *17*(3), 335–339.

Searles, H. (1979). *Countertransference and related subjects*. New York, NY: International Universities Press.

Searls, D. (2017). *The inkblots: Hermann Rorschach, his iconic test, and the power of seeing*. New York, NY: Broadway Books.

Segal, H. (1964). *Introduction to the work of Melanie Klein*. New York, NY: Basic Books.

Seligman, M. (1995a). The effectiveness of psychotherapy: The Consumer Reports study. *American Psychologist*, *50*, 965–974.

Seligman, M. (1995b). *The optimistic child*. New York, NY: Houghton Mifflin.

Selman, R. L. (1980). *The growth of interpersonal understanding*. New York, NY: Academic Press.

Shah, I. (1970). *Tales of the dervishes*. New York, NY: E.P. Dutton.

Shantz, C. A., & Hartup, W.W. (1992). *Conflict in child and adolescent development*. New York, NY: Cambridge University Press.

Shapiro, D. (1965). *Neurotic styles*. New York, NY: Basic Books.

Shapiro, D. (1981). *Autonomy and rigid character*. New York, NY: Basic Books.

Shapiro, D. L. (2010). Relational identity theory: A systematic approach for transforming the emotional dimension of conflict. *American Psychologist*, *65*(7), 634–645.

Shaver, K. G. (2016). *An introduction to attribution processes*. New York, NY: Routledge.

Shaver, P. R., Mikulincer, M., & Cassidy, J. (2019). Attachment, caregiving in couple relationships, and prosocial behavior in the wider world. *Current Opinion in Psychology*, *25*, 16–20.

Sherman, L. J., Rice, K., & Cassidy, J. (2015). Infant capacities related to building internal working models of attachment figures: A theoretical and empirical review. *Developmental Review*, *37*, 109–141.

Shevrin, H., & Dickman, S. (1980). The psychological unconscious: A necessary assumption for all psychological theory? *American Psychologist, 35,* 421–434.

Sidman, M. (1960). *Tactics of scientific research.* New York, NY: New York Basic Books.

Singer, J. L. (1990). Repressive personality style: Theoretical and methodological implications for health and pathology. In J. L. Singer (Ed.), *Repression and dissociation* (pp. 435–470). Chicago, IL: University of Chicago Press.

Skinner, B. F. (1953). *Science and human behavior.* New York, NY: Macmillan Co.

Slade, A. (2016). Attachment and adult psychotherapy: Theory, research and practice. In J. Cassidy & P. R. Shaver (Eds.), *Handbook of attachment: Theory, research, and clinical applications, 3rd ed.* (pp. 759–779). New York, NY: Guilford Press.

Smith, B. L., & Evans, F. B. (2017). Collaborative/therapeutic assessment in multimethod forensic evaluations. In R. E. Erard & F. B. Evans (Eds.), *The Rorschach in multimethod forensic assessment: Conceptual foundations and practical applications* (pp. 297–315). New York, NY: Routledge/Taylor & Francis Group.

Smith, G. S. (1972). Personal communication. Somerset, NJ.

Smith, M., Glass, G., & Miller, T. (1980). *The benefit of psychotherapy.* Baltimore, MD: Johns Hopkins University Press.

Smollar, J., & Youniss, J. (1982). Social development through friendship. In K. H. Rubin & H. S. Ross (Eds.), *Peer relations and social skills in childhood* (pp. 279–298). New York, NY: Springer-Verlag.

Soldz, S., Budman, S., Demby, A., & Merry, J. (1995). A short form of the Inventory of Interpersonal Problems Circumplex scales. *Assessment, 2*(1), 53–63.

Solomon, J., & George, C. (1999). The development of attachment in separated and divorced families: Effects of overnight visitation, parent and couple variables. *Attachment & Human Development, 1*(1), 2–33.

Solomon, J., & George, C. (Eds.). (2011). Disorganized *attachment* and *caregiving.* New York, NY: The Guilford Press.

Solomon, J., & George, C. (2016). The measurement of attachment security in infancy and childhood. In J. Cassidy & P. R. Shaver (Eds.), *Handbook of attachment: Theory, research, and clinical applications, 3rd ed.* (pp. 366–398). New York, NY: Guilford.

Spearman, C. (1923). *The nature of "intelligence" and the principles of cognition.* London, UK: Macmillan and Co.

Spearman, C. (1930). *Creative mind.* London, UK: Cambridge University Press.

Spieker, S. J., & Crittenden, P. M. (2018). Can attachment inform decision-making in child protection and forensic settings? *Infant Mental Health Journal, 39*(6), 625–641.

Spitz, R. (1945). Hospitalism: An inquiry into the genesis of psychiatric conditions in early childhood. *Psychoanalytic Study of the Child, 2,* 53–73.

Spitz, R. (1946). Anaclitic depression: An inquiry into the genesis of psychiatric conditions in early childhood, II. *Psychoanalytic Study of the Child, 3,* 53–73.

Spitz, R. (1965). *The first year of life.* New York, NY: International Universities Press.

Sroufe, L. A. (2016). The place of attachment in development. In J. Cassidy & P. R. Shaver (Eds.), *Handbook of attachment: Theory, research, and clinical applications* (pp. 997–1011). New York, NY: Guilford Press.

Stanton, A. H., & Schwartz, M. S. (1949). The management of a type of institutional participation in mental illness. *Psychiatry, 12,* 13–26.

Stanton, A. H., & Schwartz, M. S. (1954). *The mental hospital*. New York, NY: Basic Books.

Starr, R. H., MacLean, D. J., & Keating, D. P. (1991). Life-span developmental outcomes of child maltreatment. In R. H. Starr & D. A. Wolfe (Eds.), *The effects of child abuse and neglect*. New York, NY: The Guilford Press.

Steele, C. M. (2011). *Whistling Vivaldi: How stereotypes affect us and what we can do*. New York, NY: W.W. Norton & Company.

Steenkamp, M. M., & Litz, B. T. (2013). Psychotherapy for military-related posttraumatic stress disorder: Review of the evidence. *Clinical Psychology Review, 33*(1), 45–53.

Stern, A. (1938). Psychoanalytic investigation and therapy in the borderline group of neuroses. *Psychoanalytic Quarterly, 7*, 467–489.

Stern, D. (1985). *The interpersonal birth of the infant*. New York, NY: Basic Books.

Stern, D. B. (2017). *The interpersonal perspective in psychoanalysis, 1960s–1990s*. New York, NY: Routledge.

Sternberg, R. J., Grigorenko, E. L., & Kidd, K. K. (2005). Intelligence, race, and genetics. *American Psychologist, 60*(1), 46–59.

Stotland, E., & Kobler, A. L. (1965). *Life and death of a mental hospital*. Seattle, WA: University of Washington Press.

Stovall-McClough, K.C., & Dozier, M. (2016). Attachment states of mind and psychopathology in adulthood. In J. Cassidy & P. R. Shaver (Eds.), *Handbook of attachment: Theory, research, and clinical applications, 3rd ed.* (pp. 715–738). New York, NY: Guilford Press.

Strachey, J. (1934). The nature of therapeutic action of psychoanalysis. *International Journal of Psychoanalysis, 15*, 127–159.

Strupp, H. H., & Binder, J. L. (1984). *Psychotherapy in a new key: A guide to time-limited dynamic therapy*. New York, NY: Basic Books.

Sulloway, F. (1979). *Freud: Biologist of the mind*. New York, NY: Basic Books.

Suomi, S. J. (1984). The development of affect in rhesus monkeys. In F. N. Davidson (Ed.), *The psychobiology of affective development* (p. 119). Hillsdale, NJ: Lawrence Erlbaum Associates.

Suomi, S. J. (2005). Mother–infant attachment, peer relationships, and the development of social networks in rhesus monkeys. *Human Development, 48*(1–2), 67–79.

Szasz, T. S. (1957). On the theory of psycho-analytic treatment. *International Journal of Psychoanalysis, 38*, 166–182.

Szasz, T. S. (1961). *The myth of mental illness: Foundations of a theory of personal conduct*. New York, NY: Harper and Row.

Taylor, S. E. (1989). *Positive illusions: Creative self-deception and the healthy mind*. New York, NY: Basic Books.

Tharinger, D. T, Rudin, D. I., Frackowiak, M., & Finn, S. E. (2022). *Therapeutic Assessment with children: Enhancing parental empathy through psychological assessment*. New York, NY: Routledge.

Thompson, C. (1943). Penis envy in women. *Psychiatry, 6*, 123–125.

Thompson, C. (1949). Harry Stack Sullivan, the man. *Psychiatry, 12*, 435–437.

Thompson, C. (1964). Sullivan and psychoanalysis. In C. Thompson. (Ed.), *Interpersonal psychoanalysis*. New York, NY: Basic Books.

Thompson, C. (1964). *Interpersonal psychiatry*. New York, NY: Basic Books.

Thompson, R. A. (2016). Early attachment and later development: Reframing the questions. In J. Cassidy & P. R. Shaver (Eds.), *Handbook of attachment: Theory, research, and clinical applications, 3rd ed.* (pp. 63–88). New York, NY: Guilford Press.

Tinbergen, N. (1950). *The study of instinct.* New York, NY: Oxford University Press.

Tobin, R. M., & Graziano, W. G. (2010). Delay of gratification: A review of fifty years of regulation research. In R. H Hoyle (Ed.), *Handbook of personality and self-regulation* (pp. 47–63). Oxford, UK: Blackwell.

Toch, H. (1992). *Violent men: An inquiry into the psychology of violence.* Washington, DC: American Psychological Association.

Townsend, M., McCracken, H., & Wilton, K. (1988). Popularity and intimacy as determinants of psychological well-being in adolescent friendships. *Journal of Early Adolescence, 8,* 421–436.

Van de Leemput, J., Hess, J. L., Glatt, S. J., & Tsuang, M. T. (2016). Genetics of schizophrenia: Historical insights and prevailing evidence. *Advances in Genetics, 96,* 99–141.

van der Kolk, B. A. (1987). *Psychological trauma.* Washington, DC: American Psychiatric Association Press.

Van der Kolk, B. A. (2015). *The body keeps the score: Brain, mind, and body in the healing of trauma.* New York, NY: Penguin Books.

Van IJzendoorn, M. H., & Bakermans-Kranenburg, M. J. (1997). Intergenerational transmission of attachment: A move to the contextual level. In L. Atkinson & K. J. Zucker (Eds.), *Attachment and psychopathology* (pp. 135–170). New York, NY: Guilford.

Van Os, J., Kenis, G., & Rutten, B. P. (2010). The environment and schizophrenia. *Nature, 468*(7321), 203–212.

Volkart, E. (Ed.). (1951). *Social behavior and personality: Contributions of W. I. Thomas.* New York, NY: Social Science Research Council.

Wachtel, P. L. (1977). *Psychoanalysis and behavior therapy: Toward an integration.* New York, NY: Basic Books.

Wachtel, P. L. (1982). Interpersonal therapy and active intervention. In J. C. Achin & D. J. Kiesler (Eds.), *Handbook of interpersonal psychotherapy* (pp. 46–63). New York, NY: Pergamon Press.

Wake, N. (2006). "The full story is by no means all told": Harry Stack Sullivan at Sheppard-Pratt, 1922–1930. *History of Psychology, 9*(4), 325.

Wake, N. (2008). On our memory of gay Sullivan: A hidden trajectory. *Journal of Homosexuality, 55*(1), 150–165.

Wake, N. (2019). Homosexuality and psychoanalysis meet at a mental hospital: An early institutional history. *Journal of the History of Medicine and Allied Sciences, 74*(1), 34–56.

Watzlawick, P., Beavin, J. H., & Jackson, D. D. (1967). *Pragmatics of human communication: A study of interactional patterns, pathologies, and paradoxes.* New York, NY: W.W. Norton & Company.

Wake, N. (2022). Personal communication. email 12/2/2022.

Weigert, E. (1960). Loneliness and trust: Basic factors in human existence. *Psychiatry, 23,* 121–131.

Weigert, E. (1970). *The courage to love.* New Haven, CT: Yale University Press.

Weinmeyer, R. (2014). The decriminalization of sodomy in the United States. *AMA Journal of Ethics, 16*(11), 916–922.

Westland, G. (2015). *Verbal and non-verbal communication in psychotherapy.* New York, NY: W.W. Norton & Company.

White, R. K. (1988). The stream of thought, the lifespace, selective inattention, and war. *Journal of Humanistic Psychology, 28*(2), 73–86.

White, R. W. (1959). Motivation reconsidered: The concept of competence. *Psychological Review, 66,* 297–333.

White, W. A. (1933). *Crime and criminals.* New York, NY: Farrar and Rinehart.

White, W. A. (1935). *Outlines of psychiatry.* Washington, DC: Nervous and Mental Disease Publishing Co.

Wiggins, J. S. (1991). Agency and communion as conceptual coordinates for the understanding and measurement of interpersonal behavior. In W. M. Grove & D. Cicchetti (Eds.), *Thinking clearly about psychology, Vol. 2: Personality and psychopathology* (pp. 89–113). Minneapolis, MN: University of Minnesota Press.

Wiggins, J. S. (1995). *Interpersonal Adjective Scales Professional Manual.* Lutz, FL: Psychological Assessment Resources.

Wiggins, J. S. (1996). An informal history of the interpersonal circumplex tradition. *Journal of Personality Assessment, 66*(2), 217–233.

Will, O. A. (1954). Introduction. In H. S. Sullivan (Ed.), *The psychiatric interview.* New York, NY: W.W. Norton & Company.

Will, O. A. (1961). Process, psychotherapy, and schizophrenia. In A. Burton (Ed.), *Psychotherapy of the psychoses* (pp. 10–42). New York, NY: Basic Books.

Winnicott, D. W. (1947). Hate in the countertransference. In D. W. Winnicott (Ed.), *Through pediatrics to psychoanalysis* (pp. 69–74). New York, NY: Basic Books.

Winnicott, D. W. (1958). *Through pediatrics to psychoanalysis.* New York, NY: Basic Books.

Winnicott, D. W. (1960). Ego distortion in terms of true and false self. In D.W. Winnicott (Ed.), *The maturational process and the facilitating environment* (pp. 140–152). New York, NY: International Universities Press.

Winnicott, D. W. (1965). *The maturational process and the facilitating environment.* New York, NY: International Universities Press.

Woodhouse, S. S., Powell, B., Cooper, G., Hoffman, K., & Cassidy, J. (2018). The circle of security intervention: Design, research, and implementation. In H. Steele & M. Steele (Eds.), *Handbook of attachment-based interventions* (pp. 50–78). The Guilford Press.

Wright, A. G., Pincus, A., & Hopwood, C. J. (2020, June 28). Contemporary integrative interpersonal theory: Integrating structure, dynamics, temporal Scale, and levels of analysis. *American Psychologist.* 10.31234/osf.io/fknc8.

Wright, A. G., Ringwald, W. R., Hopwood, C. J., & Pincus, A. L. (2022, May 5). It's time to replace the personality disorders with the interpersonal disorders. *Journal of Psychopathology and Clinical Science.* 10.31234/osf.io/7syvf.

Yaholkoski, A., Hurl, K., & Theule, J. (2016). Efficacy of the circle of security intervention: A meta-analysis. *Journal of Infant, Child, and Adolescent Psychotherapy, 15*(2), 95–103.

Yalom, I. D. (1975). *The practice of group psychotherapy, 2nd ed.* New York, NY: Basic Books.

Yalom, I. D. (1980). *Existential psychotherapy*. New York, NY: Basic Books.

Youniss, J. (1980). *Parents and peers in social development: A Sullivan–Piaget perspective*. Chicago, IL: University of Chicago Press.

Youniss, J., & Smollar, J. (1985). *Adolescent relations with mothers, fathers, and friends*. Chicago, IL: University of Chicago Press.

Youniss, J., & Volpe, J. (1978). A relational analysis of children's friendships. In W. Damon (Ed.), *Social cognition* (pp. 1–22). San Francisco, CA: Jossey-Bass.

# Index

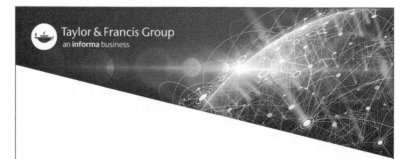